Youth Internet Habits and Mental Health

Editors

KRISTOPHER KALIEBE
PAUL WEIGLE

CHILD AND ADOLESCENT PSYCHIATRIC CLINICS OF NORTH AMERICA

www.childpsych.theclinics.com

Consulting Editor
TODD E. PETERS

April 2018 • Volume 27 • Number 2

ELSEVIER

1600 John F. Kennedy Boulevard • Suite 1800 • Philadelphia, Pennsylvania, 19103-2899

http://www.theclinics.com

CHILD AND ADOLESCENT PSYCHIATRIC CLINICS OF NORTH AMERICA Volume 27, Number 2
April 2018 ISSN 1056–4993, ISBN-13: 978-0-323-58298-8

Editor: Lauren Boyle
Developmental Editor: Kristen Helm

Child and Adolescent Psychiatric Clinics of North America (ISSN 1056-4993) is published quarterly by Elsevier Inc., 360 Park Avenue South, New York, NY 10010-1710. Months of issue are January, April, July, and October. Business and Editorial Offices: 1600 John F. Kennedy Boulevard, Suite 1800, Philadelphia, PA 19103-2899. Periodicals postage paid at New York, NY and additional mailing offices. Subscription prices are $322.00 per year (US individuals), $594.00 per year (US institutions), $100.00 per year (US students), $382.00 per year (Canadian individuals), $723.00 per year (Canadian institutions), $200.00 per year (Canadian students), $439.00 per year (international individuals), $723.00 per year (international institutions), and $200.00 per year (international students). International air speed delivery is included in all *Clinics* subscription prices. All prices are subject to change without notice. **POSTMASTER:** Send address changes to *Child and Adolescent Psychiatric Clinics of North America*, Elsevier Health Sciences Division, Subscription Customer Service, 3251 Riverport Lane, Maryland Heights, MO 63043. **Customer Service: 1-800-654-2452 (U.S. and Canada); 314-447-8871 (outside U.S. and Canada). Fax: 314-447-8029. E-mail:** JournalsCustomer Service-usa@elsevier.com **(for print support) or** journalsonlinesupport-usa@elsevier.com **(for online support).**

Reprints. For copies of 100 or more of articles in this publication, please contact the Commercial Reprints Department, Elsevier Inc., 360 Park Avenue South, New York, New York 10010-1710 Tel.: 212-633-3874; Fax: 212-633-3820, E-mail: reprints@elsevier.com.

Child and Adolescent Psychiatric Clinics of North America is covered in *MEDLINE/PubMed (Index Medicus), ISI, SSCI, Research Alert, Social Search, Current Contents,* and *EMBASE/Excerpta Medica.*

Contributors

CONSULTING EDITOR

TODD E. PETERS, MD, FAPA
Assistant Chief Medical Informatics Officer/Customer Relationship Manager, Vanderbilt University Medical Center, Associate Chief of Staff, Department of Psychiatry and Behavioral Sciences, Vanderbilt University Medical Center, Medical Director for Inpatient Services, Vanderbilt Psychiatric Hospital, Assistant Professor of Psychiatry and Behavioral Sciences, Vanderbilt University, Nashville, Tennessee, USA

EDITORS

KRISTOPHER KALIEBE, MD
Associate Professor, Department of Psychiatry, University of South Florida Morsani College of Medicine, Tampa, Florida, USA

PAUL WEIGLE, MD
Associate Medical Director, Department of Psychiatry, Natchaug Hospital, Hartford HealthCare, Mansfield, Connecticut, USA

AUTHORS

ERIN L. BELFORT, MD
Maine Medical Center, Portland, Maine, USA; Assistant Clinical Professor of Psychiatry, Tufts University School of Medicine, Boston, Massachusetts, USA

ORFEU M. BUXTON, PhD
Associate Professor, Department of Biobehavioral Health, The Pennsylvania State University, Pennsylvania, USA; Division of Sleep Medicine, Harvard Medical School, Division of Sleep and Circadian Disorders, Departments of Medicine and Neurology, Sleep Health Institute, Brigham and Women's Hospital, Department of Social and Behavioral Sciences, Harvard T.H. Chan School of Public Health, Boston, Massachusetts, USA

NICHOLAS J. CARSON, MD, FRCPC
Medical Director, Child and Adolescent Outpatient Psychiatry, Clinical Research Associate, Health Equity Research Lab, Department of Psychiatry, Cambridge Health Alliance, Cambridge, Massachusetts, USA

TOLGA ATILLA CERANOGLU, MD
Clinical Instructor, Department of Psychiatry, Director of Psychiatry Services, Shriners Hospitals for Children, Alan and Lorraine Bressler Clinical and Research Program for Autism Spectrum Disorder, Massachusetts General Hospital, Boston, Massachusetts, USA

ANNE-MARIE CHANG, PhD
Assistant Professor, Department of Biobehavioral Health, College of Nursing, The Pennsylvania State University, Pennsylvania, USA

MONICA DAIGLE, DO
Child and Adolescent Psychiatrist, Department of Mental Health and Detox, St. Mary's
Health System, Lewiston, Maine, USA

KRISTIN A. DALOPE, MD, MEd
Assistant Professor, Department of Child and Adolescent Psychiatry, University of
Pittsburgh Medical Center, Western Psychiatric Institute and Clinic, Children's Hospital of
Pittsburgh, Pittsburgh, Pennsylvania, USA

ELIZABETH K. ENGLANDER, PhD
Director, Massachusetts Aggression Reduction Center, Professor of Psychology,
Bridgewater State University, Maxwell Library, Bridgewater, Massachusetts, USA

SANDRA L. FRITSCH, MD, MSEd, DFAACAP
Associate Professor, Department of Psychiatry, Medical Director, Pediatric Mental Health
Institute, Children's Hospital Colorado, University of Colorado School of Medicine,
Aurora, Colorado, USA

MEREDITH GANSNER, MD
Child and Adolescent Psychiatry Fellow, Department of Psychiatry, Cambridge Health
Alliance, Cambridge, Massachusetts, USA

MICHELLE M. GARRISON, PhD
Research Associate Professor, Division of Child and Adolescent Psychiatry, University
of Washington School of Medicine, Department of Health Services, University of
Washington School of Public Health, Seattle, Washington, USA

ROSLYN L. GERWIN, DO
Assistant Clinical Professor, Department of Psychiatry, Tufts University School of
Medicine, Boston, Massachusetts, USA; Director, Pediatric Psychiatry Consultation
Service, Department of Child and Adolescent Psychiatry, The Barbara Bush Children's
Hospital at Maine Medical Center, Portland, Maine, USA

JENNA GLOVER, PhD
Director of Psychology Training, Pediatric Mental Health Institute, Children's Hospital
Colorado, Assistant Professor, University of Colorado School of Medicine, Aurora,
Colorado, USA

MICHAEL GRADISAR, PhD
Professor, Department of Psychology, Flinders University, Adelaide, Australia

DAVID N. GREENFIELD, PhD, MS
Assistant Clinical Professor, Department of Psychiatry, University of Connecticut, School
of Medicine, Farmington, Connecticut, USA; Founder/CCO, The Center for Internet and
Technology Addiction, West Hartford, Connecticut, USA

McLEOD FRAMPTON GWYNETTE, MD
Department of Psychiatry and Behavioral Sciences, Associate Professor, Medical
University of South Carolina, Founder and Director, Project Rex, Charleston, South
Carolina, USA

LAUREN HALE, PhD
Professor, Program in Public Health, Department of Family, Population, and Preventive
Medicine, Stony Brook Medicine, Stony Brook, New York, USA

JAMES M. HARPER, MD
Medical Director, Adolescent Inpatient Psychiatric Unit, Dominion Hospital, Falls Church, Virginia, USA; Private Practice, Child and Adolescent Psychiatrist, Columbia Associates in Psychiatry, Arlington, Virginia, USA

KRISTOPHER KALIEBE, MD
Associate Professor, Department of Psychiatry, University of South Florida Morsani College of Medicine, Tampa, Florida, USA

JEANE KHANG
Harvard University, Cambridge, Massachusetts, USA

GREGORY W. KIRSCHEN, PhD
MD Candidate, Medical Scientist Training Program, Stony Brook Medicine, Stony Brook, New York, USA

HOWARD KIRSCHEN, MD
Child, Adolescent, Adult Psychiatry and Psychotherapy Private Practice, Jericho, New York, USA

MONIQUE K. LeBOURGEOIS, PhD
Assistant Professor, Department of Integrative Physiology, University of Colorado Boulder, Boulder, Colorado, USA

AMY MAYHEW, MD, MPH
Clinical Instructor, Psychiatry, Medical Director, Psychiatry Access Service, Cambridge Health Alliance, Cambridge, Massachusetts, USA; Harvard Medical School, Boston, Massachusetts, USA

SUSAN M. McHALE, PhD
Distinguished Professor, Department of Human Development and Family Studies, The Pennsylvania State University, Pennsylvania, USA

LINDSEY MILLER, MD
Maine Medical Center, Portland, Maine, USA

HAWLEY MONTGOMERY-DOWNS, PhD
Associate Professor, Department of Psychology, West Virginia University, Morgantown, West Virginia, USA

DALE PEEPLES, MD
Associate Professor, Medical College of Georgia, Augusta University, Augusta, Georgia, USA

MANUEL D. REICH, DO
Associate Medical Director, Beacon Health Options, Trafford, Pennsylvania, USA; Medical Director, Persoma, Monroeville, Pennsylvania, USA; American Academy of Child and Adolescent Psychiatry, Media Committee Member, Washington, DC, USA; Pittsburgh Psychiatric Society, Past President, Harrisburg, Pennsylvania, USA

RACHEL F. RODGERS, PhD
Associate Professor, Department of Applied Psychology, Northeastern University, Boston, Massachusetts, USA; Department of Psychiatric Emergency & Acute Care, Lapeyronie Hospital, CHRU Montpellier, Montpellier, France

JENNIFER S. SAUL, MD, DFAACAP
Child & Adolescent Psychiatry Consulting, LLC, Marshfield, Wisconsin, USA

SHAWN S. SIDHU, MD, FAPA
Assistant Professor, Department of Psychiatry, Attending Psychiatrist, The University of New Mexico, Albuquerque, New Mexico, USA

JESSICA L. STAHL, MD
Fellow, Pediatric Nephrology, University of Washington, Seattle, Washington, USA

CLIFFORD J. SUSSMAN, MD
Private Practice, Child and Adolescent Psychiatrist Specializing in Internet and Video Addiction, Clinical Assistant Professor, Department of Psychiatry, The George Washington University School of Medicine & Health Sciences, Washington, DC, USA

PAUL WEIGLE, MD
Associate Medical Director, Department of Psychiatry, Natchaug Hospital, Hartford HealthCare, Mansfield, Connecticut, USA

LEONARD J. WOODS, LCSW
Director of Family Therapy Training, Center for Children and Families, University of Pittsburgh Medical Center, Western Psychiatric Institute and Clinic, Pittsburgh, Pennsylvania, USA

JENNIFER YEN, MD
Clinical Assistant Professor of Psychiatry and Behavioral Health, Baylor College of Medicine, Houston, Texas, USA

Contents

Digital media (also called "new media") have become an important ecosystem in which adolescents develop biologically, psychologically, and socially. When assessing adolescents in the psychiatric interview, a nuanced understanding of digital media use can inform a more accurate formulation. However, there are few published resources to help the psychiatrist assess the impact of digital media during the initial adolescent interview. The authors propose an innovation on the traditional psychiatric assessment that addresses teen Internet use and digital media habits. Through this enhanced assessment, mental health clinicians can improve upon current interviewing practices of twenty-first century adolescents.

Family dynamics are increasingly being influenced by digital media. Three frameworks are described to help clinicians to understand and respond to this influence. First, a social-ecologic framework shows how media have both a direct and indirect impact on individuals, relationships, communities, and society. Next, family systems theory is introduced to demonstrate digital media–related interactions within families. Finally, a developmental framework explores the role of digital media in shaping parenting. These theories are then integrated into practical strategies that clinicians can use, including recommendations and resources from the American Academy of Pediatrics.

Media have changed the daily lives of most Americans, especially adolescents. The interplay between development and media habits is complex. There is a link between excessive media use and risk-taking behaviors, with an alarming increase in adolescent nonsuicidal self-injury, suicidal behavior, and completed suicide. The link is complex and not necessarily causal. Clinicians should routinely take a media history that distinguishes types and extent of use, content, and psychological impact. Media are a significant part of adolescents' lives, and exploring their engagement with media is a critical piece of the initial assessment, risk assessment, and ongoing treatment.

> This article reviews the available literature regarding the interaction between child and adolescent anxiety and electronic media. It reviews current research contributing to the understanding of the correlation of youth anxiety with engagement in social media and other online platforms, including risk and protective factors. mHealth and eHealth prevention and treatment options, available via various digital resources, are discussed. Suggestions for mental health clinicians' assessment of client's online behaviors and a review of novel treatment options are provided. The article concludes with proposing healthy online technology interventions, including pop-ups for overuse and identification of digitally enhanced posts.

> As digital media (DM) access among youths continues to surge, caregivers and clinicians are concerned about problems associated with their excessive use. Children with attention-deficit/hyperactivity disorder (ADHD) have an increased risk of experiencing negative effects on sleep, academic achievement, attention, and cognitive skills. ADHD symptom severity and circumstances of DM access are among the factors that mediate these negative effects. Key interventions for parents and clinicians to assist youths with problematic DM habits and opportunities for advocacy groups and the DM industry for public health interventions are discussed.

> A robust body of scientific research explores the effects of violent media on youths. For practitioners, the volume of interdisciplinary research and controversial findings can be confusing and difficult to generalize for best practice. This article briefly reviews the literature and presents guidelines for parenting and treating youths exposed and enmeshed in violent media. Attention is given to at-risk populations and children presenting with aggressive, violent, and antisocial behavior. Guidelines assume a family-based, cognitive-behavioral approach suitable for the eclectic practitioner, with a focus on the complex, developmental, and ecologic factors that contribute to presenting symptoms.

> Electronic and social media play a prominent role in the lives of children and teenagers. Evidence suggests youth with autism spectrum disorder (ASD) use media differently than typically developing peers, and some of these differences place them at greater risk for negative health outcomes related to unhealthy and improper use of media. Such outcomes include physiologic, cognitive, social, emotional, and legal/safety problems. However, several technology-aided interventions have emerged to help youth with

ASD across multiple domains. Parents of youth with ASD may benefit from several recommendations and resources from the American Academy of Pediatrics and the American Academy of Child and Adolescent Psychiatry.

Jennifer S. Saul and Rachel F. Rodgers

The proliferation of social media and rapid increase in the use of the Internet by adolescents generates new dynamics and new risks for the development and maintenance of eating disorders. Here, the authors review different types of online content and how they are relevant to eating disorders within different theoretic frameworks, before examining the empirical evidence for the risks posed by online content in the development and maintenance of eating disorders. They describe pro-eating disorder content specifically and examine the research related to it, before considering its implications, and consider directions for future research and prevention and intervention strategies.

Lauren Hale, Gregory W. Kirschen, Monique K. LeBourgeois, Michael Gradisar, Michelle M. Garrison, Hawley Montgomery-Downs, Howard Kirschen, Susan M. McHale, Anne-Marie Chang, and Orfeu M. Buxton

With the widespread use of portable electronic devices and the normalization of screen media devices in the bedroom, insufficient sleep has become commonplace. In a recent literature review, 90% of included studies found an association between screen media use and delayed bedtime and/or decreased total sleep time. This pervasive phenomenon of pediatric sleep loss has widespread implications. There is a need for basic, translational, and clinical research examining the effects of screen media on sleep loss and health consequences in children and adolescents to educate and motivate clinicians, teachers, parents, and youth themselves to foster healthy sleep habits.

Dale Peeples, Jennifer Yen, and Paul Weigle

The Internet changed the way the global community interacts and communicates. This cultural shift allows like-minded individuals to connect and share ideas. It creates spaces for stigmatized communities to gather in a virtual presence. Youth now have greater options to explore identity and to reach peers with niche interests. From a clinical perspective, it is helpful to understand the nature of communities our patients join on the Internet. This article focuses on the broad umbrella of "geek" culture, exploring a variety of interests such as cosplay, fanfiction, and gaming.

Amy Mayhew and Paul Weigle

Clinicians who work with youth should understand how they engage with screen media, including differences between ethnic groups, and how to maximize their positive potential and minimize negative consequences. This article presents data summarizing patterns of media use by youth, with an emphasis on European Americans, African Americans, and Hispanic Americans. The authors explain how identity formation and social identity theory relate to online influences, benefits, and risks of online engagement, including those specific to minority populations. The authors clarify how child mental health professionals may use this information to better treat patients and their families.

This article reviews cyberbullying and sexting research and presents new research exploring relatively neglected areas of cyberbullying and cell phone ownership among children and outcomes following sexting in college. Two samples are studied: 4584 elementary school children and 1332 college freshman. Findings included the following: owning a cell phone increased the risk of becoming involved in cyberbullying in grades 3, 4, and 5 and, of college freshman who sexted, 61% reported no outcomes, 19% reported negative outcomes, 13% reported positive outcomes, and 7% reported mixed outcomes. This information may be useful when considering discussing these digital technology risks with patients.

In the past 2 decades, there has been a substantial increase in the availability and use of digital technologies, including the Internet, computer games, smartphones, and social media. Behavioral addiction to use of technologies spawned a body of related research. The recent inclusion of Internet gaming disorder as a condition for further study in the DSM-V invigorated a new wave of researchers, thereby expanding our understanding of these conditions. This article reviews current research, theory, and practice regarding the diagnosis, epidemiology, and neurobiology of Internet and video game addictions.

Internet and video game addiction has been a steadily developing consequence of modern living. Behavioral and process addictions and particularly Internet and video game addiction require specialized treatment protocols and techniques. Recent advances in addiction medicine have improved our understanding of the neurobiology of substance and behavioral addictions. Novel research has expanded the ways we understand and apply well-established addiction treatments as well as newer therapies specific to Internet and video game addiction. This article reviews the etiology, psychology, and neurobiology of Internet and video game addiction and presents treatment strategies and protocols for addressing this growing problem.

Roslyn L. Gerwin, Kristopher Kaliebe, and Monica Daigle

Today's youth develop immersed in a digital media world, and the effects are specific to their developmental stage. Clinicians and caretakers should be mindful regarding digital media use patterns; however, this complex and reciprocal relationship defies simple linear descriptions. The impacts of digital media can be powerful. It is important to be cautious but not over-pathologize media use because digital media enable social connections, allow self-soothing in some children, and fill needs for stimulation and self-expression. Young children or those with psychiatric disorders or developmental delays should be considered vulnerable to harmful effects of media content and overuse.

CHILD AND ADOLESCENT PSYCHIATRIC CLINICS

FORTHCOMING ISSUES

July 2018
Emergency Child and Adolescent Psychiatry
Vera Feuer, *Editor*

October 2018
Dealing with Death and Dying
David Buxton and Natalie Jacobowski, *Editors*

January 2019
Neuromodulation in Child and Adolescent Psychiatry
Jonathan Essary Becker, Christopher Todd Maley, and Todd E. Peters, *Editors*

RECENT ISSUES

January 2018
Co-occurring Medical Illnesses in Child and Adolescent Psychiatry: Updates and Treatment Considerations
Matthew D. Willis, *Editor*

October 2017
Pediatric Integrated Care
Tami D. Benton, Gregory K. Fritz, and Gary R. Maslow, *Editors*

July 2017
Early Childhood Mental Health: Empirical Assessment and Intervention from Conception through Preschool
Mini Tandon, *Editor*

ISSUE OF RELATED INTEREST

Pediatric Clinics of North America, April 2017 (Vol. 64, No. 2)
Adolescent Sexuality
Marianne E. Felice, *Editor*
Available at: http://www.pediatric.theclinics.com/

AACAP Members: Please go to www.jaacap.org for information on access to the Child and Adolescent Psychiatric Clinics. *Resident* Members of AACAP: Special access information is available at www.childpsych.theclinics.com.

THE CLINICS ARE AVAILABLE ONLINE!
Access your subscription at:
www.theclinics.com

Preface

Child Psychiatry in the Age of the Internet

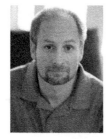 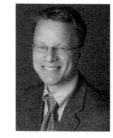

Kristopher Kaliebe, MD   Paul Weigle, MD
Editors

Experienced child and adolescent psychiatrists currently enjoy a unique but awkward position. We are part of what may be the most significant generation gap in history. We experienced life before the Internet, the revolution that changed how we interact with one another and the world we share.

We witnessed the emergence and disappearance of VCRs, audio cassettes, and pagers, as well as several generations of home computers, printers, mobile phones, and video game consoles. We recall when children played together outside, and "there's nothing on TV" meant that after the Johnny Carson show, the TV screen literally went blank until the morning. We know the pleasure of quickly writing progress notes with pen and paper and the horrors of reviewing illegible charts.

The development of the World Wide Web and the massive proliferation of Internet-connected devices are the greatest changes yet. The Web itself has exploded in content to a zettabyte of information, over 5 billion times the sum of every book ever written. Constant connectivity to essentially limitless data has swept through our personal and professional lives. Unlike future generations, we bear witness to all that childhood has gained and what has been lost, for better and worse.

As physicians and mental health professionals, we are tasked with expertly assessing and treating children and adolescents who have never known a world without perpetual interconnection. Cyber-socialization occurs ever earlier in children's lives, meaning exposure to known dangers online and the "unknown unknowns" of how daily Internet habits affect brain maturation. The Internet grants access to a myriad of amusements, teachings, and wonders of democratized human creativity. It fills social needs previously unmet in developed postindustrial societies and promises to empower more effective mental health treatments. In a world where youth development is intertwined with the vast expanse of the World Wide Web, we rely on our collective intelligence more than ever. No busy practitioner can possibly make the time to

Child Adolesc Psychiatric Clin N Am 27 (2018) xiii–xv
https://doi.org/10.1016/j.chc.2017.12.001
1056-4993/18/© 2017 Elsevier Inc. All rights reserved.

childpsych.theclinics.com

stay current with the latest online fads: which YouTubers are popular with 8 year olds, what it's like to play the new multiplayer game, and how youth share mental health concerns on Facebook. However, we should stay abreast of major online trends and synthesize the latest research into actionable assessment and treatment of our young patients.

This issue of *Child and Adolescent Psychiatric Clinics of North America* endeavors to provide a thorough and balanced update of the intersection of the digital media habits and mental health in youth.

The modern psychiatric assessment must incorporate the considerable influence of an individual's online habits on his or her mental functioning. Dr. Carson and colleagues describe how to do so by adapting the traditional biopsychosocial formulation to encompass modern media use.

Digital media is a Pandora's Box for so many modern families: easy to incorporate but subsequently difficult to control. For parents, failure to create a plan for media rules is akin to planning to fail. Drs. Dalope and Woods review how to work with families to set up a media plan and provide a social-ecologic framework for understanding mental health effects of media and its influences on family dynamics.

Internet habits create various risks and opportunities for our young patients suffering from mental illnesses. Youth suffering from depression are more and more frequently communicating distress, cutting habits, and suicidal thoughts online. Social media use is linked to both nonsuicidal self-injury and suicidal ideation, although the relationship is more complex than one might think. Drs. Belfort and Miller examine how depressed teens use social media, and how that use affects their course of illness and high-risk behaviors.

Children and teens suffering from anxiety disorders are also heavy users of social media, often preferring the perceived safety of interacting with peers online rather than in-person. Drs. Glover and Fritsch describe both prospects and perils for anxious youth online as well as the potential of innovative apps and online programs to prevent and treat anxiety.

Dr. Ceranoglu reviews the interplay between attention-deficit/hyperactivity disorder (ADHD) and digital media. Children and adolescents with ADHD are particularly drawn to electronic entertainment and have reduced capacity to resist its temptations. They consume more screen media than their peers, which potentially further degrades their capacity for attention. The research is reviewed, and clinical implications are explained.

Behaviorally disordered youth are often heavy users of digital media, and violent media in particular. Do violent video games and movies worsen their behavior? How should parents respond when their children engage in violent media? Dr. Reich explores how clinicians can respond.

Autism spectrum disorders are in part defined by a lack of social skills and narrow circumscribed interests. In modern times, autistic patients' preoccupations and splinter skills often relate to digital devices. Dr. Gwynette and colleagues review both the risk and the promise of electronic media for these populations.

For decades, concerns have been raised about the effects of media exposure on the developing minds of children, including distortion of body image potentially leading to eating disorders. Drs. Saul and Rodgers explore how children's use of social media interacts with eating-disordered behavior, and how online influences provide helpful support or toxic "thinspiration."

As more and more time in children's lives is devoted to online entertainment, important activities are often displaced or disrupted. Dr. Hale and colleagues explore the effects of screen habits on the sleep of children and adolescents and describe how and why clinicians should help families to prioritize adequate sleep for youth.

The Internet has the capacity to connect likeminded young people in a manner unprecedented in human history, essentially defining modern youth culture. Dr. Peeples and colleagues describe how the Internet united youth with niche interests to give birth to modern "geek culture" in its many forms: from cosplay to fanfiction, gamers to furries.

In contrast to its ability to bring people together, the Internet also has the capacity to spread hatred and dissention. Drs. Mayhew and Weigle examine the online habits and experiences of racial and ethnic minority youth, including the formation of a positive self-image despite the consequences of widespread online discrimination and racism.

Two of the most notorious activities made possible for today's youth by social media are cyberbullying and sexting. Dr. Englander summarizes her own research and that of others, to convey just how often they occur in the lives of youth, their psychological impact, and how clinicians can protect our patients. The results are both surprising and clinically useful.

Screen media habits among youth range from simple use to overuse and even to frank abuse. An unfortunate few engage in excessive, uncontrollable use of screen media, to the detriment of their real-life functioning. The DSM-5's inclusion of Internet gaming disorder as a potential diagnosis lent legitimacy in the West to a syndrome considered a major public health problem in China and South Korea. Dr. Sussman and colleagues review the substantial literature describing Internet gaming disorder and other online addictions, including diagnosis, epidemiology, and neurobiologic underpinnings. Dr. Greenfield compares Internet and video game addiction to substance use disorders and gives an extensive review of contemporary psychotherapeutic and psychopharmacologic treatment options for this modern clinical dilemma.

Drs. Gerwin and colleagues review recent trends in digital media use among youth and summarize available research to guide professionals and caretakers regarding the types and amounts of media content most appropriate for each developmental stage. Young children need tight controls and supervision. On the other hand, today's children and adolescents need enough gradual autonomy to develop self-regulation skills sufficient to balance their offline and virtual lives.

In the years to come, the power of the Internet will further shape the landscape of childhood and adolescence. Child and adolescent psychiatrists must understand the ways digital media influences the mental health of our patients, in order to prevent unhealthy use and correct such behavior once in place. We also need to make better use of online resources. These articles offer practitioners a means to reach across the generation gap and guide treatment of today's digital natives.

Kristopher Kaliebe, MD
Department of Psychiatry
University of South Florida Medical School
3515 East Fletcher Avenue, MDC 14
Tampa, FL 33613, USA

Paul Weigle, MD
Natchaug Hospital
189 Storrs Road, PO Box 260
Mansfield Center, CT 06250-0260, USA

E-mail addresses:
kkaliebe@health.usf.edu (K. Kaliebe)
paul.weigle@hhchealth.org (P. Weigle)

Assessment of Digital Media Use in the Adolescent Psychiatric Evaluation

Nicholas J. Carson, MD, FRCPC[a],*, Meredith Gansner, MD[b],
Jeane Khang[c]

KEYWORDS

- Adolescent • Assessment • Evaluation • Internet • Mental health • Psychiatry
- Social media

KEY POINTS

- Twenty-first century adolescents are growing up in an increasingly digital world, and their use of technology has an impact on their biological, psychological, and social development.
- This article encourages a new approach to the traditional psychiatric assessment that incorporates an evaluation of digital media use, which more accurately captures the experiences and interests of today's adolescents.
- The assessment of digital media includes how teens access media, what content they consume and create, and the related positive and negative impacts on their mental health across all domains of the traditional assessment.

INTRODUCTION

At its heart, the practice of adolescent psychiatry begins with, and is defined by, an interview of an adolescent and, when available, a family. This interview covers a set of domains that organizes the psychiatrist's understanding of the family's concerns and the formulation of the information discussed. Child psychiatrists view their patients as embedded in systems and cultures: kinship and peer networks, school

Disclosure Statement: Drs N. Carson and M. Gansner are employees of the Cambridge Health Alliance. Otherwise, the authors have no direct commercial or financial conflicts of interest nor any funding sources to report.
[a] Child and Adolescent Outpatient Psychiatry, Health Equity Research Lab, Department of Psychiatry, Cambridge Health Alliance, 1493 Cambridge Street, Cambridge, MA 02139, USA;
[b] Department of Psychiatry, Cambridge Health Alliance, 1493 Cambridge Street, Cambridge, MA 02139, USA; [c] Harvard University, 1493 Cambridge Street, Cambridge, MA 02139, USA
* Corresponding author.
E-mail address: ncarson@cha.harvard.edu

Child Adolesc Psychiatric Clin N Am 27 (2018) 133–143
https://doi.org/10.1016/j.chc.2017.11.003
1056-4993/18/© 2017 Elsevier Inc. All rights reserved.

childpsych.theclinics.com

systems, neighborhood dynamics, and ethnic cultures.[1] These systems and cultures are important domains in a psychiatric assessment for their deep influence on both the adolescent's expression of mental illness and the families help seeking. The authors suggest that online social media and other "new media" enabled by the Internet are modern examples of such systems and cultures, with potentially potent influences on child and adolescent development. This article therefore aims to describe an approach to the psychiatric assessment of such media use by adolescents to help psychiatrists appreciate its meaning in their patients' lives. The authors apply the traditional framework of the adolescent psychiatric assessment[2] that is well known to mental health clinicians to innovate from within the typically covered domains. The authors focus on adolescents specifically because issues surrounding their digital media use are better elucidated, but clinicians may also find this approach relevant to younger children, especially as children get access to more sophisticated technology at earlier ages.[2,3]

The rapid evolution of digital media devices and content ensures that the psychiatric evaluation of their use by teens will continue to evolve, and current approaches will become outdated. Thus, the authors' description of this approach is scaffolded by their clinical and research experience (N.C., M.G.) in adolescent development. Where available, research data have supplemented the authors' experience, clinical recommendations, and analysis.

Why Should the Psychiatrist Assess Internet Use by Adolescents?

The technology available to adolescents changes so rapidly that it is worth summarizing current trends in adolescent media use to convey how technology is affecting the biology, psychology, and social lives of twenty-first century teens.[4] Recent national surveys reveal a consistent trend: both the amount of time spent online and the number of devices and platforms adolescents use continue to increase. As mobile smartphones become more available, access to the Internet is all too easy, with 92% of teens going online daily, and 24% who go online almost all the time.[5] Screen time is no longer limited to a television or computer: watching shows, playing video games, texting, using social media, and even listening to music involve some form of screen-based technology. Most of these media are social, allowing communication with others and sharing one's own content. Not including academic computer use, American adolescents average close to 9 hours of entertainment media use per day.[3] Clinicians working in lower-income and culturally diverse settings should also be sensitive to how media habits vary by cultural background and socioeconomic status (SES). The recent Common Sense Media survey suggests that African American and lower SES teens spend more time on social media than their counterparts (white and Hispanic teens, and middle and higher SES teens, respectively).[3]

Potential risks and benefits of media on psychological functioning and development exist for all teens, although youth with psychiatric distress may be particularly vulnerable.[4] Some of the most concerning associations involve worse executive functioning, increased aggressive behavior due to violent media content, higher risk of depression for high users, and decreased sleep quality due to screen time.[6] The Common Sense survey reported a correlation between lower social-emotional well-being and higher use of online social media (1:27 h/d vs 55 min/d among youth with higher well-being). Equally, digital media can help teens maintain social connections, foster creative endeavors and civic engagement, develop identity and worldviews, and learn about their health.[6] Although many of these associations have yet to be studied prospectively, they validate one pressing message: teens in the twenty-first century are shaped and impacted by their digital lives. In the following sections, the authors describe an approach to guide assessment and treatment planning with this in mind. The authors have distilled the approach into specific questions (**Table 1**) to ask of patients and caregivers.

CHILD INTERVIEW
The Chief Complaint

When asking caregivers and teens to describe their chief concerns, the psychiatrist should expect on occasion to hear histories of Internet-related conflict, risk disclosure, or overuse. A teen's depression and anxiety might be related to cyberbullying, and teens might disclose unsafe thoughts exclusively through texting or social media. These chief complaints may come as a result of peers notifying school staff of worrisome online activities, which precipitates a request for psychiatric evaluation. Families may also present for evaluation after children become aggressive when their technology use is limited. To give a rough sense of how often Internet-related presentations occur, in the authors' unpublished survey of 241 adolescents hospitalized for psychiatric reasons, more than 20% thought their admission was "related to something that happened online or texting with others."[7]

History of Presenting Illness, Review of Psychiatric Symptoms, Past Psychiatric History

Traditional screening for psychiatric symptoms remains largely unchanged in a new media-related framework, with a focus on timing, onset, and severity of symptoms. The ways in which online interactions play a significant role in a teen's expression or exploration of their symptoms warrant exploration. As noted by Cuffe and Desai[2] in their guide to adolescent psychiatric assessment, the history of presenting illness involves a dialectic of rapport building and data collection, often with an unwilling interviewee. The psychiatrist who expresses interest in a teen's online life may accomplish both tasks by conveying an authentic concern about the teen's inner life, interests, and closest relationships, which sometimes are best found in online spaces.

For example, social media (as of 2017, popular sites include Facebook, YouTube, Twitter, Instagram, Snapchat) can be seen as a safe space to disclose internalizing symptoms or risky behaviors in order to elicit peer support. This behaviour appears to be more common among adolescent girls and may lead to "co-rumination," where peers exacerbate each other's distress.[8] The clinician might therefore ask patients if they feel supported or isolated online. Note that online "support" can be double-edged: adolescents may disclose that social networks help them feel healthy, playful, and connected, but others may use online communities to learn about and engage in risky behaviors, for example, self-injury,[9,10] restricted eating,[11] and even suicide.[12] Clinicians should keep an open mind when inquiring about new media, without assuming benefit or risk, but being attentive to both possibilities.

When assessing for risky behaviors, it is also necessary to inquire about the pressing public health problems of online conflict, such as cyberbullying (lifetime prevalence of 23% in high school students)[13] and problematic Internet use (prevalence ranging up to 26.3% in US youth).[14] Detailed screening tools exist, but given time pressures of the initial assessment, high-yield questions should explore online "drama" as well as the desire to cut back on Internet use, the urge to use the Internet, and tension or anxiety that can only be relieved by Internet use.[15] Further assessment should include the teen's access to devices and how caregivers supervise their use. Identifying problematic Internet use or Internet addiction can be an important proxy for anxiety, depression, or online risk behaviors like cyberbullying or meeting strangers online.[16]

Table 1
Screening questions for further study

Interview Domain	Screening Questions
Chief complaint	• Do you think your main concern today is related to something that happened online?
History of presenting illness/psychiatric review of systems	• Do you ever post online about your current problem? How so, and where? • Have you been involved in any online bullying or "drama"? • Do you think using the Internet has been helpful or harmful to your current situation? • Do you ever go online to learn about the problems you've been experiencing?
Past psychiatric history	• Have you/has your child ever been diagnosed with or treated for Internet addiction or problematic Internet use?
Past medical history	• Do you go online before you fall asleep? • Would you say your (media use) affects your sleep? • Do you go online to learn about physical health?
School history	• Do you use your cell phone in the classroom? • Would you say your media use affects your ability to get your schoolwork done?
Social history	• Who do you talk to online, and how do you interact with them? • What are your favorite Web sites and apps? • What kind of things do you post online, and what kind of feedback do you get? Have you gotten in trouble for it? • Is anyone bothering you online? Are *you* bothering anyone online?
Developmental history	• (Caregiver) What kind of screen time was allowed during the early years? How did you supervise this? • (Adolescent) What are you good at online? What is your favorite thing to do online? • (Adolescent) Do you feel like you belong to something online? • (Adolescent) Does going online help you figure out the kind of person you want to be?
Sexual history	(Adolescent only) • Do you go online to start romantic or sexual relationships? Did you meet these people in person? • Have you sent sexually explicit texts to anyone? Were there positive or negative consequences? • Do you go online to view sexual content, such as pornography? If so, how often? • Has going online helped you explore your gender or sexuality?
Mental status examination	(Questions for psychiatrist to ask self during interview) • What does the adolescent do with their device before, during, and after the interview? • Does the adolescent reference online content or platforms repeatedly? (Questions for provider to ask patient) • Sometimes people prefer to say how they are feeling online rather than face to face. Is there anything that you have posted online that you think might help me understand who you are or how you have been feeling? • Is anything from online constantly in your thoughts?

(continued on next page)

Table 1 (continued)	
Interview Domain	**Screening Questions**
Caregiver interview/family history	• How many devices are in the home, and who owns them? • How do you talk about Internet use in your family? • Has there been conflict among family members related to devices or the Internet? • How many hours of screen time are allowed on school days and on weekends? • Does your family have rules for using devices? • Do you discuss what your teen is watching and doing online? • Do you think your teen's digital media use is having a positive or negative impact?

Medical/Physical History and Review of Systems

As adolescent obesity reaches epidemic proportions, and given the effects of certain psychiatric medications on appetite and sleep, metabolic health is often a major concern in the adolescent psychiatric assessment. "High screen users" have less physical activity than low screen users, and recent Youth Risk Behavior Survey analyses link screen time greater than 5 h/d with inadequate physical activity and sleep.[3,17] The authors also know that furtive smartphone use makes it easy for most adolescents to sleep with their devices in their bedrooms, another contributor to inefficient sleep.[18–20] The authors recommend exploring how screen time might be displacing other healthy activities (like exercise) or interfering with healthy sleep habits.[21] Note that nearly a third of teens use the Internet to learn about health-related information.[22] Clinicians can support this positive habit by reviewing which sites they are consulting and suggesting trusted online resources.[23]

School History

Academics are another prime candidate for displacement by screen time. As schools increasingly use computers in the classroom and share information with caregivers online, Internet literacy is an important developmental achievement for adolescents, and those who are strongest at this benefit academically.[24] Thus, it is worth exploring with caregivers and teachers whether they perceive a teen's Internet use to help or impede school performance. Frequent cell phone use in the classroom may signal concern, especially because many schools prohibit them. At the same time, the clinician should explore how school pressures interact with unhealthy Internet habits. Teachers might be able to shed light on links between academic stress, negative emotions, and problematic Internet use (overuse or online conflict).[25]

Social History

The social history characterizes the adolescent's neighborhood and school relationships, communities, extracurricular interests and strengths, as well as risk behaviors (sex, substance use). As adolescents connect via Facebook, Tinder, Instagram, and other social media applications, their social lives will involve digital media to varying degrees. The clinician should be curious about how often the adolescent uses the Internet to talk to others, what kinds of people he or she networks with online, and whether these online social circles are having a positive or negative effect on well-being. Although some adolescents may identify with online peer groups as much as they do with their families,[26] the benefits are primarily dependent on the quality of feedback they receive.[27] Some distressed adolescents may seek offline contact with strangers they meet through social media; this habit is associated with cyberbullying and can leave a teen vulnerable to victimization.[16] Thus, the clinician should be curious about the quality of online feedback, and whether such contact puts the teen at risk for trauma.

When exploring substance use, the clinician should ask about "displays" of substance use on social media. Teens with high Internet use are more likely to have substance use disorders, especially when they post online about their use (eg, profile picture or videos).[28] A teen admitting to such posts should prompt more intensive screening surrounding drug and alcohol use.

Developmental History

Assessing exposure to screens as part of a developmental history can help the clinician assess attachment and caregiving approaches. Virtually all children less than the age of 2 are exposed to screen time, and a third of children less than the age of 3 have televisions in their room.[6] The focus here should be on how engaged a caregiver was when allowing devices for play, learning, or communication (eg, with family separated by long distances). This parental scaffolding is an important mediator of positive outcomes for children using devices.

As adolescence looms, the clinician can apply developmental theories (eg, Erikson's stages) to assess how media take on different purposes and meanings over time.[29] The task of "industry versus inferiority" can be explored by asking how the patient is allowed to use devices at home and school, both for play and for learning, with an ear to problematic uses (eg, excessive/inappropriate video game play). Older adolescents might be very open to discussions of how they use digital media to communicate with peers, explore romantic relationships, participate in cultural movements or subgroups, and share their lives through text, pictures, and video. All of these online activities can be understood in the frame of "identity versus isolation," and the clinician should be attentive to both feelings of connection or loneliness in online activities.

Sexual History

Although most teenagers continue to seek sexual or romantic partners offline, a quarter of teens "dating" are reported to have met a partner through digital media.[5,30] Teens have also adopted the use of apps specifically created for finding romantic or sexual partners; nearly 10% of Tinder users, for example, are teenagers.[31] However, the search for intimate relationships via the Internet can expose a teen to new potential threats: unwanted exposure to sexual material, harassment, or the risk that a sexually suggestive or explicit text ("sext") is shared beyond its intended recipient.[32,33] For these reasons, the clinician should ask how the adolescent uses the Internet to find relationships or share sexual feelings and behaviors, including viewing of pornography. If sexting is endorsed, a high-yield follow-up is to ask whether the adolescent felt *pressured* to sext. Most adolescents appear to use new media safely to express sexuality and build intimacy in new romantic relationships with peers, but those pressured to share sexual material more often experience dating violence, "self-cyberbullying," and have the sext shared with greater than 3 others.[34]

The Internet can be a safe space for adolescents to express and understand their gender and sexuality. Not all LGBTQ (lesbian, gay, bisexual, transgender, queer or questioning) adolescents may feel safe exploring in-person relationships, especially in more heteronormative communities. Such adolescents meet others online within the community and gain support in the coming-out process.[35,36] This particular use of digital media is just one important example of how clinicians can learn about adolescent identity development by inquiring about media use.

Trauma History

Clinicians who care for traumatized adolescents may want to take particular care in asking about media use among their patients. The research tells us that teens exposed to sexual or physical abuse or high parental conflict are more likely to engage in aggressive behavior online, receive sexual solicitation online, and have difficulties controlling their Internet use.[37] Conversely, clinicians should not miss those traumatic experiences that occur through a digital screen. As noted above, the prevalence of cyberbullying is high and takes many forms: verbal harassment through texting or social media platform, or the spread of sensitive information to a wider peer network. Youth with intellectual and developmental disabilities appear to be at particular risk for online victimization, given their cognitive vulnerabilities and their frequent preoccupation with digital media.[38] Clinicians should inquire about parental supervision of media use, which moderates the impact of childhood trauma on Internet risk behaviors and offline sexual meetings.[39]

MENTAL STATUS EXAMINATION

There is much to learn about the importance of technology in a family's life through careful observation during the psychiatric interview. Does the teen or their caregiver use a device in the waiting room or office, and how is it used? This observation can be a quick way to determine how a family uses technology for distraction or learning. The clothing choices of patients will often speak volumes about their cultural interests, some of which may represent obsessions (eg, the favorite television show of a patient with autism) or passions (eg, music bands, video games, or other brands). Once in the room, patients may text, take calls, or be preoccupied with phone games during the session and may even ask the psychiatrist to allow recording of pictures, audio, or video during the assessment.[40] These small requests and distractions may be signs of the patient's defensiveness, anxiety, boredom, or other internal distractions. Some patients will feel compelled to use the psychiatrist's computer to search for favorite Web sites or products, or even to read documentation in the electronic record, such that all devices might need to be turned off during the evaluation. The patient's language might be full of references to media content (eg, a patient with autism who scripts a favorite film or anime; a patient with psychosis who has ideas of reference regarding online content).

When describing thought content, the patient may disclose a broad range of media-related concerns: intense craving for video games or social networks, conflict with peers online, or obsessions indulged through hours of Web surfing. Adolescent patients may disclose a "fear of missing out (FOMO)"[41] on the latest in their peer network, which may signal insecurity. Some teens may even find it easier to "let the phone talk for them" by showing relevant texts, posts, or videos in their online social profiles directly revealing thought content. This willingness of youth to share their devices in session is no surprise given research that suggests "Facebook activates the ideal self."[42] The clinician may find this a high-yield opportunity to notice how the patient's history differs from, or confirms, the way they present themselves online.

Disclosure of dangerous thoughts or actions in online spaces may not be readily obvious in the examination room, but rather in the history gathered from the patient, caregiver, and collateral sources (eg, unsafe texts seen by teachers). The psychiatrist should look for indications of the patient's insight that their distress is connected to use of the Internet, or that they can use online resources to improve their health. A patient's judgment in relation to Internet use can be seen in the way they use technology in the office, or in other domains in life as revealed through the history of presenting illness and the social history.

CAREGIVER INTERVIEW

Time spent with the caregiver can be a crucial way to validate and clarify the history received from the adolescent. Media use can be explored with caregivers by asking about what devices are in the home, who uses them, and for how long (school days and weekends). This query may quickly reveal a caregiver who is at wit's end trying to rein in their teen's (or spouse's) problematic phone or computer use. It may equally show a family whose time is well balanced across online and offline activities, with healthy monitoring and engagement in the teen's online activities. It is important to ask for the caregiver's perspective on their teen's positive and negative uses of technology; both may often be present. A parent's perception of these positive and negative uses may provide helpful information about the parent-child dyad. For example, a caregiver who is entirely unaware of a child's online presence, as well as one who knows all too much, may represent broader problematic attachment styles within the family.[43] It is therefore worth getting a sense of the caregiver's digital literacy. In divided households, poor communication between the parent who pays the cell phone bill and the parent who sets limits on cell phone use may create triangulation within the family.

BIOPSYCHOSOCIAL FORMULATION

Once the assessment is complete, the formulation is wherein the psychiatrist integrates the media-related aspects of the history and examination into an overall explanatory model of the adolescent's presentation. The authors have presented a framework for a "media formulation" in prior work.[4] The clinician considers how Internet and technology use affect the adolescent's biology (eg, sleep disruption by devices in the bedroom), psychology (eg, online self-disclosure and identity, sexuality, and intimacy),[27] and social functioning (eg, online sharing or conflict). It can be useful to consider how media use interacts with biopsychosocial factors affecting mental health (eg, unmonitored access to social networks can increase the risk for bullying or academic problems, which can worsen depression). The Diagnostic and Statistical Manual of Mental Disorders, 5th edition cultural formulation[44] is a practical interview guide that can help formulate the media-related context of illness experience. It covers domains of explanatory models, stressors and supports, cultural identity, and help seeking that can all be asked with new media concerns in mind.

ETHICAL CONSIDERATIONS

After the in-person family interview is over, it may be tempting for clinicians to search for a patient's online activities to verify the history. The authors are not the first to suggest a cautious consideration of the impact on the physician-patient relationship. The family may consider this a breach of trust. Even when the adolescent extends an explicit invitation to view their content in or out of session, there is still a good chance the clinician may view content that requires unanticipated action (eg, informing parents of inappropriate, risky, or suicidal posts).[45] Clinton and colleagues[46] suggest a pragmatic framework to guide clinicians through this process, and DeJong[47] discusses the broader implications for professionalism. The authors agree that informed consent and assent be used to frame the risks and benefits of reviewing the patient's online content in and outside of the clinical session. Careful consideration of how to view digital media in an adolescent's assessment can strengthen the therapeutic alliance while deepening the psychiatrist's understanding of the patient.

SUMMARY

The online social networks that are popular today will likely soon fade in importance as newer services take their place, offering different technological capabilities. Such rapid change will require psychiatrists to constantly reevaluate digital media's relevance to diagnosis, treatment, and broader social concerns, such as privacy. Providers in different clinical settings (inpatient, community, emergency room care) will need to adapt this approach to their specific context. Now that digital technology is such an intimate aspect of adolescent culture, the inclusion of a media-related framework in the psychiatric assessment will likely become ever more relevant because the physical and digital worlds continue to blur. The psychiatrist will be challenged to explain a teen's individualized relationship with digital media in the formulation and treatment, in a way that respects the youth's digital autonomy and reinforces responsible and healthy behaviors.

REFERENCES

1. Storck MG, Stoep AV. Fostering ecologic perspectives in child psychiatry. Child Adolesc Psychiatr Clin N Am 2007;16(1):133–63.
2. Cuffe S, Desai C. Assessing adolescents. In: Dulcan MK, editor. Dulcan's textbook of child and adolescent psychiatry. Arlington (VA): American Psychiatric Pub; 2015. p. 73–88.
3. Rideout V. The common sense census: media use by tweens and teens. 2015.
4. Rafla M, Carson NJ, DeJong SM. Adolescents and the internet: what mental health clinicians need to know. Curr Psychiatry Rep 2014;16(9):472.
5. Lenhart A. Teens, Social Media and Technology Overview 2015: Smartphones Facilitate Shifts in Communication Landscape for Teens. 2015.
6. Reid Chassiakos Y, Radesky J, Christakis D, et al. Children and Adolescents and Digital Media. Elk Grove Village (IL): The American Academy of Pediatrics; 2016.
7. Gansner M, Cook B, Webster C, et al. Problematic internet use in psychiatrically hospitalized adolescents. Poster presented at 2017 Harvard Psychiatry Research Day, Boston (MA), April 12, 2017.
8. Ehrenreich SE, Underwood MK. Adolescents' internalizing symptoms as predictors of the content of their Facebook communication and responses received from peers. Transl Issues Psychol Sci 2016;2(3):227–37.
9. Whitlock JL, Powers JL, Eckenrode J. The virtual cutting edge: the internet and adolescent self-injury. Dev Psychol 2006;42(3):407–17.
10. Lewis SP, Seko Y. A double-edged sword: a review of benefits and risks of online nonsuicidal self-injury activities. J Clin Psychol 2016;72(3):249–62.
11. Custers K, Van den Bulck J. Viewership of pro-anorexia websites in seventh, ninth and eleventh graders. Eur Eat Disord Rev 2009;17(3):214–9.
12. Mok K, Jorm AF, Pirkis J. Suicide-related internet use: a review. Aust N Z J Psychiatry 2015;49(8):697–705.
13. Hamm MP, Newton AS, Chisholm A, et al. Prevalence and effect of cyberbullying on children and young people. JAMA Pediatr 2015;169(8):770–7.
14. Moreno MA, Jelenchick L, Cox E, et al. Problematic internet use among US youth. Arch Pediatr Adolesc Med 2011;165(9):797–805.

15. Liu TC, Desai RA, Krishnan-Sarin S, et al. Problematic internet use and health in adolescents: data from a high school survey in Connecticut. J Clin Psychiatry 2011;72(6):836–45.
16. Gámez-Guadix M, Borrajo E, Almendros C. Risky online behaviors among adolescents: longitudinal relations among problematic internet use, cyberbullying perpetration, and meeting strangers online. J Behav Addict 2016;5(1):100–7.
17. Kenney EL, Gortmaker SL. United States adolescents' television, computer, videogame, smartphone, and tablet use: associations with sugary drinks, sleep, physical activity, and obesity. J Pediatr 2017;182:144–9.
18. Gamble AL, D'Rozario AL, Bartlett DJ, et al. Adolescent sleep patterns and nighttime technology use: results of the Australian Broadcasting Corporation's Big Sleep Survey. PLoS One 2014;9(11):e111700.
19. Van den Bulck J. Adolescent use of mobile phones for calling and for sending text messages after lights out: results from a prospective cohort study with a one-year follow-up. Sleep 2007;30(9):1220–3.
20. Fobian AD, Avis K, Schwebel DC. Impact of media use on adolescent sleep efficiency. J Dev Behav Pediatr 2016;37(1):9–14.
21. Kaliebe K. Rules of thumb: three simple ideas for overcoming the complex problem of childhood obesity. J Am Acad Child Adolesc Psychiatry 2014;53(4):385–7.
22. Lenhart A, Purcell K, Smith A, et al. Social media & mobile internet use among teens and young adults. Pew Internet Am Life Proj 2010. Available at: https://files.eric.ed.gov/fulltext/ED525056.pdf. Accessed December 4, 2017.
23. Gray NJ, Klein JD, Noyce PR, et al. Health information-seeking behaviour in adolescence: the place of the internet. Soc Sci Med 2005;60(7):1467–78.
24. Leung L, Lee PSN. Impact of internet literacy, internet addiction symptoms, and internet activities on academic performance. Soc Sci Comput Rev 2012;30(4):403–18.
25. Jun S, Choi E. Academic stress and internet addiction from general strain theory framework. Comput Hum Behav 2015;49:282–7.
26. Davis K. Friendship 2.0: adolescents' experiences of belonging and self-disclosure online. J Adolesc 2012;35(6):1527–36.
27. Valkenburg PM, Peter J. Online communication among adolescents: an integrated model of its attraction, opportunities, and risks. J Adolesc Health 2011;48(2):121–7.
28. Moreno MA, Cox ED, Young HN, et al. Underage college students' alcohol displays on Facebook and real-time alcohol behaviors. J Adolesc Health 2015;56(6):646–51.
29. Erikson EH. Identity: youth and crisis (No. 7). New York: WW Norton & Company; 1994.
30. Blunt-Vinti HD, Wheldon C, McFarlane M, et al. Assessing relationship and sexual satisfaction in adolescent relationships formed online and offline. J Adolesc Health 2016;58(1):11–6.
31. Duan N. Swipe right for prom: how teens are using Tinder. The Guardian 2017.
32. Ybarra ML, Mitchell KJ. How risky are social networking sites? A comparison of places online where youth sexual solicitation and harassment occurs. Pediatrics 2008;121(2):e350–7.
33. Strassberg DS, McKinnon RK, Sustaíta MA, et al. Sexting by high school students: an exploratory and descriptive study. Arch Sex Behav 2013;42(1):15–21.
34. Englander E. Low risk associated with most teenage sexting: a study of 617 18-year-olds. 2012. Available at: http://webhost.bridgew.edu/marc/sexting%20and%20coercion%20report.pdf. Accessed December 4, 2017.

35. Harper GW, Serrano PA, Bruce D, et al. The internet's multiple roles in facilitating the sexual orientation identity development of gay and bisexual male adolescents. Am J Mens Health 2016;10(5):359–76.
36. Ybarra ML, Mitchell KJ. A national study of lesbian, gay, bisexual (LGB), and non-LGB youth sexual behavior online and in-person. Arch Sex Behav 2016;45(6): 1357–72.
37. Wells M, Mitchell KJ. How do high-risk youth use the internet? Characteristics and implications for prevention. Child Maltreat 2008;13(3):227–34.
38. Normand CL, Sallafranque-St-Louis F. Cybervictimization of young people with an intellectual or developmental disability: risks specific to sexual solicitation. J Appl Res Intellect Disabil 2016;29(2):99–110.
39. Noll JG, Shenk CE, Barnes JE, et al. Association of maltreatment with high-risk internet behaviors and offline encounters. Pediatrics 2013;131(2):e510–7.
40. Elwyn G, Barr PJ, Castaldo M. Can patients make recordings of medical encounters?: what does the law say? JAMA 2017;318(6):513–4.
41. Przybylski AK, Murayama K, Dehaan CR, et al. Motivational, emotional, and behavioral correlates of fear of missing out. Comput Hum Behav 2013;29(4): 1841–8.
42. Gonzales AL, Hancock JT. Mirror, mirror on my Facebook wall: effects of exposure to Facebook on self-esteem. Cyberpsychol Behav Soc Netw 2011;14(1–2): 79–83.
43. King DL, Delfabbro PH. My Facebook family: should adolescent psychiatric evaluation include information about online social networks? Aust N Z J Psychiatry 2014;48(9):805–8.
44. American Psychiatric Association. Cultural formulation. The diagnostic and statistical manual of mental disorders. 5th edition. 2013. Available at: http://dsm.psychiatryonline.org/doi/full/10.1176/appi.books.9780890425596.Cultural Formulation. Accessed July 13, 2017.
45. Gabbard GO, Kassaw KA, Perez-Garcia G. Professional boundaries in the era of the internet. Acad Psychiatry 2011;35(3):168–74.
46. Clinton BK, Silverman BC, Brendel DH. Patient-targeted googling: the ethics of searching online for patient information. Harv Rev Psychiatry 2010;18(2):103–12.
47. DeJong SM. Blogs and tweets, texting and friending: social media and online professionalism in health care. San Diego (CA): Academic Press; 2013.

Digital Media Use in Families

Theories and Strategies for Intervention

Kristin A. Dalope, MD, MEd[a],*, Leonard J. Woods, LCSW[b]

KEYWORDS

- Digital media • Families • Social-ecological • Family systems • Developmental
- Parenting

KEY POINTS

- Digital media is changing the lives of individuals and families.
- A social-ecological framework shows how media has both a direct and indirect impact on individuals, relationships, communities, and society.
- Family systems theory demonstrates how digital media is incorporated into family dynamics.
- A developmental framework explores the role of digital media in shaping parenting.
- Practical strategies and resources (eg, the Family Media Use Plan from the American Academy of Pediatrics) are available and discussed.

INTRODUCTION

When a child, adolescent, or family presents to a professional with concerns about digital media use, there are three frameworks that can be useful in determining where and how to intervene. The social-ecological model illustrates the direct and indirect impact of media on individuals, relationships, communities, and society. Family systems theory demonstrates the integration of digital media-related issues into family dynamics. A developmental framework explores the role of digital media in shaping parenting. These theories can inform practice by providing clinicians a variety of strategies, including recommendations and resources (eg, Family Media Use Plan) from the American Academy of Pediatrics (AAP).

Disclosure Statement: None.
[a] Department of Child and Adolescent Psychiatry, University of Pittsburgh Medical Center, Western Psychiatric Institute and Clinic, Children's Hospital of Pittsburgh, Merck Clinic, Franklin Building, 1st Floor, 1011 Bingham Street, Pittsburgh, PA 15203, USA; [b] Child and Adolescent Psychiatry, Center for Children and Families, University of Pittsburgh Medical Center, Western Psychiatric Institute and Clinic, Merck Clinic, Franklin Building, 1st Floor, 1011 Bingham Street, Pittsburgh, PA 15203, USA
* Corresponding author.
E-mail address: dalopek@upmc.edu

Child Adolesc Psychiatric Clin N Am 27 (2018) 145–158
https://doi.org/10.1016/j.chc.2017.11.001
1056-4993/18/© 2017 Elsevier Inc. All rights reserved.

childpsych.theclinics.com

Terms of Reference

Digital media is a generic term for any content in electronic form. Common examples of digital media include:

- Text
- Audio
- Photographs
- Videos (eg, broadcast television, streaming video services)
- Software (eg, mobile apps and video games)
- Messaging and chat (eg, email, instant messaging, video chat)
- Web sites and online services (eg, social media, discussion forums, newspapers, blogs).

Digital media is accessed, consumed, created, modified, shared, used, or interacted with on a constantly evolving set of technology platforms. These technologies may be:

- Hand-held, mobile devices (eg, smartphones, mobile gaming consoles, tablets, e-readers)
- General purpose laptops or computers
- Gaming consoles
- Televisions.

Most of these technology platforms have Internet connectivity. Due to the pervasive and growing use of digital media by children, adolescents, and parents on these technology platforms, it is helpful to understand how digital media can have such a significant impact on families. With that in mind, three models and theories are presented here.

FAMILY MODELS AND THEORIES
Social-Ecological Model

The Center for Disease Control uses a 4-stage, social-ecological model to describe how an individual exists within a variety of systems.[1] This model (**Fig. 1**) describes an individual (eg, child or adolescent) who has a variety of relationships (eg, family and peers), which are present within a community (physically and virtually), which all exist within a society (with overarching laws and norms). The concentric nature of the model illustrates how factors at any level can have a direct or indirect impact on the other levels.

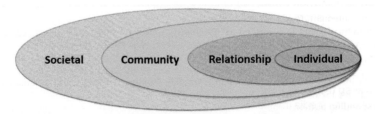

Fig. 1. Social-ecological model. (*Adapted from* Centers for Disease Control and Prevention (CDC). Violence prevention. The social-ecological model: a framework for prevention. Available at: https://www.cdc.gov/violenceprevention/overview/social-ecologicalmodel.html. Accessed May 30, 2017; with permission.)

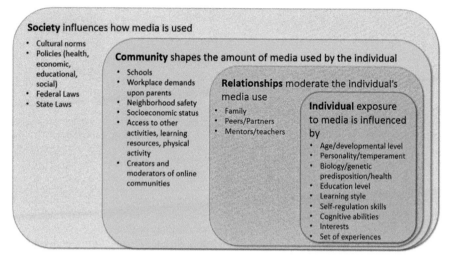

Fig. 2. Social-ecological model: expanded. (*Data from* Centers for Disease Control and Prevention (CDC). Violence prevention. The social-ecological model: a framework for prevention. Available at: https://www.cdc.gov/violenceprevention/overview/social-ecologicalmodel.html. Accessed May 30, 2017.)

The model can also help frame the ways in which digital media and technology are directly and indirectly shaping individuals and family systems[2] (**Fig. 2**). These influences are further expanded on here.

Individual exposure to media is influenced by a variety of factors ranging from the biological to education levels and interests. Relationships moderate the individual's media use through modelling, access, and expectations. Community shapes the amount of media used by the individual through school, work, neighborhoods, socioeconomic status, local and online resources. Society influences how media is used via local, state, and federal policies and laws. Federal laws include the Children's Online Privacy Protection Act (COPPA), which does not allow direct advertising to children younger than 13 years of age.[3–5] State laws include varied legal consequences for sexting, which is pertains to the sending of sexually explicit images or texts by mobile phone.

Consider the situation of a 13-year-old with an elevated body mass index comes in for an appointment (**Fig. 3**). During the interview with the teenage patient (individual) and parent (family), questions are asked about diet, exercise, and media. The clinican hears that the teenager spends several hours after school with a smartphone, tablet, and laptop, while doing homework, watching videos, using social media, and playing video games. The time spent with media displaces time that could include physical activity.

In asking more about this teen's life, additional information comes to light. This teen (individual) has a single working parent (family) who is spending more time at work and answering work emails from home. The parent does not want this individual unsupervised in the neighborhood (community) after school, so the parent permits the use of media to keep the teen physically safe indoors. Although the teen is using various modalities of digital media (multitasking is a social norm in society), there are frequent advertisements for various types of junk food (because the teen is no longer under the limited protection of COPPA). This relationship that the adolescent (or even the parent) has with electronics has not been planned, managed, or regularly teen reassessed by the family, and yet it is having a significant impact on this teen's life.

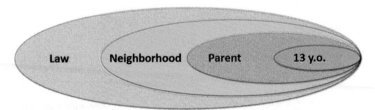

Fig. 3. Social-ecological model: example. y.o., years old. (*Adapted from* Centers for Disease Control and Prevention (CDC). Violence prevention. The social-ecological model: a framework for prevention. Available at: https://www.cdc.gov/violenceprevention/overview/social-ecologicalmodel.html. Accessed May 30, 2017; with permission.)

Possible interventions (**Fig. 4**) could go beyond focusing on diet, activity, and limiting digital media (at an individual level). Interventions could include limiting digital media for the parent (family or relationship), encouraging participation through afterschool or mentorship programs (neighbourhood or community), and engaging in advocacy locally for healthier choices, or advocacy nationally for less direct-to-consumer advertising (society).

This social-ecological model helps clinicians identify individual, relationship, community, and social influences and interventions pertaining to digital media. As providers examine the family relationship, family systems theory can be informative.

Family Systems Theory

Family systems theory looks beyond the digital media issues. The model considers the individual and focuses on the family dynamics. It considers the individual and the relationships within the family, and acknowledges that each person who exists within a family has their own unique temperament which frames how engagement occurs.

Table 1 illustrates an example of digital media–related interactions within a family. Consider the situation of an early adolescent who is experimenting with different profiles or avatars on social media sites and complaining about family. A parent learns about this behavior; confiscates the individual's smartphone; reads all the texts, emails, instant messages, and more; and becomes upset. Another parent gets pulled into the conflict and tries to play the role of a "peacemaker." The parents argue about what to do with the technology, especially with regard to societal expectations. The individual becomes anxious or depressed, and the family then presents to a clinician.

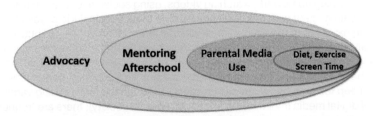

Fig. 4. Social-ecological model and interventions. (*Adapted from* Centers for Disease Control and Prevention (CDC). Violence prevention. The social-ecological model: a framework for prevention. Available at: https://www.cdc.gov/violenceprevention/overview/social-ecologicalmodel.html. Accessed May 30, 2017; with permission.)

Table 1
Examples of digital media–related interactions within a family

Concept	Explanation	Behavioral Examples Involving Technology
Nuclear Family Emotional System	Each family has implicit roles for each member. These implicit roles influence how each person acts and shapes how they deal with conflict.	A parent assuming the role of a protector reads and comments on a child's or adolescent's texts, emails, and social media use
Differentiation of Self	An individual decides how to become their own person while being influenced by the family Decisions are made not as a reaction against to the family or emotional pressures but thoughtfully and reflectively	Adolescent on social media tries out different profiles, but parent sees a profile, is not comfortable with it, and limits access to Web site or app, causing conflict between parent and teen
Triangles	Strong feelings between two members becomes too much and a third person is engaged to help diffuse the emotion This situation is problematic if those involved do not revisit the initial, unresolved conflict	Parent and teen argue over media sanctions and another parent gets pulled in to attempt to mediate the intense conflict Parents then argue over the appropriate handling of the situation and come to a stalemate where they are unable to agree on the situation Original conflict remains unaddressed
Emotional Cutoff	Describes how some family members deal with anxiety in relationships Family member retreats from physical and/or emotional contact with another family member and does not resolve the underlying conflict	To stop conflict, protector parent distances self from media issues leaving it up to the other parent to address, in effect cutting himself or herself off from both teen and other parent
Multigenerational Transmission Process	Family emotional processes, values and roles are transferred and maintained over generations in a varety of ways	Grandparents who lived through a time of scarcity, taught frugality to parents who, in reaction, either do not buy the adolescent a smartphone like their peer group or gives the adolescent everything they did not have
Societal-Emotional Process	Similar to social-ecological theory, families are overtly and covertly influenced by the societal expectations and values about race, class, gender, sexual orientation, culture, and technology	Access to smartphones, Internet, tablets, and laptops often depends on socioeconomic status Peer pressure exists related to these status symbols Communication is influenced by technology (texting instead of calling) Many relationships are in cyberspace not in person

Data from Nichols, MP. Bowen Family Systems Therapy. In: The Essentials of Family Therapy, 6th edition. New York: Pearson, Inc; 2013.

To reframe this digital media–focused situation within family systems theory, the individual is attempting to differentiate but, in doing so, violated the expectations and values within the nuclear family (nuclear family emotional system). The conflict between the parent and individual is so strong that another parent is pulled into the conflict (triangulation), which helps to diffuse the situation slightly, but results in a stalemate between parents. The parent pulls who engaged the adolescent first pulls away and reactively distances himself or herself, leaving it between the second parent and the teen to work out. This distancing can cut off the original parent emotionally from the relationships with the teen and the second parent as a method of modulating the strong emotions in this conflict. The original parent and child do not talk about the original conflict, thus stopping a healthy differentiation process.

The unconscious approach toward technology may have been consistent with how the parents were raised by grandparents who taught frugality, or a response in the opposite direction to give the teenager all the advantages unavailable to the parents (multigenerational transmission process). When limiting access to digital media, the family is then influenced by the social realities outside of the home (societal emotional process). The school is expecting online access to do schoolwork, digital media is accessible in every library, and ease of access to digital media is in almost all social settings. Thus, there is another, external set of pressures to allow the individual to continue using digital media; that is, to be plugged in.

The goal of family systems therapy is to help family members better understand their interactions and increase awareness of how they solve problems, either reactively in response to strong emotional influences or in a more consciously reflective manner. If clinicians want to examine parenting itself, then the developmental model provides a useful construct.

Developmental Model

The developmental model synthesizes parenting stages[6] with typical media use at certain ages[7,8] to describe how digital media can influence parenting and family dynamics throughout the years. **Fig. 5** illustrates these evolving developmental stages of parents compared with against digital media use and its impact on families.

Parenting infants and young toddlers (0–18 months old)

For parents, the time from birth to 18 months of age is a nurturing stage in which they get to know the individual child's personality and bond. Parents question their priorities and how to allocate their time; ie, how much time should be spent caring for the child in relation to work or pursuing other interests.

When digital media is inserted in between the caregiver-child, then the interaction is interrupted. One extreme example is of parents who neglect their infants to engage in online activities. More commonly, parents engage in the use of digital technology for a variety of reasons (eg, boredom, social support, shopping) and, in doing so, may miss cues from their child or be late in acknowledging their child's needs. This phenomenon has been termed technoconference or the ways in which digital and mobile technology interrupt everyday interpersonal interactions.[9] With frequent interruptions, there is less eye contact and less sustained speech.[10] Play is less interactive or displaced by the digital media use.[11] Instead of becoming more attuned to each other through small, focused, and frequent interactions, they can become less responsive to each other. The attachment process is influenced indirectly by digital media.

In terms of direct interactions with digital media, parents often allow infants and toddlers to video chat with family members who are geographically distant, thus increasing opportunities for the young children to meet with and bond with others.

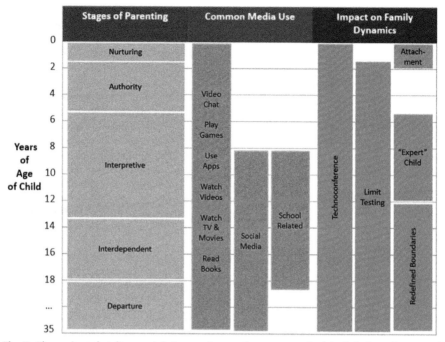

Fig. 5. The various developmental stages of parenting compared with digital media use and their impact on families. (*Data from* Galinsky E. In: the six stages of parenthood. Reading (United Kingdom): Perseus Books; 1987; and Common Sense Media. Zero to Eight: Children's Media Use in America, 2011. Available at: https://www.commonsensemedia.org/research/zero-to-eight-childrens-media-use-in-america.)

As the toddlers mature, parents may allow additional use of technology, using educational apps, reading e-books, playing games, and watching videos, television, and movies.

Parenting older toddlers and preschoolers (18 months–5 years old)

Starting at about age 2 years, parents decide what kind of authority figure to be. Parents develop, set, and enforce explicit rules and limits.

Parents may allow toddlers to use digital media, but the reasons behind this use may evolve. Mobile technology helps to keep young children calm[12] or distracted while a parent tends to certain tasks (eg, dishes, showering, phone calls, errands, eating out).[13] It is common for conflict to arise when the parent tries to end media use, with the child testing limits and the parent maintaining limits. How the media conflict is resolved depends on the temperaments of the parent and the child, as well as the parenting style.

In addition, many parents see a child's engagement with mobile technology as good parenting because it can be a source of educational activities or child-led endeavors.[14] Parents may not see that screen time can displace language and play-based interactions.[11]

Parenting school-age children (6–12 years old)

When children are in school, their parents decide how to interpret experiences and reality for their children. This is called the parental interpretive stage. Parents decide what values are important to teach, the level of involvement in sibling or peer interactions, and the degree of independence to allow. Many parents continue to believe that their child's engagement with technology is beneficial.[15]

At this age, there may be more external factors increasing digital media exposure, such as schools and peers. Many schools may request that parents and students use more technology (for homework assignments or cyberschool). Due to the increasing importance of peers, this is also a time when many children ask for increasing access to mobile phones and social media so that they can stay connected to their peers.

Parents often believe they are not able to keep up with the rapid changes in technology and media.[16] A child may even become the technology "expert" within the family. This role may lead to a shift in the power dynamic between the child and parent, whereby the child seems to have more authority. When children ask for their own mobile devices because other children have them, parents may then defer to the family "expert" or give in to peer pressure. However, parents are sometimes not aware of the amount of maturity that is needed when making decisions online or when using digital technology. If there is a mismatch between maturity and decision making, this can then have implications on how the child interacts with digital media.

Parenting adolescents (12–18 years old)

As adolescents mature, parents give guidance and prepare for the individual to separate from the family. Parents are interdependent with their adolescents, often spending a significant amount of time redefining boundaries with each other and redefining the parent-child relationship.

Social media plays a larger role because it is another (virtual) environment where adolescents can explore. If appropriate behaviors or explicit boundaries have not been defined before social media use, then adolescents may delve into this online world and mimic the behaviors they see without understanding the potential long-term consequences or repercussions.

In many respects, the family interactions that are common during this stage (in terms of ie, negotiating new boundaries and roles) are the same as they have been in the past when parents tried to understand new technology (eg, rock and roll music, television) However, the mediums in which these interactions can play out (eg, monitoring behavior online as well as offline[16]), and the magnitude of the impact of decisions and actions online, can be multiplied by the use of digital media.

Parenting young adults (older than 18 years old)

With young adults, parents are at a departure stage, when they evaluate how they did as parents, and if they negotiated an appropriate and desired parent and (grown) child relationship. They find new ways to define themselves as parents or as part of a family, even if the child is no longer at home.

Digital media can serve to isolate or connect the young adult to parents. In terms of the parent and young adult relationship, this negotiation may play out as some parents continue to email professors when the young adult is away at college (thus impeding independence) or as parents ask to friend their young adult through social media (to stay connected). This relationship may also need to be renegotiated if the young adult moves back into the home after a period of independence. Families have to decide what behaviors are acceptable and appropriate, for both the parents and the young adult.

When families present to providers with digital media issues, having an understanding of the parental stages of development can be informative for clinicians as they decide what kind of strategies or approaches to use.

CLINICIAN STRATEGIES

By incorporating these three theories into practice, interdisciplinary teams can intervene with different family members, at a variety of levels, with interventions focusing on knowledge, skills, or both. These interventions are summarized in **Table 2**.

Intervention with an Individual

Working with an individual, the provider (mental health or primary care) can assess the child's developmental level and the level of knowledge that the child has about technology and media, then determine if there is a good fit between them.

Intervention with a Parent

For parents who do not have the knowledge to keep up with the rapidly changing technology, the provider (mental health or primary care) can provide education about what is developmentally appropriate and information about how to help manage digital media (see later discussion of AAP guidelines).

Consultation

At a one-time, consultative level, the clinician (mental health, primary care provider, or family therapist) can meet with the family, to gather information about what is effective, assess the knowledge base of the parent with digital media, and determine the developmental level of the individual. This consultation may result in a brief problem-solving session to address the immediate problem.

Stabilizing a Crisis

It is not uncommon for some behavior or activity to come to light (eg, sexting, pornography, involvement in worrisome online activities), that creates a crisis in the family due to the transgression of a family value or a legal situation. At these times, a clinician may assist the family in navigating the situational crisis by providing feedback and psychoeducation, and assisting the family with devising a plan for the next steps in addressing the issue.

Family Therapy

More formal family therapy would not only provide information about digital media but also help the family learn and practice skills to better negotiate various family roles and problem-solving situations.

RESOURCES FROM THE AMERICAN ACADEMY OF PEDIATRICS

Parents have voiced the need for guidance about media use in their families.[14] To meet this need, in 2012, the American Academy of Pediatrics (AAP) made the issue of children, adolescents, and the media a priority in their Agenda for Children. In 2015, the AAP convened a Growing Up Digital: Media Research Symposium.[17] In October, 2016, the AAP published a technical report, *Children and Adolescents and Digital Media*.[18] They also published 2 policy statements: *Media and Young Minds*[19] and *Media Use in School-Age Children and Adolescents*.[20] In addition, the AAP updated their guidelines about media use.

Table 2
Providers can work with families using various interventions to set limits and become more literate with digital media

Level of Intervention	Possible Providers			Type of Intervention		Evaluation or Intervention
	Medical Health Clinician	Primary Care Provider	Family Therapist	Knowledge	Skill	
Individual	●	●	—	●	—	Assess developmental level and knowledge of technology or media to determine if they match
Parental	●	●	—	●	—	Provide education about what is developmentally appropriate and how to manage technology
Consultation	●	●	—	●	—	Assess what is or is not working, parental knowledge level, and individual's developmental level / Brief problem-solving session
Crisis Stabilization	●	●	●	●	●	Assist the family to navigate the situational crisis, provide feedback and psychoeducation, and assist the family with devising a plan for the next steps in addressing the issue which led to the crisis
Family Therapy	●	—	●	●	●	All of the previous, plus help family navigate roles and conflicts around technology

●, applicable; —, not applicable.

Common themes that arose from the symposium, reports, policy statements, and guidelines included

- The importance of sleep and physical exercise
- An introduction to the topic of high-quality programming
- Incorporation of limit-setting regarding time with media
- Designation of media-free times and locations at home
- A discussion of online citizenship and safety.

AMERICAN ACADEMY OF PEDIATRICS GUIDELINES

The AAP created a set of recommendations for families and professionals. These recommendations can be divided into three broad categories: limit-setting, media literacy, and collaboration.

American Academy of Pediatrics and Limit-Setting

Within the broad category of limit-setting, families are encouraged to limit digital media in 3 different dimensions: time, space, and use. Media-free times and locations are designed to encourage direct, nondistracted family interactions via play, discussions over meals, and bedtime routines. Families are asked to prioritize play, meals, schoolwork, physical exercise, and sleep over digital media use. These recommendations are modified as children age (**Fig. 6**).

American Academy of Pediatrics and Media Literacy

Media literacy refers to the process by which parents evaluate and supervise their children with digital media, so that the media use is in line with the values of the family. Once parents are ready to introduce developmentally appropriate media and have determined what kind of digital media to use. They start by using it together and graduating to varying degrees of supvervision. Parents can reevaluate the arrangement and (if desired) start the process again to refine it. Because digital media is constantly changing, this evaluation-supervision process is an interactive cycle (**Fig. 7**).

American Academy of Pediatrics and Collaboration

Families are encouraged to collaborate with professionals to set limits and become more literate with digital media. There are various ways in which families can work with providers (see **Table 2**).

One tool that parents and clinicians can use to implement the AAP guidelines is the AAP Family Media Use Plan.

AMERICAN ACADEMY OF PEDIATRICS FAMILY MEDIA USE PLAN

To provide parents with mechanisms to implement these guidelines, the AAP developed the Family Media Use Plan, found at www.healthychildren.org/MediaUsePlan. This plan provides a free, customizable online tool for parents and family members. It is also a reference that clinicians can share with their patients or clients. Families can decide which aspects of the plan are realistic and attainable for their families. This plan can:

- Be individualized
- Identify an appropriate balance between screen time or online time and other activities
- Set boundaries for accessing content

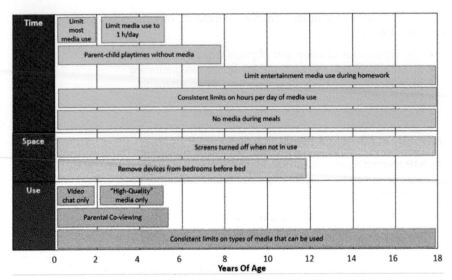

Fig. 6. Digital media limit-setting. (*Data from* Reid Chassiakos YL, Radesky J, Christakis D, et al. Children and adolescents and digital media. Pediatrics 2016;138(5):[pii:e20162593].)

- Guide displays of personal information
- Encourage age-appropriate critical thinking and digital literacy
- Support open family communication and implementation of consistent rules about media use.

Feedback About the American Academy of Pediatrics Family Media Use Plan

Since October, 2016, the AAP Family Media Use Plan has been recommended to parents who have expressed concerns about digital media. Themes from informal, anecdotal reports from individuals, families, and clinicians include the following:

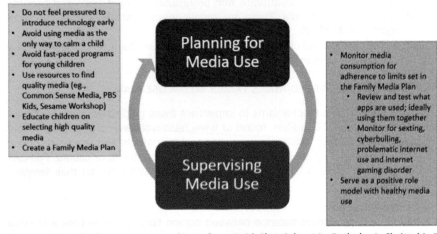

Fig. 7. AAP media literacy process. (*Data from* Reid Chassiakos YL, Radesky J, Christakis D, et al. Children and adolescents and digital media. Pediatrics 2016;138(5):[pii:e20162593].)

- Many parents appreciate having a resource to help them manage media use in their homes.
- Many parents talk about feeling empowered with the recommendations and the plan from the AAP.
- Some providers have found that it can be very helpful to use the AAP Family Media Use Plan as an actionable goal that families can explore and use as part of media management.
- After recommending the Family Media Plan and revisiting the topic with families, clinicians can use motivational interviewing to determine what stage parents are at with managing digital media. Motivational interviewing can lead to lasting changes with media use.[21] Some families need support with moving from the precontemplation or contemplation stages regarding media management. Others want assistance with moving from the preparation and action stages. For those individuals and families that need more formal assistance with digital media management, they have sometimes been referred for individual therapy, parent management training, and/or family therapy.

The Family Media Use Plan can be a helpful tool for a provider to have, at the individual, parental, consultative, crisis management, or family therapy levels of intervention.

SUMMARY

Three frameworks were provided to help inform clinicians when individuals or families presented with digital media concerns. The social-ecological model illustrates how media has direct and indirect effects at individual, relationship, community, and societal levels. The family systems theory demonstrates that conflicts around digital media use are rooted in family dynamics. The developmental framework shows how parenting is being shaped by digital media use. These theories are used as a foundation from which clinicians can identify possible strategies for interventions, including use of the 2016 recommendations and the Family Media Use Plan from the AAP.

REFERENCES

1. Center for Disease Control. The social-ecological model: a framework for prevention 2015. Available at: https://www.cdc.gov/violenceprevention/overview/social-ecologicalmodel.html. Accessed May 30, 2017.
2. Radesky JS. The social-ecological context of media use and school success. J Pediatr (Rio J) 2015;91:318–9.
3. The Child Online Privacy Protection Act. Available at: https://www.ftc.gov/system/files/2012-31341.pdf.
4. Erikson E. Identity: youth and crisis. New York: WWNorton; 1968.
5. Nichols MP. Bowen family systems therapy. In: Dodge A, editor. The essentials of family therapy. 6th edition. Upper Saddle River (NJ): Pearson, Inc; 2014. p. 69–87.
6. Galinsky E. The six stages of parenting. Reading (MA): Perseus Books; 1987.
7. Rideout V. Zero to eight: children's media use in America 2013: a common sense media research study. Common sense media. 2013. Available at: www.commonsensemedia.org. Accessed June 29, 2017.
8. Rideout V. The common sense census: media use by tweens and teens: a common sense media research study. Common sense media. 2015. Available at: www.commonsensemedia.org. Accessed June 29, 2017.

9. McDaniel BT, Radesky JS. Technoference: parent distraction with technology and associations with child behavior problems. Child Dev 2017. https://doi.org/10.1111/cdev.12822.

10. Radesky J, Miller AL, Rosenblum KL, et al. Maternal mobile device use during a structured parent-child interaction task. Acad Pediatr 2015;15(2):238–44.

11. Radesky JS, Schumacher J, Zuckerman B. Mobile and interactive media use by young children: the good, the bad, and the unknown. Pediatrics 2015;135(1):1–3.

12. Radesky JS, Peacock-Chambers E, Zuckerman B, et al. Use of mobile technology to calm upset children: associations with social-emotional development. JAMA Pediatr 2016;170(4):397–9.

13. Radesky JS, Kistin CJ, Zuckerman B, et al. Patterns of mobile device use by caregivers and children during meals in fast food restaurants. Pediatrics 2014;133(4): e843–9.

14. Radesky JS, Eisenberg S, Kistin CJ, et al. Overstimulated consumers or next-generation learners? Parent tensions about child mobile technology use. Ann Fam Med 2016;14(6):503–8.

15. Anderson M. Parents, teens, and digital monitoring. Pew Research Center; 2016. Available at: http://www.pewinternet.org/2016/01/07/parents-teens-and-digital-monitoring/. Accessed June 27, 2017.

16. Radesky JS, Kistin C, Eisenberg S, et al. Parent perspectives on their mobile technology use: the excitement and exhaustion of parenting while connected. J Dev Behav Pediatr 2016;37(9):694–701.

17. Shifrin D, Brown A, Hill D, et al. Growing up digital: media research symposium. American Academy of Pediatrics; 2015. Available at: https://www.aap.org/en-us/Documents/digital_media_symposium_proceedings.pdf. Accessed June 29, 2017.

18. Reid Chassiakos YL, Radesky J, Christakis D, et al, Council on Communications and Media. Children and adolescents and digital media [review]. Pediatrics 2016;138(5) [pii:e20162593].

19. Council on Communications and Media. Media and young minds [review]. Pediatrics 2016;138(5) [pii:e20162591].

20. Council on Communications and Media. Media use in school-aged children and adolescents [review]. Pediatrics 2016;138(5) [pii:e20162592].

21. Garkin SL, Finch SA, Ip EH, et al. Is office-based counseling about media use, timeouts, and firearm storage effective? Results from a cluster-randomized, controlled trial. Pediatrics 2008;122(1):e15–25.

Relationship Between Adolescent Suicidality, Self-Injury, and Media Habits

Erin L. Belfort, MD*, Lindsey Miller, MD

KEYWORDS

- Social media • Adolescence • Suicidality • Nonsuicidal self-injury (NSSI)
- Contagion

KEY POINTS

- Adolescents grow up immersed in media, which will continue to be ubiquitous in their lives.
- A significant body of research demonstrates links between social media or Internet use and risk-taking behaviors among adolescents.
- Social media is linked to nonsuicidal self-injury and suicidal ideation, but the relationship is complex and not necessarily a causal one.
- Mental health practitioners must partner with adolescents to take a screen media history that distinguishes types and extent of use, content, and psychological impact.

CASE PRESENTATION

Emma, a 15-year-old white girl living with her mother and younger sister, presented to a local emergency room after posting a suicidal statement on Facebook. A friend saw the message shortly after it was posted and told her own mother, who called Emma's mother out of concern. This prompted the emergency room visit and Emma's first psychiatric assessment. In the course of the evaluation, it was determined that Emma met criteria for major depressive disorder and had been struggling with depressive symptoms for the last 6 months in the context of several social stressors. Her parents had divorced at the beginning of her freshman year of high school and she had had a falling out with a childhood best friend. In the emergency room, she reported weeks of increasing suicidal thoughts, including some planning and intent to end her life. She and her mother agreed to a voluntary psychiatric admission and she was transferred to the adolescent inpatient unit.

The authors have no conflicts of interest.
Department of Psychiatry, Maine Medical Center, 66 Bramhall Street, Portland, ME 04101, USA
* Corresponding author.
E-mail address: ebelfort@mmc.org

Child Adolesc Psychiatric Clin N Am 27 (2018) 159–169
https://doi.org/10.1016/j.chc.2017.11.004
1056-4993/18/© 2017 Elsevier Inc. All rights reserved.

On the unit, she worked closed with a child psychiatry fellow who discovered that Emma had increasingly withdrawn from friends and family in recent months. She had stopped participating in her usual extracurricular activities. Emma reported spending most of her time alone in her room, using her smartphone almost constantly, and feeling panicked and empty when she did not have access to it. She communicated via text and private messaging on Facebook with 1 or 2 friends, sending hundreds of messages a day. Emma became increasingly anxious about missing out on social activities and would obsessively comb through Facebook to see if there were photos of parties or events she had not been invited to. A few months before, she searched the word "cutting" online and found how-to videos on YouTube that were very appealing to her. Emma identified with the emo culture she discovered and started following related blogs, occasionally posting an anonymous comment. She admitted to superficially cutting her thighs for the last 3 months, which she felt relieved her emotional pain, though she was ashamed and embarrassed about her behavior. Emma reported that a main source of stress at home was arguments with her mother around household chores. She felt incapable of doing the assigned chores due to her depression, and her mother often took away her phone as punishment when they were left undone. This led Emma to feel worse and further disconnected from the few social supports she relied on.

In addition to starting a selective serotonin reuptake inhibitor for her depression, Emma engaged in family sessions while on the adolescent unit, facilitated by a child psychiatry fellow. She identified her use of her smartphone and other screens had become problematic, worsening her mood and interfering with healthier coping strategies. Emma liked some of the dialectical behavioral therapy skills that she had learned on the unit and agreed to work with a therapist after discharge. She decided she would stop visiting cutting blogs and videos on YouTube, and agreed that her mother might have a supportive role. Emma and her mother renegotiated the rules around her smartphone, she agreed to turn her phone in at 9 PM every night, and her mother agreed to use alternative consequences for undone chores rather than taking away her cell phone. Both wanted better communication and a closer relationship, and agreed to make this a goal of Emma's treatment planning.

Discussion of Emma's use of screens and social media became a central part of the assessment and treatment provided to Emma and her family during her hospitalization. Allowing Emma to be ambivalent about her social media use and then to self-identify the ways in which her use was problematic facilitated her to join with her mother to be a part of the problem-solving. Additionally, Emma's family could help her fight social media fire with social media water. For example, instead of following blogs and posting anonymous comments, perhaps she could create her own private supportive blog and the team could enlist family to support her both offline and online.[1]

INTRODUCTION

Americans, adolescents in particular, are more engaged with media than ever before. Concern around adolescent overuse of media is not a new phenomenon. In the past, parents may have worried about the amount of time their children watched television or the content of the shows, movies, or music consumed. Now, fears have shifted to concerns about violent video game use, Internet addiction, social media use, sexting, online pornography exposure, and cyberbullying. Many of these topics are addressed in related articles in this issue.

More than 90% of teens report daily Internet use and 22% reported using the Internet almost constantly.[2] A Common Sense Media report from 2015, notes that, on average, American teens engage in 9 hours of entertainment screen media per day. Media diets vary widely and several distinct use patterns have emerged, including mobile gamers, social networkers, heavy viewers, video gamers, readers, light users, and gamer or computer users. There are clear gender differences regarding how adolescents engage with media. For example, boys spend roughly twice as much time playing video games as girls. Girls outpace boys in their use of text messaging and use of visual social media platforms.[2] There are also socioeconomic differences in media use. Teens from low-income families spend an average of 2 hours and 45 minutes more time on screens each day than those from higher-income families. Twenty percent of youth in upper income homes have a television in their bedroom before the age of 8 years compared with 64% from lower income homes.[3] Given that average teens engage with media for more than 9 hours a day, the definition of excessive use or problematic use becomes somewhat difficult for parents and clinicians working with adolescents.

Key finding: Adolescents are growing up immersed in screen media in various degrees and ways, which will continue to be ubiquitous in their lives.

ADOLESCENT IDENTITY DEVELOPMENT IN A DIGITAL WORLD

The developmental tasks of adolescence are relatively unchanged over time, although some new challenges are created by the digitally saturated culture. The interplay between adolescent development and media habits is complex. Developmental tasks of adolescence include identity consolidation and navigating intimacy and sexuality. There is no clear link in the literature between online activity and self-concept clarity, which is the extent to which one's beliefs and opinions about oneself are clearly defined and stable over time. Adolescents do clearly use social media to explore and experiment with their self-concept. Regarding intimacy, some researchers hypothesize that socially anxious or awkward teens benefit from social relationships mediated through online platforms. However, although internalizing teens typically prefer the controlled nature of online communication, this strategy does not necessarily translate to more or better friendships.[4] An alternative hypothesis suggests that through social media the adage of rich get richer seems to have more empirical support. Those teenagers with well-developed social skills capitalize effectively on social media to further support their social lives and build social capital, whereas teens with poor social skills typically fail to make gains on social media. In fact, teenagers who used Facebook to compensate for poor social skills demonstrated increased loneliness over 5 months.[5]

Some groups benefit more than others from Internet and social media access. Social media may allow social connections among marginalized youth, such as the lesbian, gay, bisexual, transgender, and questioning (LGBTQ) population.[6] (See Amy Mayhew and Paul Weigle's article, "Media Engagement and Identity Formation Among Minority Youth," in this issue.) Youth with mental illness report greater social connectedness and feelings of group belonging when social media is used in this way. They are able to share personal stories and coping skills, avoid feared stigma or judgment, gain additional information, and increase their social networks by connecting to peers with similar experiences. Risks include misinformation, negative communications with peers, unhealthy influences, or behaviors and delays in seeking out traditional medical resources.[7,8]

Neuroanatomical maturation of the adolescent brain adds complexities to the phenomenon. The frontal lobes of the brain continue to mature, via myelination, through adolescence into the age of the mid-20s, which helps to explain how otherwise bright teenagers can at times exhibit poor judgment, difficulty assessing consequences, and significant impulsivity. In the context of social media, this effect may be implicated when adolescents make risky social media posts without considering future implications.

College admissions officers and employers are increasingly conducting online searches of applicants to review their digital footprint, so such posts can have unintended long-term consequences. This is especially important to keep in mind as young people are sharing more and more of their lives on online forums. Youth do not always understand and use privacy-protecting tools. A digital taskforce in England concluded that youth typically consent to social networking sites terms and agreements with no real understanding of what their privacy rights and options are. The taskforce asked teens to read and interpret Instagram's privacy policy and afterward teens reported little understanding of what they read. Quotes from teens included, "It doesn't make any sense," "This is boring," and "I don't know due to the sheer amount of writing and lack of clarity within the document."[9]

LINKS BETWEEN MEDIA HABITS AND RISK-TAKING BEHAVIOR

A significant body of research documents links Internet and social media use with risk-taking behaviors among adolescents. Several online communities glorify, normalize, and even encourage behaviors such as nonsuicidal self-injury (NSSI), suicide, disordered eating, and substance abuse. Some smartphone or mobile apps can be vehicles for cyberbullying and sexting. Although the psychological effects of Internet pornography are poorly studied, engagement may contribute also to negative attitudes about gender roles and relationships, and encourage unhealthy sexual practices.[10]

Distinguishing between types of media use, content of media consumption, and their psychological impact on the particular adolescent patient is important in clinical work. For example, some adolescents, primarily gamers, may use little social media and interact minimally with other players. Others, primarily social media users, may spend hours each day engaged in Facebook, Instagram, and Snapchat, and regard this habit as a crucial part of their social capital. Various platforms and content have different psychological effects for individual adolescents. For example, passive consumption of social media has been linked with increased feelings of loneliness, whereas 2-way online communication with friends is not.[11] The adolescent who actively chats with close friends from school via social media may report different psychological effects compared with the one who obsessively scans Facebook to ensure they have not missed out on something, termed the fear of missing out (FOMO), which can lead to loneliness and distress. Therapists working with young patients regarding behaviors related to Internet use suggest that they "fear the sort of relentlessness of on-going messaging [...] but concurrently with that is an absolute terror of exclusion."[12]

The content of media use is also important to elucidate. Many adolescents use the Internet to search for information about particularly sensitive topics, such as mental health symptoms, depression, safe sexual practices, or contraception. More than 90% of teenagers with mental illness seek help online due to perceived accessibility and anonymity.[13] The content and veracity of information found can vary widely from potentially helpful (a suicide prevention Web site with a hotline) to harmful (a how-to site for self-injury or suicide).

SUICIDALITY AND NONSUICIDAL SELF-INJURY

Adolescent suicide is a major public health crisis and represents a leading cause of death in young people, second only to accidents.[14] The suicide rate among youngsters ages 10 to 14 years has been increasing in recent years.[15] According to the national Youth Risk Behavior Survey data, approximately 20% of adolescents from a nonclinical high school sample reported they had seriously considered suicide in the past year. Of these, approximately 14% reported having a suicide plan and approximately 8% reported have made a suicide attempt.

The literature suggests that there is a complex indirect association between Internet use and suicidal behavior.[16] The content of information sought and viewed is important to consider for a particular adolescent. Studies analyzing Web content using keyword searches related to suicide found that approximately half of Web sites were either neutral or pro-suicide in tone.[17,18] Similarly, a 2008 content analysis found an equal number of suicide prevention Web sites as pro-suicide Web sites, but the pro-suicide Web sites were more often visited.[19]

Recently, an online phenomenon called the Blue Whale Challenge has allegedly led to the death of dozens of youth in Russia and around the world. The challenge involves 50 days of increasingly dangerous and escalating tasks, including self-injurious behavior ultimately culminating in suicide on the last day of the challenge. The original creator has been jailed but teens may still search social media sites for an administrator who assigns daily tasks. It is important for clinicians to be aware, consider asking about it among youth who self-harm or are experiencing suicidal ideation, and inform parents of those at risk.[5]

Exposure to suicide or suicidal behaviors within one's family, peers, or through media can result in an increase in suicide and suicidal behaviors, an effect called contagion. Information about a suicide may be particularly virulent when transmitted via social media, which allows for the instantaneous spread of information to a potentially large audience. The ways in which adolescents learn about a completed suicide may influence their own suicidal thoughts and feelings. One study interviewed more than 700 youth ages 14 to 24 years on 2 occasions, 1 year apart, and found that learning about a suicide on a social networking site was not linked with increased suicidal thinking 1 year later; however, learning about a suicide on an online discussion forum was. Social networking allows for an instantaneous spread of information to a potentially wide audience, which may allow for greater access to support and connectedness. This is in contrast to forums that offer greater anonymity and, therefore, potentially less support.[19] The degree of connectedness, or perceived connectedness, to others may be an important consideration for assessing the impact of various media phenomena on adolescents. Social media interventions may have utility for suicide prevention, though further research is necessary to consider user behavior, risk-assessment in this platform, privacy and confidentiality, and the possibility of contagion.[20]

NSSI is a separate, though related, phenomenon. This behavior is relatively common, with approximately 12% of adolescents from a community sample endorsing engagement in NSSI in the past year.[21] Each year, approximately 157,000 youth ages 10 to 24 years, receive emergency room care for self-inflicted injuries. A minority of youth with NSSI, approximately 6%, seek professional help for self-injury.[22] Though most adolescents who self-injure do so without suicidal intent, those who engage in NSSI are also more likely to make a suicide attempt.[23] The reasons for NSSI are complex but may more frequently represent a mechanism for coping with stress than a failed suicide attempt, or a way to seek attention.[22] Some experts note that youth who self-injure tend to be particularly emotionally sensitive and vulnerable, and suffer from an emotional illiteracy. Unable to name their feelings, they are ineffective in coping with them and use NSSI to this end.

Virtual communities supporting NSSI can be quite attractive and potentially dangerous for adolescents considering or engaging in self-injury. Self-harm is searched 42 million times per year and these searches typically lead to false information. Ninety-one percent of searches related to NSSI lead to sites that are not endorsed by a health or educational institution.[24] Greater exposure to NSSI in the media and seeking out NSSI content were related to higher frequency self-injurious behavior in 1 study.[25] A content analysis of self-injury videos on YouTube found that they are typically viewed by adolescent girls, have very high viewership, and overall are rated positively by viewers.[26] Furthermore, adolescents who self-harm have higher rates of Internet use than their peers.[27]

Vulnerable adolescents, particularly those with internalizing mental health disorders such as depression, may be more likely than their peers to seek information and support from the Internet rather than from mental health professionals. These adolescents typically prefer nonprofessional, unmoderated sites offering anonymity, which may delay or prevent needed treatment.[28] Youth who experience significant distress may be more likely to use the Internet as a coping tool to manage their problems.[29] One way youth communicate NSSI online is to discuss or post pictures of their self-injury for a variety of reasons, including seeking help to change, seeking reassurance or care from others, or seeking approval from peers.

Web sites devoted to NSSI have pros and cons. The anonymity offered by some online forums and groups may allow adolescents who would not otherwise seek help to do so. One study found that most teens engaging in a self-harm discussion group reported a subsequent reduction rather than an increase in NSSI. These teens expressed that the groups were helpful for receiving validation, crisis support, and as a place to vent frustrations. However, many of these online forums are unmoderated, and offer amateur support that may normalize or encourage NSSI. These sites, even those intending to help teens curb NSSI, may serve as a trigger for adolescents to engage in new or continued NSSI.[22]

One study looking at NSSI first aid videos on YouTube found that, although the content was generally neutral and neither encouraged nor discouraged NSSI, few encouraged seeking help for this behavior. Such videos are generally favorably perceived by viewers. The investigators hypothesize that many teens prefer to access information and support from these videos rather than to seek help from a mental health professional.[30]

As adolescents increasingly prefer texting and social media to other forms of communication, clinicians have noted increasing numbers of adolescents communicating distress, specifically suicidal ideation, via electronic means. A retrospective chart review of adolescent emergency room visits for suicidality between 2005 and 2009 found increasing numbers of initial communications of suicidality via texting or social media posts.[31] These electronic communications are increasingly received by peers rather than parents or adults. Teens typically prefer to handle situations like this on their own, with only a minority disclosing the information to an adult.[32,33] This phenomenon risks delaying or preventing access to needed care for teens in crisis.

A recent Netflix television series entitled "13 Reasons Why" has received significant attention in the press and among providers of adolescent mental health services. The series portrays a teenage girl driven to suicide via mistreatment by her peers, including sexting, bullying, and sexual assault. The protagonist, who kills herself, tells her story in a series of cassette tapes left behind, effectively blaming 13 people. The series is very popular and was recently renewed for a second season (and presumably a second suicide). The series producers expressed that the series is intended to start important conversations about mental health and reduce stigma; however, the series does little to encourage help-seeking behavior. On the contrary, the adults in the show are uniformly unavailable, disinterested, or ineffective. The show seems to glorify suicide as the ultimate revenge fantasy and further exacerbate the misconception among teens that death is an acceptable response to mistreatment, as well as an effective retribution. Such dramatic portrayals of suicide may contribute to suicide contagion among youth.

Cyberbullying linked (directly or indirectly) to suicide has been referred to as cyberbullicide. This growing phenomenon has garnered significant media attention in the coverage of numerous cases around the country. In a survey of 2000 middle school children, victims of cyberbullying were almost twice as likely to attempt suicide. Cyberbullying offenders themselves were also at elevated risk of having attempted suicide.[16,34] A meta-analysis examining the relationship between traditional bullying (physical, verbal, and via social exclusion) with cyberbullying found that cyberbullying was more strongly related to suicidal ideation and suicide attempts.[35] Cyberbullying is especially challenging as perpetrators can bully youth anywhere and at any time of the day, and information is spread rapidly online.

There are many studies linking excessive engagement with social media with negative mental health outcomes. Particular platforms, such as Facebook, have been linked to negative outcomes. An important caveat to note is that the associations are largely correlational, so causality cannot necessarily be inferred. For instance, a 2011 study by Moreno and colleagues[36] concluded that college students commonly express symptoms consistent with depression on Facebook.[37] One result of such reports is that the popular press coverage at times inappropriately ascribes causality, for example indicating that Facebook use causes depression. A Google search of "Facebook depression" leads to numerous articles on NPR, Forbes.com, and Parenting.com, with titles such as "Facebook may make you depressed and jealous, but we still love it",[38] "Research links heavy Facebook and social media usage to depression,"[39,40] and "Social Networking Among Teens Can Lead to 'Facebook Depression.'"[38] One article reports, "Facebook depression is an affliction that results from establishing a presence on social networking sites, spending a great deal of time on these sites and then feeling unaccepted among peers online."[39] This approach can be misleading and risks trivializing the diagnosis of major depressive disorder.

WORKING WITH ADOLESCENTS AND FAMILIES AROUND MEDIA

Clinicians working with adolescents and their families should be cautioned against uniformly vilifying social media inappropriately. Whether one believes social media is harmful or not, it remains a significant part of the fabric of adolescents' lives and an important element of their social capital. Exploring how adolescents use social media and engage with the virtual world is an important part of the initial psychiatric assessment and ongoing work with teens. Inquiring about these topics can be a good way to join with adolescents early in the interview process. Rather than starting with a chief complaint, joining with an adolescent positively around their interests and friendships can pave the way for a constructive therapeutic alliance. Allowing the adolescent take the role of an expert and to teach the clinician about their virtual world can help the teen feel comfortable and ease into an exploration of psychiatric symptoms and risk-taking behaviors both on and offline.

A major cause of conflict in families who present for treatment by child psychiatrists concerns media rules and limits. Many adolescents consider Internet access (via smartphone, IPad, or computer) as their right rather than a privilege, and this attitude often brings them into conflict with parents who have the opposite view. Working with families of young children to closely monitor their media habits, and teach and encourage appropriate habits, helps shape healthy adolescents capable of being good digital citizens. Families who do not monitor and set limits around their child's social media use are often surprised to discover their child's online experiences. This frequently happens in the context of a crisis, such as admission to an emergency room or inpatient unit.

Often, with some room for reflection, adolescents themselves can identify ways in which their social media habits displace healthy ones or interfere with their social, academic, or family roles. Once a problem has been identified and some motivation for positive change is elicited, the adolescent can then partner with the clinician and family to reach this goal. Risky behaviors online are likely to be mirrored in similar offline behaviors, and helping families navigate appropriate limits regarding media use, complete with appropriate rewards and consequences, is an important and fruitful role for mental health providers. Risky behavior both offline and online warrants additional supervision and limitations placed by caregivers.

DISCUSSION

The use of screens and social media is ubiquitous in the lives of adolescents today and, regardless of clinicians' feelings about it, it is here to stay. There is an extensive body of literature linking excessive media use and screen time with risk-taking behaviors and mental health symptoms, such as depression, suicidality and suicide contagion, NSSI, and cyberbullying.

Adolescents needing mental health services may be less likely to seek out help from adults or professionals, and prefer instead to turn to their peers via texting or social media or to informal online sources of support. Social media is linked to NSSI and suicidal ideation, but the relationship is complex and not necessarily a causal one. Vulnerable adolescents, such as those prone to internalizing disorders, may be susceptible to online communities that normalize or glorify self-destructive behaviors. The sense of connectedness may be an important factor for adolescents, such that social media sites or Web sites promoting anonymity may be more concerning.

The lives of adolescent patients are often saturated by media, adding further complexity and nuance to the already difficult tasks of adolescent growth and development. Mental health providers working with adolescents must explore the virtual world of adolescent patients to be effective in building a therapeutic alliance and enacting appropriate treatment. All clinicians working with children and teens should routinely inquire about screen time and media habits. (See Nicholas Carson and colleagues' article, "Assessment of Digital Media Use in the Adolescent Psychiatric Evaluation," in this issue.) Complaints such as inattention, depression, or fatigue may in fact be linked to too much screen time, which can interfere with sleep, academic studies, physical exercise, or socialization. Risk assessments usually include a detailed exploration of offline or real-world risk-taking behaviors and this inquiry should extend to online risk-taking behaviors.

REFERENCES

1. Sivashanker K. Cyberbullying and the digital self. J Am Acad Child Adolesc Psychiatry 2013;52(2):113–5.

2. Lenhart A. Teens, social media & technology overview 2015. Pew Research Center; 2015. p. 9. Available at: http://www.pewinternet.org/2015/04/09/teens-social-media-technology-2015/. Accessed November 29, 2017.
3. Media CS, Rideout V. Zero to eight: children's media use in America. Common Sense Media; 2011. Available at: https://www.commonsensemedia.org/research/zero-to-eight-childrens-media-use-in-america. Accessed November 29, 2017.
4. Amichai-Hamburger Y, Wainapel G, Fox S. "On the internet no one knows I'm an introvert": extroversion, neuroticism, and internet interaction. Cyberpsychol Behav 2002;5(2):125–8.
5. Teppers E, Luyckx K, Klimstra TA, et al. Loneliness and Facebook motives in adolescence: a longitudinal inquiry into directionality of effect. J Adolesc 2014; 37(5):691–9.
6. Valkenburg PM, Peter J. Online communication among adolescents: an integrated model of its attraction, opportunities, and risks. J Adolesc Health 2011; 48(2):121–7.
7. Reid Chassiakos YL, Radesky J, Christakis D, et al. Children and adolescents and digital media. Pediatrics 2016;138(5) [pii:e20162593].
8. Felt L, Robb M. Technology addiction: concern, controversy, and finding a balance. San Francisco (CA): Common Sense Media; 2016.
9. Children's Commissioner. Growing up digital: a report of the growing up digital taskforce. 2017:1–24. Available at: https://www.childrenscommissioner.gov.uk/wp-content/uploads/2017/06/Growing-Up-Digital-Taskforce-Report-January-2017_0.pdf. Accessed November 29, 2017.
10. Stanley N, Barter C, Wood M, et al. Pornography, sexual coercion and abuse and sexting in young people's intimate relationships: a European study. J Interpers Violence 2016. [Epub ahead of print].
11. Hökby S, Hadlaczky G, Westerlund J, et al. Are mental health effects of internet use attributable to the web-based content or perceived consequences of usage? A longitudinal study of European adolescents. JMIR Ment Health 2016;3(3):e31.
12. Kuss D, Griffiths M. Internet addiction in psychotherapy. Basingstoke: Palgrave Macmillan; 2014.
13. Burns JM, Durkin LA, Nicholas J. Mental health of young people in the United States: what role can the internet play in reducing stigma and promoting help seeking? J Adolesc Health 2009;45(1):95–7.
14. Prevention CfDCa. Adolescent Health National Center for Health Statistics. 2017. Available at: https://www.cdc.gov/nchs/fastats/adolescent-health.htm. Accessed June 19, 2017.
15. Prevention CfDCa. QuickStats: death rates for motor vehicle traffic injury, suicide and Homicide among children and adolescents aged 10-14 years-United States, 1999-2014. 2016. Available at: https://www.cdc.gov/mmwr/volumes/65/wr/mm6543a8.htm?s_cid=mm6543a8_w. Accessed June 19, 2017.
16. Luxton DD, June JD, Fairall JM. Social media and suicide: a public health perspective. Am J Public Health 2012;102(S2):S195–200.
17. Biddle L, Donovan J, Hawton K, et al. Suicide and the internet. BMJ 2008; 336(7648):800.
18. Recupero PR, Harms SE, Noble JM. Googling suicide: surfing for suicide information on the Internet. J Clin Psychiatry 2008;69(6):878–88.
19. Dunlop SM, More E, Romer D. Where do youth learn about suicides on the Internet, and what influence does this have on suicidal ideation? J Child Psychol Psychiatry 2011;52(10):1073–80.

20. Robinson J, Cox G, Bailey E, et al. Social media and suicide prevention: a systematic review. Early Interv Psychiatry 2015;10(2):103–21.
21. Nock MK. Self-injury. Annu Rev Clin Psychol 2010;6:339–63.
22. Messina ES, Iwasaki Y. Internet use and self-injurious behaviors among adolescents and young adults: an interdisciplinary literature review and implications for health professionals. Cyberpsychol Behav Soc Netw 2011;14(3):161–8.
23. Klonsky ED, May AM, Glenn CR. The relationship between nonsuicidal self-injury and attempted suicide: converging evidence from four samples. J Abnorm Psychol 2013;122(1):231.
24. Lewis SP, Mahdy JC, Michal NJ, et al. Googling self-injury: the state of health information obtained through online searches for self-injury. JAMA Pediatr 2014; 168(5):443–9.
25. Zhu L, Westers NJ, Horton SE, et al. Frequency of exposure to and engagement in nonsuicidal self-injury among inpatient adolescents. Arch Suicide Res 2016; 20(4):580–90.
26. Lewis SP, Heath NL, St Denis JM, et al. The scope of nonsuicidal self-injury on YouTube. Pediatrics 2011;127(3):e552–7.
27. Daine K, Hawton K, Singaravelu V, et al. The power of the web: a systematic review of studies of the influence of the internet on self-harm and suicide in young people. PLoS One 2013;8(10):e77555.
28. Gould MS, Munfakh JLH, Lubell K, et al. Seeking help from the internet during adolescence. J Am Acad Child Adolesc Psychiatry 2002;41(10):1182–9.
29. Trefflich F, Kalckreuth S, Mergl R, et al. Psychiatric patients' internet use corresponds to the internet use of the general public. Psychiatry Res 2015;226(1): 136–41.
30. Lewis SP, Knoll AK. Do it yourself: examination of self-injury first aid tips on YouTube. Cyberpsychol Behav Soc Netw 2015;18(5):301–4.
31. Belfort EL, Mezzacappa E, Ginnis K. Similarities and differences among adolescents who communicate suicidality to others via electronic versus other means: a pilot study. Adolesc Psychiatry 2012;2(3):258–62.
32. Dunham K. Young adults' support strategies when peers disclose suicidal intent. Suicide Life Threat Behav 2004;34(1):56–65.
33. Young R, Subramanian R, Miles S, et al. Social representation of cyberbullying and adolescent suicide: a mixed-method analysis of news stories. Health Commun 2017;32(9):1082–92.
34. Hinduja S, Patchin JW. Cyberbullying fact sheet: identification, prevention, and response. Cyberbullying Research Center; 2014. Available at: http://cyberbullying.org/Cyberbullying_Identification_Prevention_Response.pdf. Accessed November 29, 2017.
35. Van Geel M, Vedder P, Tanilon J. Relationship between peer victimization, cyberbullying, and suicide in children and adolescents: a meta-analysis. JAMA Pediatr 2014;168(5):435–42.
36. Moreno MA, Jelenchick LA, Egan KG, et al. Feeling bad on Facebook: depression disclosures by college students on a social networking site. Depress Anxiety 2011;28(6):447–55.
37. O'Keeffe GS, Clarke-Pearson K. The impact of social media on children, adolescents, and families. Pediatrics 2011;127(4):800–4.
38. Tahnk JL. Social Networking among teens can lead to 'Facebook depression. [Parenting Magazine]. Available at: http://www.parenting.com/blogs/screen-play/jeana-lee-tahnk/social-networking-among-teens-can-lead-facebook-depression. Accessed June 19, 2017.

39. Chaudry A. Research links heavy Facebook and social media usage to depression. Forbes; 2016. Available at: https://www.forbes.com/sites/amitchowdhry/2016/04/30/study-links-heavy-facebook-and-social-media-usage-to-depression/#3fe138534b53. Accessed November 29, 2017.
40. Jacobson C, Bailin A, Milanaik R, et al. Adolescent health implications of new age technology. Pediatr Clin North Am 2016;63(1):183–94.

#KidsAnxiety and Social Media: A Review

Jenna Glover, PhD, Sandra L. Fritsch, MD, MSEd*

KEYWORDS

- Child anxiety • Adolescent anxiety • Social media • Internet • Online gaming
- Cyberbullying

KEY POINTS

- Currently, there is limited research guiding clinician's understanding of child or adolescent anxiety and the negative and positive impact social media may have for youth with anxiety.
- Socially anxious youth may find a social media presence helpful in developing relationships.
- Problematic Internet use in children and adolescents has significant impact on sleep, anxiety, and depression.
- There are emerging prevention and treatment tools through eHealth and mHealth technologies for childhood anxiety.

INTRODUCTION

Anxiety is the most common mental health condition in childhood, with prevalence rates ranging from 5% to 10% in children and up to 25% in teens.[1,2] Untreated anxiety in youth can lead to other mental health conditions, including depression and substance use disorders. Common presentations in younger children include fear of separation from a caregiver, social worries, specific phobias, and anxiety with novel situations. A child's world is filled with new social tasks that are potentially anxiety-provoking: separating from parents to attend school, making friendships and managing peer relationships, learning, active class participation, and pursuing interests or socializing beyond the school setting. In adolescence, developing complex peer relationships, including romantic relationships, as well as planning for adulthood can cause or exacerbate anxiety. Over the past 10 years, social media has become a prominent component of our youth's lives, with use peaking in 16 to 24 year olds.[3]

Disclosure Statement: The authors have nothing to disclose.
Pediatric Mental Health Institute, Children's Hospital Colorado, University of Colorado School of Medicine, 13123 East 16th Avenue, B130, Aurora, CO 80045, USA
* Corresponding author:
E-mail address: Sandra.fritsch@childrenscolorado.org

Child Adolesc Psychiatric Clin N Am 27 (2018) 171–182
https://doi.org/10.1016/j.chc.2017.11.005
1056-4993/18/© 2017 Elsevier Inc. All rights reserved.

childpsych.theclinics.com

Younger children are also increasingly exposed to the digital world and social media. This article reviews current understanding of how childhood anxiety disorders interact with electronic media, including risks and protective factors, challenges faced by caretakers navigating the digital world of youth, and the current and potential future digital applications to treat anxiety in children and adolescents.

RISK FACTORS ASSOCIATED WITH COMPUTER HABITS

The ubiquitous nature of digital technology in the everyday life of modern youth makes it essential for clinicians to understand the potential risks these mediums pose. Limited research on the relationship between technology and anxiety in children and adolescents suggests there are associations between computer habits and symptoms of anxiety.[4] To best understand the implications of these relationships, the following are important:

1. Understand how the developmental tasks of youth are affected by technology habits.
2. Recognize how digital communication differs from face-to face-interactions for anxious youth.
3. Identify individual factors associated with anxiety and problematic Internet use (PIU) in youth.
4. Examine unique features of social media that may serve to worsen anxiety in young people.

Developmental Tasks

One of the major tasks of childhood and adolescence is the creation and maintenance of significant relationships. Friendship in childhood is followed by increasingly intimate relationships in adolescence. Modern life has changed the nature of play in the lives of youth. Most parents no longer consider wandering local neighborhoods to be safe for their children, thus virtual worlds provide an alternate setting for play.[5] The sense of safety provided by the digital world has enabled shy youth to explore friendships in games geared toward children as young as 5 years. Games and Web sites, such as SecretBuilders, Disney Fairies, Angelina Ballerina, and ZuluWorld, are developed for younger children and allow limited social networking.[6] Grom Social is a social networking site for children ages 10 years and older described as safe but flawed because links sometimes lead to inappropriate sites.[6] There is little research evidence to date regarding the potential of social media to facilitate friendships in younger children. Minecraft is a popular video game played by latency-aged children that can facilitate engagement with peers in person and virtually.[7] Inherent risks of heavy digital technology engagement for latency-age anxious children include sleep impairment, use of the virtual world to avoid healthy exposures in the real world, inadequate exercise, and development of problematic overuse.

Important tasks of adolescence include the development of identity and managing relationships with peers. Self-presentation is the process by which individuals selectively manage the image and identity shown to others. Self-disclosure involves sharing one's thoughts, feelings, and behaviors.[8] Both self-presentation and self-disclosure are critical in the exploration of identity and relationships with others. However, anxiety may interfere with an adolescent's self-presentation efficacy, leading to avoidance of social interactions with peers. Computer-mediated communication (CMC) offers an alternative platform to engage with others that is typically perceived by socially anxious youth as safer than face-to-face contact.

Computer-Mediated Communication

Social anxiety involves fear of negative evaluation by others, so socially anxious youth avoid experiences they believe are likely to result in unfavorable impressions.[9] CMC allows for text-based conversations without need of traditional audio or visual cues, a comforting alternative for youth fearing judgements about their appearance, speech, and physiologic signs of anxiety (eg, blushing).[10] CMC also enables asynchronized communication, allowing participants to take more time to construct and edit messages before sending them. Asynchronicity especially appeals to youth who are self-conscious, easily embarrassed, or likely to withdraw in face-to-face settings.[8]

Social anxiety is positively related to preference for the freedom from nonverbal cues provided by CMC, according to a recent meta-analytic review of 22 studies. The review found that socially anxious individuals prefer online interaction to in-person interaction, and are more likely than peers to consider it an effective medium for developing relationships.[10] With the greater comfort and perceived increase in self-presentational efficacy provided by CMC, the socially anxious individual's preference for online social interactions may be a risk factor for the development of PIU.[11]

Problematic Internet Use

PIU consists of cognitive and behavioral symptoms that result in distress and impairment in functioning.[9] PIU may also be called Internet and video game addiction (IVGA), Internet addiction, virtual addiction, and technology addiction. PIU-IVGA involves difficulty controlling the amount of time an individual spends online and distress when Internet access is unavailable.[10]

A history of psychological illness is associated with PIU-IVGA. Users with psychological problems may use online activity to escape negative feelings and increase positive ones, potentially creating a pattern of compulsive use.[4] Research has found that socially anxious young adults needing social assurance are more likely to develop addiction to social media than those with little need for such assurance.[12] Socially anxious youth seeking to manage anxiety through external validation also seem to be at greater risk for developing problematic use than those with less need for social approval. These results reflect the importance of understanding individual cognitions and attitudes about online engagement because individuals are affected differently by Internet habits.[13]

Engagement in pathologic video gaming has also been identified as a risk factor in the development of anxiety in youth. In a longitudinal study, pathologic gaming (ie, use that disrupts interpersonal, psychological, and/or academic functioning) was found to predict increases in depression, anxiety, and social phobia. Children and adolescents who were able to stop pathologic gaming showed a reduction in all 3 areas compared with peers who remained pathologic gamers.[14] These results are notable because this is the first research to demonstrate that pathologic gaming is predictive of later-onset and maintenance of mental health disorders.

Social Media and Anxiety

Social media sites are designed to allow users to share content, interact with others, and disseminate information about themselves and their world.[15] Numerous social media platforms are used by both children and adolescents (eg, Club Penguin, Facebook, Instagram, Snapchat). Social media sites play an important role in self-presentation.[16]

Platforms such as Facebook and Instagram allow users to develop a digital identity that can be carefully constructed and digitally enhanced to the point of idealization, potentially creating a culture of unrealistic comparisons. Many youth feel the need to be on social media at all times to be part of their peer group, and may use social networking sites to alleviate the fear of missing out (FOMO). FOMO is worry about missing connections that peers are enjoying without you, potentially risking loss of social status. Youth indicate that FOMO often results in anxiety and feelings of inadequacy.[3] High levels of FOMO in youth mediated the relationship between anxiety symptoms and negative consequences (eg, impairment in academic and/or social functioning), according to a large survey of Latin American teens accessing social media via mobile devices.[4] Thus, anxious youth, who also have heightened FOMO are more likely to experience problems in functioning related to their use of social media. Unlimited access to many idealized representations of peers via social media can lead youth to believe that peers are leading better, happier, and more fulfilled lives. This engenders anxiety, self-consciousness, and perfectionism, which, in turn, triggers compulsive use of social networking sites.[3,17]

Maintaining multiple social media accounts simultaneously is commonplace among youth and has been positively correlated with anxiety.[15] Youth who operate multiple social media sites may feel social pressure to sustain a carefully crafted online identity on multiple fronts, resulting in preservative thoughts and behaviors. Engagement with multiple social media platforms also increases demands for multitasking, which has been found to worsen mood and anxiety.[15] Adolescents plugged in to social media late at night displace needed sleep. One in 5 youth report waking during the night to check messages on social media.[3] Having multiple social media accounts seems to increase cognitive demands, impair restorative sleep, and increase risk for anxiety and obsessive Internet habits.

Some youth use social media as a maladaptive coping strategy to avoid unpleasant emotions and real-world stressors through distraction, excessive viewing of others' social media profiles (eg, passively viewing Instagram profiles, known as Instastalk), or posting complaints. Lonely teens may use social media, a more comfortable mechanism for expression, as an emotion-regulation strategy.[4] This can lead to PIU-IVGA impairing real-world relationships, especially in lonely individuals who prefer socializing online.[9] Similarly, shy youth are more likely to post negative content on social media sites than peers. Those who do so endorse greater feelings of loneliness, which can lead to the development of PIU-IVGA.[18] Young people often use social media to gain relief from distress (eg, loneliness, anxiety) but overuse increases the risk of a cyclic pattern of avoidant coping and social isolation, addictive use of social media, and ultimately exacerbated loneliness and social anxiety[19] (**Fig. 1**).

Limitations

Research in this area is continuing to develop but several limitations exist currently. First, most aforementioned studies are based on cross-sectional designs, of which causality is unclear.[15] For example, associations between social anxiety and social media use may indicate that individuals with anxiety tend to use social media more, or that increased use of social media worsens anxiety, or both. Additional research using experimental design is needed to establish the direction of these relationships. Second, most studies have focused on older adolescents and young adults, so there is limited research on the relationship of social media use and anxiety among preadolescent children.[13] Third, most research is focused on community-based populations, and more work is needed studying these relationships in clinical populations.[15]

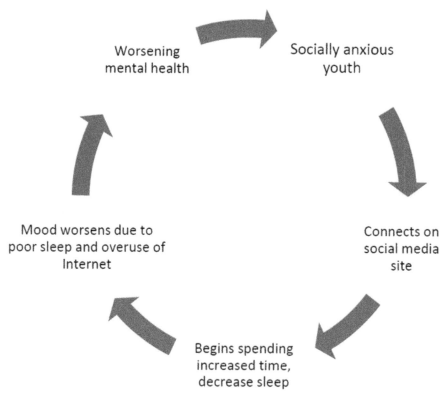

Fig. 1. Cycle of socially anxious youth and social media.

BENEFITS AND PROTECTIVE FACTORS

There are several means by which online activities can benefit children and teens. The online world of youth is typically intertwined with their offline lives. Both can work in conjunction to support individual and interpersonal development.[16] Social media provides an opportunity for young people to share their own creations: videos, pictures, blogs, and tweets. Status updates allow practice expressing self-disclosure skills, permitting communication that might otherwise be impossible. Social media is a platform for adolescent self-expression that can help scaffold the development of identity[3] and offers countless opportunities to connect with others of similar interests, and enhance real-world social relationships. Preadolescents and adolescents interact online to remain connected to their real-world friends, which confers important benefits for communication, according to research.[13]

The Internet also provides access to potential networks of support. Most teenagers surveyed endorsed having received support via social media during times of distress.[3] Online sources of support may be a particularly helpful for youth whose anxiety interferes with their ability to seek support face-to-face. Specialized social media sites related to mental health (eg, Big White Wall, Half of us, To Write Love on Her Arms) provide a platform for youth to access information and potential support from peers encountering similar problems, which may help alleviate stigma related to seeking help for mental health issues.[15] However, it is important for providers to understand potential risks associated with use of these sites.

Youth who are part of marginalized groups are at higher risk for developing mental health problems, may find safety, support, and information through online interactions and social networking. For example, lesbian, gay, bisexual, transgender, and questioning (LGBTQ) youth are able to connect, discuss aspects of gender and sexuality, possibly receive affirmation and support, and practice coming out.[8] Research has found that adolescent mothers' use of social networking sites is related to reduced anxiety and improved confidence.[20] An overview of risk and protective factors related to online engagement and anxiety is summarized in **Table 1**.

PARENTING AN ANXIOUS CHILD IN THE DIGITAL AGE

Children today are digital natives, whereas most of their parents are not. Parents often lack the technical abilities to keep pace with their children's, and may be unaware that passwords or filters are easily bypassed by savvy youth.[21] Parents and grandparents providing supervision are frequently naïve to the concept that children's offline lives intertwine with their online lives and that social media can also facilitate healthy socialization.[22] Managing the online behaviors of a socially anxious child is particularly challenging, particularly in balancing the need to limit the child's time spent online and protecting him or her from online risks with the potential benefits of increased socialization. Parents may struggle to reconcile this mixed picture when video games such as Minecraft are incorporated into school curricula, when providers recommend treatment apps for anxiety, and when they have their own maladaptive Internet habits.

Providers need working knowledge and skills to support families as they navigate these complex issues. For example, youth may engage excessively with computers (eg, playing videogames) to avoid anxious thoughts, feelings, and physiologic symptoms that are triggered by real-world activities (eg, going to school, social activities with peers). When socially anxious youth refuse to go to school, caregivers should be advised to limit or restrict media and Internet use until successful attendance occurs. Providers should advise caregivers to not allow youth with significant anxiety symptoms to participate in online schooling that provides no face-to-face peer interactions because this reinforces avoidant coping. For anxious youth, behavior plans that grant online entertainment as a positive reward for exposure to and engagement in real-world activities promote the practice of active rather than avoidant coping. Several online resources (**Table 2**) are available to support family's management of their children's computer habits.

Table 1 Risk and benefits of online habits for youth with anxiety	
Risks for Developing Problematic Internet Use	**Benefits of Online Engagement**
History of Psychopathology	Identity exploration and expression
Loneliness	Practice with self-disclosure
Shyness	Increased creativity
Preference for online social interactions	Augmenting real-world social relationships
Great need for social assurance	Access to health-related information
High levels of FOMO	Increased availability of mental health treatments
Use social media for 2+ h daily	Destigmatizing mental health forums
Multiple social media accounts	Companionship for members of marginalized groups

Table 2
Resources for families

Resource	Potential Use
American Academy of Child & Adolescent Psychiatry's Facts for Families: http://www.aacap.org/AACAP/Families_and_Youth/Facts_for_Families/FFF-Guide/FFF-Guide-Home.aspx	Downloadable materials to guide parents, including Internet Use in Children, Social Networking and Children, Children and Video Games, and Watching TV/Screen Time and Children
American Academy of Pediatrics HealthyChildren.org: https://www.healthychildren.org/English/family-life/Media/Pages/How-to-Make-a-Family-Media-Use-Plan.aspx	Practical guidelines and support for families around mindful media use from birth through adolescence
Common Sense Media: https://www.commonsensemedia.org/	Guidelines for parents around media use, and independent ratings of appropriateness of social media apps and games for youth of various ages

TECHNOLOGY AND TREATMENT OF ANXIETY

Youth frequently use online searches and social networking to learn about health-related topics. Teens use online resources to gather health information, share their own related experiences, learn of others' experiences, and track data related to health goals.[23] Online platforms can augment or replace conventional treatment. Mobile health (mHealth) interventions involve the use of text messaging and smart phone applications, whereas electronic health (eHealth) interventions include video-games and other computer-based interventions. Both mHealth and eHealth may augment conventional therapies or serve as stand-alone interventions for anxiety disorders and distress associated with medical procedures and conditions.[24]

There are numerous potential benefits offered by online treatment programs that may expand the scope of mental health services. Online treatments are often cost-effective and could increase accessibility for families with limited time, financial resources, and transportation options. They may also be preferable for anxious youth who desire greater autonomy and anonymity.[25] However, the efficacy of these novel treatments remains unproven and, when used in lieu of traditional care, risks delaying access to more effective treatments.

Mobile Health Apps

Mental health providers can partner with youth in using mHealth resources in a variety of ways.[26] A recent review report cited 55 apps intended to help youth with anxiety available on Google Play and the Apple App store.[27] Apps can be used to help youth better engage in treatment via reminders to take medication (eg, Round Health Medicine Reminder and Pill Tracker), track mood (eg, Moodtrack Diary), keep thought diaries (Moodnotes Thought Journal), or engage in self-regulatory skills such as mindfulness (Calm: Meditation to Relax, Focus & Sleep Better).

Despite the availability of many mHealth interventions, very little research supports the effectiveness and usability of these programs. The Reach for Success mental health application, a 6-session cognitive behavioral therapy (CBT)-based protocol designed for prevention of anxiety problems in children 8 to 12 years old, was examined for usability. Children and preadolescents rated the app as having high usability, but future research is needed determine its effectiveness.[28] A recent review of 8 mHealth intervention studies for children with mental disorders found that most assessed only feasibility and the 2 studies that assessed efficacy found no statistically significant benefit.[26] Considering that such minimal research validates the effectiveness of mental health apps for anxiety, providers should evaluate the content of individual apps before recommending use with patients.

Electronic Health Prevention and Interventions

Other programs have also been developed for prevention and treatment of anxiety disorders in children and adolescents. Prevention programs have the potential to significantly reduce the burden of mental health problems for youth. One online prevention program was adapted from a manualized face-to-face version, targeting younger children at risk for developing anxiety disorders. Researchers conducted a randomized controlled trial comparing parents of inhibited preschoolers participating in an 8-module online prevention program providing psychoeducation and skills for anxiety reduction (The Cool Little Kids) to controls. Participants reported high rates of satisfaction and the children in the intervention group showed significantly improved anxiety compared with controls.[25]

Video games have been developed to prevent anxiety by teaching youth coping skills. One example is the game Dojo developed by Game Desk (http://gamedesk.org/project/dojo), which teaches emotion regulation training using heart rate variability biofeedback. In a randomized controlled trial of adolescents, the intervention group played Dojo and the control group played the popular game Rayman 6 times over a 3-week period. Both groups showed improvement in anxiety.[29] The investigators speculated that persevering through game challenges in either condition may have alleviated worries. Further research is needed to better understand whether video games may be an effective prevention tool for adolescents.

A growing number of online programs show promise in the treatment of anxiety disorders. Some are intended to augment face-to-face psychotherapy and others are intended as stand-alone therapy. Examples include Fearfighter, Beating the Blues, and The Brave Program. Most use empirically supported CBT practices.[30] A recent review of randomized controlled trials for such programs found that Internet-delivered CBT self-help programs were highly effective in treating children and adolescents with anxiety, yielding comparable adherence and outcomes as traditional psychotherapy.[30] CBT seems to be the essential modality because programs using other interventions, such as bias modification and stress management, had nonsignificant effects. These encouraging results suggest that online CBT-based treatment programs may be a viable, affordable, and accessible option to treat youth with anxiety disorders.

Electronic Health and Anxiety Related to Other Health Conditions

Online programs and games have demonstrated effectiveness as tools for children with preoperative anxiety, anticipatory dental anxiety, and anxiety comorbid with chronic physical conditions.[31–34] Preoperative anxiety in children has been correlated with distress immediately postoperation, after which maladaptive anxiety and poor functioning may persist up to 2 weeks. Researchers have found that video-game play significantly decreases perioperative anxiety, delirium, and time to discharge when compared with treatment as usual.[31,32]

Other eHealth interventions for youth with long-term physical conditions address anxiety related to illness or treatment. A qualitative study of eHealth for youth with chronic physical illnesses revealed: "(1) Chronic illness as an anxiety-provoking journey (2) Limited access to information and eHealth interventions to support the journey (3) Desires [among patients and their families] for interventions that assist with better understanding of the illness, personal support, and peer connection (especially for illnesses that restrict contact such as cystic fibrosis)." Therefore, eHealth interventions such as Quest for the Code, Re-Mission, and SPARX may be particularly valuable.[34] eHealth interventions have significant potential to help families of youth facing chronic illness gain valuable knowledge, increase social support, and reduce anxiety associated with treatment.

POKÉMON GO: VENTURING INTO THE WORLD

This article would not be complete without a description of the phenomenon of Pokémon Go, an augmented reality (AR) smartphone game introduced in the summer of 2016. People of all ages rapidly embraced this game, which was played by an estimated 44 million people worldwide at the height of its popularity.[35,36] Pokémon Go encourages exploration and activity by requiring players to physically travel around their communities seeking virtual treasures. In a study of 399 US adults, Pokémon Go gameplay was found to be associated with increased positive affect and physical activity.[35] Another study demonstrated that young adult players increased physical movement by 955 steps daily; however, these gains became attenuated over a 6-week period.[37] Anecdotally, child mental health providers have described children with severe social phobia, separation anxiety, and agoraphobia who were motivated to leave home to play Pokémon Go. Additional research examining the role of AR games among children in teens is needed, but these results suggest that AR games may prove useful in encouraging physical activity and social engagement, and could serve to reduce symptoms of anxiety.

SUMMARY
Recommendations for Providers

Despite limitations, current research related to online habits and anxiety reveals important considerations for mental health providers. Clinicians should assess online activity beyond simply assessing total time spent online, including specific aspects of use and individual factors that inform associated risks. The following points provide guidance for providers gathering information about the Internet habits of young patients during clinical interviews:

- Type and frequency of online activities: What are the primary online activities (eg, YouTube, instant messaging [IMing], social media, gaming) and how much time is spent on each? What is the general content, and does it include age-inappropriate material or interactions? How many social media accounts are currently being used?
- Active versus passive use: How much time online is spent actively posting content (text, pictures, videos) or engaged in real-time communication (IMing, chatrooms)? How much time online is spent passively viewing content?
- Emotional valence: Is the content viewed and shared primarily positive (liking others' posts, communicating positive messages or stories about one's own life) or negative (unhappy status updates, sharing frustrations, critical or contentious interactions with others)?
- Beliefs and attitudes: Does the individual prefer online communication over face-to-face interactions? If so, why? How important are either the need for social assurance or FOMO as motivators for online engagement?

> **Box 1**
> **Related articles available in this *Clinics* issue**
>
> - Amy Mayhew and Paul Weigle's article, "Media Engagement and Identity Formation Among Minority Youth," in this issue.
> - Dale Peeples and colleagues' article, "Geeks, Fandoms, and Social Engagement," in this issue.
> - Clifford J. Sussman and colleagues' article, "Internet and Video Game Addictions: Diagnosis, Epidemiology, and Neurobiology," in this issue.
> - Erin L. Belfort and Lindsey Miller's article, "Relationship Between Adolescent Suicidality, Self-injury and Media Habits," in this issue.

- Positive or avoidant coping skills: Is the youth using online activity to extend real-life friendships, or spending time online avoiding school and other interpersonal interactions?
- Virtual gaming: Does the patient meet criteria for Internet or video game addiction? If so, providers need to prioritize treatment of IVGA because these patterns have been found to predict the subsequent development of anxiety disorders.[14]

General recommendations for policy articulated in #StatusOfMind and the European Commission reports[3,21] include the following:

- Popups should warn that Internet use has become excessive when it is accessed for more than a set amount of time per day or week.
- Social media platforms should indicate to the observer whether viewed photos have been digitally enhanced.
- Social medial platforms should identify and support users whose posts display signs of mental health problems.
- Social media training should be made available for teachers and other professionals working with youth.
- More research should explore the effects of social media on mental health of children and adolescents.
- Parents and grandparents should receive support enabling them to actively engage in digital technology with children and grandchildren.

Online resources (see **Table 2**) are available to support parents to guide children and teens in traversing the virtual world. It is important for mental health providers to acknowledge that the Internet and social media play an important role in the social development of young patients, and to advise patients and families how online habits can either exacerbate or alleviate anxiety. This is a rapidly moving digital era in which both online hazards and prospects abound. It is critical that mental health providers understand and manage the risks while embracing the potential benefits and treatment possibilities that the digital world offers patients (**Box 1**).

ACKNOWLEDGMENTS

The authors would like to acknowledge the technical support provided by Robert Evans, BS, and Paul Weigle's editorial support. Their support was invaluable in the writing of this article.

REFERENCES

1. Angold A, Costello EJ, Erkanli A. Comorbidity. J Child Psychol Psychiatry 1999; 40(1):57–87.

2. Kessler RC, Berglund P, Demler O, et al. Lifetime prevalence and age-of-onset distributions of DSM-IV disorders in the National Comorbidity survey Replication. Arch Gen Psychiatry 2005;62(6):593–602.

3. #StatusOfMind, examining the positive and negative effects of social media on young people's health. London: RSPH and Young Health Movement. Available at: https://www.rsph.org.uk/uploads/assets/uploaded/62be270a-a55f-4719-ad668c2ec7a74c2a.pdf. Accessed December 20, 2017.

4. Oberst U, Wegmann E, Stodt B, et al. Negative consequences from heavy social networking in adolescents: the mediating role of fear of missing out. J Adolesc 2017;55:51–60.

5. Bauman S, Rivers I. Virtual worlds. In: mental health in the digital age. London: Palgrave Macmillan; 2015. p. 117–40.

6. Sense C. Common Sense Media. 2017; Available at: https://www.commonsensemedia.org. Accessed June 26, 2017.

7. Zolyomi A, Schmalz M. Mining for Social Skills: Minecraft in Home and Therapy for Neurodiverse Youth. Paper presented at the proceedings of the 50th Hawaii International Conference on System Sciences. Honolulu (HI), 2017.

8. Valkenburg PM, Peter J. Online Communication among adolescents: an integrated model of its attraction, opportunities, and risks. J Adolesc Health 2011; 48(2):121–7.

9. Caplan SE. Relations among loneliness, social anxiety, and problematic internet use. Cyberpsychol Behav 2007;10(2):234–42.

10. Prizant-Passal S, Shechner T, Aderka IM. Social anxiety and internet use–a meta-analysis: what do we know? what are we missing? Comput Hum Behav 2016;62: 221–9.

11. Rauch SM, Strobel C, Bella M, et al. Face to face versus Facebook: does exposure to social networking web sites augment or attenuate physiological arousal among the socially anxious? Cyberpsychol Behav Soc Netw 2014;17(3):187–90.

12. Lee-Won RJ, Herzog L, Park SG. Hooked on Facebook: the role of social anxiety and need for social assurance in problematic use of Facebook. Cyberpsychol Behav Soc Netw 2015;18(10):567–74.

13. Wood MA, Bukowski WM, Lis E. The digital self: how social media serves as a setting that shapes youth's emotional experiences. Adolesc Res Rev 2016;1(2): 163–73.

14. Gentile DA, Choo H, Liau A, et al. Pathological video game use among youths: a two-year longitudinal study. Pediatrics 2011;127(2):e319–29.

15. Primack BA, Escobar-Viera CG. Social media as it interfaces with psychosocial development and mental illness in transitional age youth. Child Adolesc Psychiatr Clin N Am 2017;26(2):217–33.

16. Byron P, Albury K, Evers C. "It would be weird to have that on Facebook": young people's use of social media and the risk of sharing sexual health information. Reprod Health Matters 2013;21(41):35–44.

17. Chou HT, Edge N. "They are happier and having better lives than I am": the impact of using Facebook on perceptions of others' lives. Cyberpsychol Behav Soc Netw 2012;15(2):117–21.

18. Laghi F, Schneider BH, Vitoroulis I, et al. Knowing when not to use the internet: shyness and adolescents' on-line and off-line interactions with friends. Comput Hum Behav 2013;29(1):51–7.

19. Vannucci A, Flannery KM, Ohannessian CM. Social media use and anxiety in emerging adults. J Affect Disord 2017;207:163–6.

20. Nolan S, Hendricks J, Towell A. Adolescent mothers' use of social networking sites creating positive mental health outcomes. Aust Nurs Midwifery J 2016; 23(11):50.
21. Chaudron S. Young children (0-8) and digital technology a qualitative exploratory study across seven countries. Luxembourg: Publications Office; 2016.
22. O'Keeffe GS, Clarke-Pearson K. The impact of social media on children, adolescents, and families. Pediatrics 2011;127(4):800–4.
23. Radovic A, Gmelin T, Stein BD, et al. Depressed adolescents' positive and negative use of social media. J Adolescence 2017;55:5–15.
24. Lindhiem O, Bennett CB, Rosen D, et al. Mobile technology boosts the effectiveness of psychotherapy and behavioral interventions. Behav Modif 2015;39(6): 785–804.
25. Morgan AJ, Rapee RM, Salim A, et al. Internet-delivered parenting program for prevention and early intervention of anxiety problems in young children: randomized controlled trial. J Am Acad Child Adolesc Psychiatry 2017;56(5):417–25.e1.
26. Archangeli C, Marti FA, Wobga-Pasiah EA, et al. Mobile health interventions for psychiatric conditions in children: a scoping review: a scoping review. Child Adolesc Psychiatr Clin N Am 2017;26(1):13–31.
27. Whiteside SP. Mobile device-based applications for childhood anxiety disorders. J Child Adolesc Psychopharmacol 2016;26(3):246–51.
28. Stoll RD, Pina AA, Gary K, et al. Usability of a smartphone application to support the prevention and early intervention of anxiety in youth. Cogn Behav Pract 2017; 24(4):393–404.
29. Scholten H, Malmberg M, Lobel A, et al. A randomized controlled trial to test the effectiveness of an immersive 3d video game for anxiety prevention among adolescents. PLoS One 2016;11(1):e0147763.
30. Christensen H, Batterham P, Calear A. Online interventions for anxiety disorders. Curr Opin Psychiatry 2014;27(1):7–13.
31. Patel A, Schieble T, Davidson M, et al. Distraction with a hand-held video game reduces pediatric preoperative anxiety. Paediatr Anaesth 2006;16(10):1019–27.
32. Seiden SC, McMullan S, Sequera-Ramos L, et al. Tablet-based Interactive Distraction (TBID) vs oral midazolam to minimize perioperative anxiety in pediatric patients: a noninferiority randomized trial. Pediatr Anesth 2014;24(12): 1217–23.
33. Wiederhold MD, Gao K, Wiederhold BK. Clinical use of virtual reality distraction system to reduce anxiety and pain in dental procedures. Cyberpsychol Behav Soc Netw 2014;17(6):359–65.
34. Thabrew H, Stasiak K, Garcia-Hoyos V, et al. Game for health: how eHealth approaches might address the psychological needs of children and young people with long-term physical conditions. J Paediatr Child Health 2016;52(11):1012–8.
35. Bonus JA, Peebles A, Mares ML, et al. Look on the bright side (of Media Effects): Pokémon go as a catalyst for positive life experiences. Media Psychol 2017. [Epub ahead of print].
36. Dotinga R. Gotta catch 'em all: is Pokémon Go an intervention for schizophrenia? Clin Psychiatry News 2017;2017.
37. Howe KB, Suharlim C, Ueda P, et al. Gotta catch'em all! Pokémon GO and physical activity among young adults: difference in differences study. BMJ 2016;355: i6270.

Inattention to Problematic Media Use Habits

Interaction Between Digital Media Use and Attention-Deficit/Hyperactivity Disorder

Tolga Atilla Ceranoglu, MD

KEYWORDS

- ADHD • Media • Children • Adolescents

KEY POINTS

- As digital media (DM) access continues to surge among youth, caregivers and clinicians are concerned about problems associated with its excessive use.
- Children with attention-deficit/hyperactivity disorder (ADHD) are more at risk to experience negative effects on sleep, academic achievement, attention and cognitive skills.
- Youth with ADHD are more likely to use DM excessively.
- ADHD symptom severity and circumstances of DM access are among the factors that mediate these negative effects.
- Several key interventions for parents and clinicians to assist youth with problematic DM habits, and opportunities for advocacy groups and DM industry for public health interventions are discussed in light of research.

Digital media (DM) use is increasingly prevalent among youths. In the United States, the average child spends almost 10 hours a day engaging in some form of DM, which represents a longer duration than an adult's average workday.[1] Caregivers and clinicians have been concerned about the effects of heavy media engagement on adolescents.[2] These effects include problems with sleep, cognitive skills, academic vigor,

There are no conflicts of interest regarding this article.

Disclosures: Research support from the Department of Defense (W81XWH-12-1-0510), Massachusetts Department of Mental Health, Massachusetts General Hospital Department of Psychiatry, National Institutes of Health (5K23MH100450-02), Shriners Hospitals for Children, Lundbeck A/S, Pamlab LLC, Pfizer, Sunovion Pharmaceuticals Inc, Magceutics, Inc; advisor/consultant: Jack Kent Cooke Foundation; employee: Massachusetts General Hospital, Shriners Hospitals for Children–Boston.

Alan and Lorraine Bressler Clinical and Research Program for Autism Spectrum Disorder, Massachusetts General Hospital, 55 Fruit Street, Warren 624, Boston, MA 02114, USA

E-mail address: aceranoglu@mgh.harvard.edu

Child Adolesc Psychiatric Clin N Am 27 (2018) 183–191
https://doi.org/10.1016/j.chc.2017.11.009
1056-4993/18/© 2017 Elsevier Inc. All rights reserved.

childpsych.theclinics.com

and athletic participation. Factors that mediate the negative effects of media include location, timing, and duration of access.[3] More recent findings also suggest children with certain psychiatric disorders may be at increased risk of experiencing these negative effects.[4]

Attention-deficit/hyperactivity disorder (ADHD) is a neurobiologic disorder affecting up to 10% of youths across the world and is characterized by cognitive and behavioral symptoms that include inattention, impulsivity, and hyperactivity.[5] Children with ADHD face difficulties in regulating impulses and maintaining engagement in age-typical activities, including academics and social obligations. ADHD has been linked to polymorphisms of the DRD4 gene (DRDR-7 repeat allele), which has been associated with sensation-seeking behaviors and, thus, struggles with impulse control and limiting time spent on preferred activities.[6]

Hypoactivity in dorsolateral prefrontal cortex among individuals with ADHD correlates with deficits in both executive functions (EFs) and emotion regulation. Such deficits may result in increased reliance on adults to regulate the behavior of children with ADHD, including media activity, along with increased mood reactivity in response to caregiver's attempts to intervene in DM use.

In order to understand the interaction between DM use and ADHD, a review of the literature with clinical studies and surveys on PubMed and PsycInfo was carried out using the keywords *attention*, *ADHD*, *media*, *Internet*, *video games*, *social network*, and *children and adolescents*. The resulting studies were reviewed for content and relevance. Further literature identified among references was also retrieved and reviewed. In result, a total of 38 clinical studies were reviewed; a synopsis is presented next.

MEDIA USE HABITS AMONG YOUTH WITH ATTENTION-DEFICIT/HYPERACTIVITY DISORDER

Children with ADHD experience problems with impulse regulation, time management, task organization, and prioritization. These children experience more difficulty in limiting and monitoring their own media use and tend to spend more time on video games (VGs) compared with healthy children.[7] Similarly, children with ADHD tend to have more problematic play characteristics compared with the general population, resulting in frequent excessive media use. More severe ADHD symptoms correlate with lower academic achievement among participants who played VGs greater than1 h/d on average.[8] These studies tend to be cross-sectional and cannot address whether excessive media use leads to attention problems or vice versa. However, increased attention symptoms were found to predict heavier and problematic media use 1 year later in one prospective study.[9]

Sleep difficulties are often reported among youths with problematic DM use.[3] Sleep deprivation is a known risk factor for psychiatric problems, obesity, and memory deficits. In summary, ADHD poses a risk factor for excessive DM use and several biological factors seem to contribute to this heavier engagement.

The severity of ADHD symptoms has been shown to correlate with various aspects of problematic media use in children.[10] Excessive VG play is correlated with the severity of inattention symptoms rather than hyperactivity.[4] Hyperactivity/impulsivity symptom severity was linked to a 3 times more likelihood of severe reactions to attempts at limiting DM use. As a result, parents often report a reduced ability to limit, regulate, and supervise their children's DM use.[7]

Social and psychological factors mediating the relationship between media use and ADHD include frequency of interpersonal conflict.[11] Children who use DM more tend to report lower friendship trust and disrupted communication, alienation, and increase rate of conflict with peers.[12] Children experiencing dissatisfaction in their social relationships and academic performance may gravitate toward areas where their deficits will not manifest as significantly. Inhibitory processes are diminished in children with ADHD, resulting in frequent errors during tasks requiring sustained attention. Interestingly, children with ADHD present no difference in inhibitory performances compared with control groups during VG play.[13,14] As a compensatory mechanism, a child struggling with ADHD may find a more level ground for competing against peers playing VGs and may further engage in excessive use.

EFFECTS OF MEDIA USE ON ATTENTION-DEFICIT/HYPERACTIVITY DISORDER

In moderate amounts, and with appropriate supervision, DM may be a useful and convenient tool for social activity, communication, and education.[15] DM offers a platform for fast social communication. Enhanced social bonding and expression may enrich a child's social world in real life and enhance social competence.[16] Conversely, problems in real life often persist into virtual life, leading to progressive interference with overall function. Therefore, the effects of DM use on attention problems need to be better understood, as exposure to television (TV) and VGs was reported to correlate with more severe attention problems.[17] The applicability of existing research to clinical care has been limited because of a relatively smaller effect size, inconsistent use of clinically well-validated measures, and a lack of multiple informants. However, it raises valid concerns about excessive media access and the relationship to attention problems.

Persistent concerns about unsupervised DM access and exposure will remain relevant, as new forms of DM (streaming on individual devices, smart phones, tablets, laptops, and so forth) are now in mainstream use in addition to background TV at homes. The amount of screen time has consistently increased because of the ease of access and tends to begin very early in life. Problems in language development, attention problems, and behavioral disorders have been reported among children who are exposed to DM during early ages.[18–20]

The interaction between DM and attention and cognitive skill development is complex, as research has revealed several factors involved. In addition to a child's age, the circumstances of media access seem to determine the effects of DM. These factors include the duration of media use, timing of access in relation to sleep, and location of media equipment in the household.

Duration

The effects of media use on mental health and cognitive functions correlate with the average amount of media use in a dose-dependent manner. Children who played on average 96 minutes or more per day were found to perform poorly on attention tasks, compared with those who played 78 minutes. Interestingly, children who played 36 minutes per day have performed better on the same tasks. Young boys with a diagnosis of ADHD, inattentive subtype were found to be more susceptible to these effects and they tended to play longer than their peers.[21]

Location

Bedroom access to DM has been consistently shown to correlate with longer time spent and less parental supervision. The number of media items in bedrooms correlates with sleep and academic problems.[22] The location of media access is also even more significant for children with ADHD, as they are more likely to have DM in their bedrooms compared with the general population.[23]

Schedule

Time spent on media tends to displace sleep and may lead to sleep problems and worsening of attention problems. Furthermore, it may interfere with clinical interventions (eg, treatment-resistant sleep problems) and participation in educational programs.[24,25] Later sleep onset, reduced sleep, and memory deficits the following day were reported among individuals who accessed DM within 2 hours of bedtime.[26] Intense media engagement at late night may also change sleep architecture and contribute to problems with cognitive functions.[27]

Content

Violent media content has raised numerous concerns about the increased risk of violence and aggression among children. The relationship between violence in media and risk of aggression has been controversial, effects of media content on EF have been more consistent.[28,29] VGs have been widely researched in this regard, and various content and types of VG play were shown to have different effects on the EF of individuals who use them. Players who prefer VG genres that portray continuous activity on screen requiring ongoing attention were found to process a larger area and react faster to visual attention tasks with no decrease in accuracy.[30–33] Engagement style (cooperative vs competitive vs solitary play) may also have different effects on EF. Indeed, children playing cooperatively or competitively with a peer performed much better on EF tasks compared with those who played alone.[34] Interestingly, when comparing playing an exercise VG alone to playing with a peer, a recent study reported EF improvement in the EFs of children who played alone.[35] However, the investigators included children with ADHD and autism spectrum disorder; the average play session lasted 10 to 18 minutes, which may not have been sufficient to produce EF benefits of paired play. Playing VGs that require active exercise in front of a screen has also been reported to improve EF among children aged 6 to 10 years.[36] Cognitive engagement coupled with required exercise during VG play was found to be associated with further improvement in EF.[37]

INTERVENTIONS FOR EXCESSIVE MEDIA USE IN ATTENTION-DEFICIT/HYPERACTIVITY DISORDER

Psychopharmacological Treatments

Close association of excessive media use with ADHD symptoms suggests a valid opportunity for intervention. Indeed, excessive DM use among children with ADHD was shown to improve with stimulant treatment.[38] Similarly, excessive Internet gaming habits were improved in individuals who received bupropion and escitalopram treatment. Although no information was available regarding presence or rate of comorbid mood or anxiety disorder diagnoses, a greater change in bupropion group was noted to correlate with improvement in ADHD symptoms.[39] Based on available data, screening and treatment of underlying psychiatric disorders should be considered in children with excessive DM use habits.

Family Interventions

Caregiver supervision of a child's DM access remains crucial.[40] In clinical settings, screening for problematic media habits of children with risk factors, such as a diagnosis of ADHD, forms an important first step. Both the American Academy of Pediatrics (AAP) and the American Academy of Child and Adolescent Psychiatry (AACAP) provide a series of recommendations and resources to help families regulate DM access of their youths from birth to adulthood.[41-43] Despite these resources and available research, 3 important barriers seem to interfere with accurate and appropriate screening and intervention opportunities. First, most clinicians do not include systematic screening for media habits in their evaluations. This barrier may be due to the lack of availability of a widely accepted curriculum in pediatric and child psychiatry residency training programs. Second, most pediatricians consider it futile to make the AAP's recommendations to parents regarding DM access.[44] Similarly, most parents have acknowledged they are unaware of expert and consensus recommendations.[1,45] Finally, most adolescents typically underestimate how much time they spend on DM and have difficulty breaking off from them.[46,47]

Parental monitoring and modeling is associated with positive outcomes. Monitoring the amount of time spent on DM has led to better school performance.[14] Adolescents' DM use directly correlates to parental attitudes and media use habits, and the perceived relationship with parents remains the most protective factor against problematic DM use.[48,49] Restrictive mediation strategies (limiting access) by mothers and evaluative strategies (discussion of media content) by fathers were reported to influence media use of their daughters in the desired direction.[50] Despite this protective effect of monitoring circumstances of media use, only 40% of households report having rules on media access.[44] Interestingly, children even in households that use rules on media access still remain at risk of experiencing a decline in academic performance within 4 months following acquisition of new digital technologies, without any associating behavioral problems. Therefore, the need for continuous monitoring and adjustment of rules and supervision with changes to household DM seems necessary.[51]

Advocacy Groups and Public Health Interventions

In response to growing concerns about excessive media use, governments across the globe have passed laws and regulations that limit the amount of time spent on screen playing a game and have mandated media providers to implement reminders and mandatory breaks or hard stops in media format.[52] Professional societies, such as the AAP and AACAP, provide recommendations, resources, and tools aimed to inform and help caregivers to regulate their children's DM access.[41-43] Manufacturers in VG industry have long been required to put warnings for seizures in their products, similar to that placed on alcohol and tobacco products. These warnings will need to be extended to include caution against risks of academic underachievement, sleep disturbance, and worsening of attention problems associated with excessive media use.

Available research data not only reveals the circumstances the mediating effects of DM on youths but also offers important guidance on several intervention opportunities and recommendations for parents, clinicians, advocacy groups, and relevant industry. The key recommendations derived from the literature reviewed are listed in **Box 1**. In summary, moving DM equipment out of bedrooms to a common place remains an important first step. Limiting media access to daytime and having a DM curfew within 1 to 2 hours of bedtime may help avoiding sleep problems and sleep-deprivation–related cognitive deficits. Instead of one long DM access session, limiting play sessions to multiple shorter episodes spaced out with breaks and other activities would likely help with attention skills or avoid most negative effects associated with extended or excessive DM use. Finally, coviewing DM and monitoring social aspects of media use offers an important supervision and role-modeling opportunity both for adults and children.

Box 1
Key recommendations

What caregivers can do:

- Monitor the circumstances of the DM access (rule of 2s).
  - Where: Move DM out of bedrooms to a family room where a total of 2 or more people are present (child + adult).
  - How long:
    - Limit screen access of children younger than 2 years to personal communication (eg, video chatting).
    - For children younger than 5 years, limit access to high-quality programming and prioritize coviewing (2 viewers). For older children, limit to 1 to 2 hours of total daily access.
    - Limit DM access to smaller bits of multiple sessions instead of one long protracted session (eg, 2 × 30-minute sessions instead of one 60-minute sessions, separated by an independent activity).
  - When: Limit DM access close to bedtime (within 1–2 hours) to avoid sleep-onset problems.
  - With whom: For TV, encourage coviewing; for online social networks, consider monitoring or connecting to the child's activities; for VGs, encourage playing with friends in real time and in person instead of anonymously and online.
- Monitor the content of the DM accessed.
  - Check the Entertainment Software Rating Board's rating assigned to the media accessed (VGs, TV shows, movies, and so forth).
  - Monitor online social network activity and access, paying attention to the content shared (cyberbullying, sexting).

What clinicians can do

- Inform parents about problems associated with excessive DM access and intervention opportunities.
- Screen DM access among youths during clinic visits.
- Refer youths for treatment of underlying psychiatric conditions associated with excessive DM access (ADHD, mood and anxiety disorders, autism spectrum disorders).

What industry and advocacy groups can do

- Create funding for further research into the benefits and risks associated with DM access.
- Provide appropriate warnings in DM materials for caregivers similar to photogenic seizure warnings in VGs. Caution against sleep, cognitive, and academic problems and obesity in VGs and cyberbullying and sexting during communication via DM.

SUMMARY

ADHD represents a significant risk factor for excessive DM use. Following new advances in communication technology, from smart phones to virtual reality, DM has become more ubiquitous and readily available. New digital frontiers demand caution from parents of children with ADHD and clinical monitoring from mental health professionals. Emerging research now provides important information for clinicians and caregivers developing a thoughtful approach to manage DM exposure in children at risk for or diagnosed with ADHD.

Clinicians and advocacy groups have a valuable opportunity to inform the public about the effects of DM use, as caregivers form the most important interveners on regulating DM access of their children. More research is necessary to further understand the effects of media use on children, so that more targeted interventions may be designed.

REFERENCES

1. Rideout VJ, Foehr UG, Roberts DF. Generation M2: media in the lives of 8-18 year olds. Menlo Park (CA): Henry J. Kaiser Family Foundation; 2010.
2. Primack BA, Swanier B, Georgiopoulos AM, et al. Association between media use in adolescence and depression in young adulthood: a longitudinal study. Arch Gen Psychiatry 2009;66:181–8.
3. Ceranoglu T. Video games and sleep: an overlooked challenge. Adolesc Psychiatry 2014;4:104–8.
4. Mazurek MO, Engelhardt CR. Video game use in boys with autism spectrum disorder, ADHD, or typical development. Pediatrics 2013;132:260–6.
5. Faraone SV, Sergeant J, Gillberg C, et al. The worldwide prevalence of ADHD: is it an American condition? World Psychiatry 2003;2:104–13.
6. Franke B, Faraone SV, Asherson P, et al. International multicentre persistent AC. The genetics of attention deficit/hyperactivity disorder in adults, a review. Mol Psychiatry 2012;17:960–87.
7. Bioulac S, Arfi L, Bouvard MP. Attention deficit/hyperactivity disorder and video games: a comparative study of hyperactive and control children. Eur Psychiatry 2008;23:134–41.
8. Chan P, Rabinowitz T. A cross-sectional analysis of video games and attention deficit hyperactivity disorder symptoms in adolescents. Ann Gen Psychiatry 2006;5:16.
9. Ferguson CJ, Ceranoglu TA. Attention problems and pathological gaming: resolving the 'chicken and egg' in a prospective analysis. Psychiatr Q 2014;85:103–10.
10. Yoo HJ, Cho SC, Ha J, et al. Attention deficit hyperactivity symptoms and Internet addiction. Psychiatry Clin Neurosciences 2004;58:487–94.
11. Hoza B. Peer functioning in children with ADHD. Ambul Pediatr 2007;7:101–6.
12. Blais JJ, Craig WM, Pepler D, et al. Adolescents online: the importance of internet activity choices to salient relationships. J Youth Adolescence 2008;37:522–36.
13. Shaw DS, Lacourse E, Nagin DS. Developmental trajectories of conduct problems and hyperactivity from ages 2 to 10. J Child Psychol Psychiatry 2005;46:931–42.
14. Hastings EC, Karas TL, Winsler A, et al. Young children's video/computer game use: relations with school performance and behavior. Issues Ment Health Nurs 2009;30:638–49.
15. Olson CK. Children's motivations for video game play in the context of normal development. Rev Gen Psychol 2010;14:180–7.
16. Valkenburg PM, Peter J. Online communication among adolescents: an integrated model of its attraction, opportunities, and risks. J Adolesc Health 2011;48:121–7.
17. Swing EL, Gentile DA, Anderson CA, et al. Television and video game exposure and the development of attention problems. Pediatrics 2010;126:214–21.
18. Christakis DA, Zimmerman FJ. Violent television viewing during preschool is associated with antisocial behavior during school age. Pediatrics 2007;120:993–9.
19. Christakis DA, Zimmerman FJ, DiGiuseppe DL, et al. Early television exposure and subsequent attentional problems in children. Pediatrics 2004;113:708–13.
20. Zimmerman FJ, Christakis DA, Meltzoff AN. Associations between media viewing and language development in children under age 2 years. J Pediatr 2007;151:364–8.

21. Tahiroglu AY, Celik GG, Avci A, et al. Short-term effects of playing computer games on attention. J Atten Disord 2010;13:668–76.
22. Eggermont S, Van den Bulck J. Nodding off or switching off? The use of popular media as a sleep aid in secondary-school children. J Paediatr Child Health 2006; 42:428–33.
23. Engelhardt CR, Mazurek MO, Sohl K. Media use and sleep among boys with autism spectrum disorder, ADHD, or typical development. Pediatrics 2013;132: 1081–9.
24. Gaina A, Sekine M, Kanayama H, et al. Morning-evening preference: sleep pattern spectrum and lifestyle habits among Japanese junior high school pupils. Chronobiology Int 2006;23:607–21.
25. Oka Y, Suzuki S, Inoue Y. Bedtime activities, sleep environment, and sleep/wake patterns of Japanese elementary school children. Behav Sleep Med 2008;6: 220–33.
26. Dworak M, Schierl T, Bruns T, et al. Impact of singular excessive computer game and television exposure on sleep patterns and memory performance of school-aged children. Pediatrics 2007;120:978–85.
27. Higuchi S, Motohashi Y, Liu Y, et al. Effects of playing a computer game using a bright display on presleep physiological variables, sleep latency, slow wave sleep and REM sleep. J Sleep Res 2005;14:267–73.
28. Ferguson CJ. The good, the bad and the ugly: a meta-analytic review of positive and negative effects of violent video games. Psychiatr Q 2007;78:309–16.
29. Gao X, Pan W, Li C, et al. Long-time exposure to violent video games does not show desensitization on empathy for pain: an fMRI study. Front Psychol 2017;8: 650.
30. Clark K, Fleck MS, Mitroff SR. Enhanced change detection performance reveals improved strategy use in avid action video game players. Acta Psychol (Amst) 2011;136:67–72.
31. Dye MW, Green CS, Bavelier D. The development of attention skills in action video game players. Neuropsychologia 2009;47:1780–9.
32. Chisholm JD, Hickey C, Theeuwes J, et al. Reduced attentional capture in action video game players. Atten Percept Psychophys 2010;72:667–71.
33. Boot WR, Blakely DP, Simons DJ. Do action video games improve perception and cognition? Front Psychol 2011;2:226.
34. Staiano AE, Abraham AA, Calvert SL. Competitive versus cooperative exergame play for African American adolescents' executive function skills: short-term effects in a long-term training intervention. Developmental Psychol 2012;48: 337–42.
35. Flynn RM, Colon N. Solitary active videogame play improves executive functioning more than collaborative play for children with special needs. Games Health J 2016;5:398–404.
36. Best JR. Exergaming immediately enhances children's executive function. Developmental Psychol 2012;48(5):1501–10.
37. Benzing V, Heinks T, Eggenberger N, et al. Acute cognitively engaging exergame-based physical activity enhances executive functions in adolescents. PLoS One 2016;11:e0167501.
38. Han DH, Lee YS, Na C, et al. The effect of methylphenidate on Internet video game play in children with attention-deficit/hyperactivity disorder. Compr Psychiatry 2009;50:251–6.

39. Song J, Park JH, Han DH, et al. Comparative study of the effects of bupropion and escitalopram on Internet gaming disorder. Psychiatry Clin Neurosciences 2016;70:527–35.
40. Weigle P, Reid D. Helping parents promote healthy and safe computer habits. Adolesc Psychiatry 2014;4:92–7.
41. Radesky J, Christakis D. Media and young minds. Pediatrics 2016;138(5): e20162591.
42. Council on Communications and Media. Media use in school-aged children and adolescents. Pediatrics 2016;138(5) [pii:e20162592].
43. Screen time and children in facts for families. Washington, DC: American Academy of Child and Adolescent Psychiatry; 2015. Available at: http://www.aacap.org/AACAP/Families_and_Youth/Facts_for_Families/FFF-Guide/Children-And-Watching-TV-054.aspx. Accessed December 11, 2017.
44. Gentile DA, Reimer RA, Nathanson AI, et al. Protective effects of parental monitoring of children's media use: a prospective study. JAMA Pediatr 2014;168: 479–84.
45. Kutner L, Olson C. Grand theft childhood: the surprising truth about violent video games and what parents can do. New York: Simon & Schuster; 2008.
46. Tobin S, Grondin S. Video games and the perception of very long durations by adolescents. Comput Hum Behav 2009;25:554–9.
47. Rau PL, Peng SY, Yang CC. Time distortion for expert and novice online game players. Cyberpsychol Behav 2006;9:396–403.
48. Liu QX, Fang XY, Deng LY, et al. Parent-adolescent communication, parental internet use and internet-specific norms and pathological internet use among Chinese adolescents. Comput Hum Behav 2012;28:1269–75.
49. Nathanson AI. The unintended effects of parental mediation of television on adolescents. Media Psychol 2002;4:207–30.
50. Van den Bulck J, Van den Bergh B. The influence of perceived parental guidance patterns on children's media use: gender differences and media displacement. J Broadcast Electron Media 2000;44:329–48.
51. Weis R, Cerankosky BC. Effects of video-game ownership on young boys' academic and behavioral functioning: a randomized, controlled study. Psychol Sci 2010;21:463–70.
52. Davies B, Blake E. Evaluating existing strategies to limit video game playing time. IEEE Comput Graph Appl 2016;36:47–57.

The Interplay of Media Violence Effects and Behaviorally Disordered Children and Adolescents
Guidelines for Practitioners

Manuel D. Reich, DO[a,b,c,d],*

KEYWORDS

- Media violence effects • Aggression • Child development • Externalizing behaviors
- Treatment guidelines • Disordered youths

KEY POINTS

- The importance of this topic is that children and youths are immersed in media, much of it violent.
- The clinical significance is that mental health practitioners are challenged with treating children and adolescents that have extensive exposure to violent media.
- Research has demonstrated that exposure to violent media has short- and long-term effects and contributes to aggressive behaviors.

Violence is an established genre in the media dating back to ancient civilizations. The dissemination of violent themes was part of an oral tradition of storytelling. The *Epic of Gilgamesh* precedes Christ by 3000 years and has themes of demons, disaster, anxiety, death by the gods, battles, and revenge.[1] Concern about the impact of exposure to violence on youths was a matter of importance to the early philosophers. Aristotle and Plato discussed the pros and cons of exposure to emotionally charged content with regard to character development. Such concerns continue

Disclosure Statement: The author has no conflicting relationships to report.
M.D. Reich, DO graduated from the New York College of Osteopathic Medicine and completed a residency in adult psychiatry at the Downstate Medical Center/Kings County Hospital. He worked as a psychiatrist in the US Public Health Service and completed a fellowship in child and adolescent psychiatry at New York University/Bellevue Hospital.

[a] Beacon Health Options, 520 Pleasant Valley Road, Trafford, PA 15085, USA; [b] Persoma, PC 2540 Monroeville Boulevard, Monroeville, PA 15146, USA; [c] American Academy of Child and Adolescent Psychiatry, 3615 Wisconsin Avenue, NW, Washington, DC 20016, USA; [d] Pittsburgh Psychiatric Society, 777 E. Park Dr., Harrisburg, PA 17111, USA
* 2540 Monroeville Boulevard, Monroeville, PA 15146.
E-mail address: dr.manuel.reich@gmail.com

Child Adolesc Psychiatric Clin N Am 27 (2018) 193–202
https://doi.org/10.1016/j.chc.2017.11.006
1056-4993/18/© 2017 Elsevier Inc. All rights reserved.

childpsych.theclinics.com

today and manifest in a plethora of academic research as well as in public policy debates and cultural manifestations.[2]

In contemporary society, violence appears in religious texts, mythology, literature, newspapers, books, comic books, theater, film, television, cartoons, animation, radio, music, music videos, video games, and virtual reality. As a research construct, violence is usually defined as any intentionally harmful act perpetrated by one human being toward another human being, with the intention to cause significant injury or death.[3,4]

ACCESS AND CONSUMPTION

The range, quantity, and accessibility of media devices available to youths were evaluated for public policy makers by the Kaiser Family Foundation in a 2010 study.[5] Youths aged 8 to 18 years report the following devices in their homes and bedrooms, respectively: TV (99%, 71%), DVD/VCR (97%, 57%), radio (94%, 75%), computer (93%, 36%), video game console (87%, 50%), CD player (87%, 68%), TiVo/DVR (52%, 13%).[5] Usage findings are as follows: media consumption for 8 to 10 year olds is less than for 11 to 14 year olds (12 hours); boys consume more media than girls because of video game usage; white youths report lower consumption (8:36 hours) than black (12:59 hours) and Hispanic (13:00 hours) youths; at risk for higher usage are also tweens and early teens aged 11 to 14 years.[5] Huesmann,[6] a prolific researcher on media and aggression, describes this ubiquitous environment as a "saturation of our culture and daily lives."[6]

As technology has evolved, so have the media platforms that depict violence. Portable devices with Internet, photo, and video capacities provide unsupervised venues to share and observe real-time, unrated violence.[7] Viewers can select from an endless variety of real violence for viewing, including, terrorism, police shootings, sexual violence, suicides, and so forth.[7] The plethora of media genres and available outlets enables high consumption. After sleeping, media is the leading childhood activity.[5] It is not uncommon for children less than a year old to begin viewing television.[8] Children and teenagers spend more hours using media than they are in school (8–11 hours daily).[5] In terms of violent content and programming, these statistics translate into youths viewing up to 24 violent acts per hour[9]; cumulatively, by 18 years of age, a child will have watched thousands of murders and hundreds of thousands of acts of violence.

CAUSE

Since the emergence of television in the 1940s, the harmful effects of programming content have been a cause for concern.[8] Research did not emerge until the 1960s. In the early part of the decade, Alfred Bandura's research with Bobo dolls established social learning theory and the effect of role models on human behavior; children exposed to adult aggression were more likely to be aggressive.[10] By 1969, the Surgeon General's Scientific Advisory Committee on Television and Social Behavior was formed to "focus on the effects of televised violence on the behavior, attitudes, development, and mental health of children."[3] The 1972 US Surgeon General's Report established TV as a form of social learning. The study concluded viewing violent programming does not adversely affect most youths. However, it does adversely impact a small group of children with a predisposition for aggressive tendencies.[3] In 1982, the National Institute of Mental Health published a follow-up report to the surgeon general and found that children who are exposed to violent media may experience desensitization to pain and suffering of others, become fearful about the world, and behave aggressively toward others.[11]

The 1990s saw mostly agreement within the scientific community that the effect of violent media on youths is statistically significant and causes an increase in aggression and violence.[12] Research shifted to understanding the processes underlying the effects of violent media consumption on behavior.[13]

CURRENT RESEARCH FINDINGS

Child and adolescent exposure to media violence is empirically proven to have a short-term impact.[6,13–15] This finding is also acknowledged by scholars who question the validity of other research outcomes in the field.[16] Immediate consequences are verbal aggression (making mean and hurtful comments to the victim), physical aggression (pushing, shoving, assaulting, fighting), and experiencing aggressive thoughts and emotions.[12–14] A study of preschool children's play behaviors following exposure to violent media found children could become physically violent and go so far as to push another child off a game and waiting to do so until the teacher was not looking.[17] Brief exposure for children can also cause fear and anxiety as well as nightmares lasting for long periods of time.[14] Violent media also teaches viewers new ways to harm others.[14]

There is compelling evidence that long-term exposure to media violence can cause desensitization to both violence and the ramifications of violence; it can also cause lasting aggressive scripts[6,12,13]; it can increase the acceptance of violence as a way to solve conflict, increase hostile attribution biases about the world, cause aggressive and violent tendencies that can last decades,[14] and can lead to violent criminal behavior.[4] A 2-year longitudinal study found playing violent electronic video games is the strongest measured risk factor for violent criminality and that, with repeated exposure, violence and criminality increases.[18] Exposure to media with the core theme of revenge is a specific risk factor for violent behaviors in school and community settings.[18] Other long-term adverse mental health outcomes include poor academic achievement and reduced motivation.[19]

Anderson and colleagues[12] provide an exhaustive review of theoretic explanations in the research literature, which explain the underlying psychological processes manifesting in the latter outcomes. Short-term consequences relate to

- Observational learning: Children engage in imitation and learn social scripts, including how to react to conflict.
- Priming by environmental stimuli and automatization of aggressive schematic processing: When youngsters view violence, it primes thoughts, feelings, and scripts about aggression so that, as the number of aggressive cues increase, the easier associated aggressive scripts are processed. Thus, aggression becomes internalized.
- Arousal and excitation transfer: This concept refers to the exciting nature of violence, which can increase aggression in the short-term. For example, if a frustrating experience occurs after watching a violent movie, there is a greater risk for that individual to have an aggressive response to the frustration.[12] Theories about long-term outcomes are as follows.
- Emotional desensitization occurs as the more violence an individual views, the less disturbing and arousing it seems.
- Moderators of the influence of violent media on aggression include viewer characteristics (age, sex, aggressiveness, intelligence, perceptions of realism, and identification with aggressive characters); media content characteristics (characteristics of the aggressive perpetrator, portrayed justification, and consequences of the aggression); and social environment (influence of culture, neighborhood, socioeconomic status, parents).[12]

From a developmental perspective, high-risk periods for viewing violent media include preschool[20] and middle childhood (8–10 years of age).[21] Social information processing initiates when young children take in the world around them and imitate what they see. During middle childhood, behavioral norms, based on these scripts, are internalized and individual personalities emerge. Social scripts determine social adjustment, and poor adjustment can lead to aggressive behavior.[21] Also, children become adept at self-comparison and more proficient at using peer comparison to rank individual abilities.[22] Self-esteem becomes enmeshed with peer response to behavior. Social rejection and poor self-esteem also contribute to maladaptive externalizing behaviors and can, for example, fuel identification with media role models who engage in negative behavior, often without consequences. Furthermore, developmental pathways established in early childhood have been found to impact well-being in middle childhood; early exposure has diverse negative impacts, including reduced classroom engagement, poorer math scores, increased victimization by peers, less physical activity, higher consumption of soft drinks, and a higher body mass index.[19] Study limitations include not knowing media content and relying on teacher reports (not achievement tests) for academic performance.

Compelling evidence does exist to show reducing violent media consumption can reduce later aggressive tendencies.[14] Furthermore, there are group effects that can draw antisocial or violent youths together, creating subcultures especially at risk from the effects of media violence.

A QUESTION OF CATHARSIS

For some youths with aggressive behaviors, violent media, including violent video games, may actually reduce aggression and provide a distraction or acceptable and enjoyable activity when upset. During middle childhood, as the social world becomes more complex and difficult to maneuver, violent media can offer relief.[23] However, viewing violence is not therapeutic purging but simply a distraction from what is bothering the viewer.[23] This point does not imply all violent media is void of benefits. Violent programming can highlight negative consequences and offer positive themes that promote learning, positive values, and feelings of safety.[24]

CRITICISM OF RESEARCH

In a culture awash with digital media violence, episodes such as mass shootings lead to an emotionally charged reevaluation of media violence, as we collectively look for answers as to why these events occur. At these times the critics of our current media habits have a more prominent place in the public forum than is typical. Violent media can easily play the role of scapegoat.[16] A more nuanced look at media research is often beyond the scope of news programming, which often seeks out sensationalistic or provocative viewpoints.[15] Intense periods of public discussion can be useful to bring the issue of media violence into the discussion, but these complex matters can confuse caregivers and increase anxiety and concern beyond what is warranted. The cause of violence is multifactorial; collectively, over time, viewing violent media is one of many potential risk factors that contribute to aggressive and violent behaviors.[6]

BEHAVIORALLY DISORDERED YOUTHS

Youth presenting with maladaptive and disruptive, externalizing behaviors represent anywhere from one-third to one-half of all clinical referrals.[25] Fortunately, there is a growing body of evidence-based psychotherapy research for the treatment of this population and their caregivers.[26] Although treatments vary to accommodate different age groups, symptom severity, and caregiver availability, the guiding principles share common themes. First, there are 2 distinct problem areas: disruptive child behavior and ineffective parenting styles. Second, children with aggression and conduct problems are at risk for having cognitive biases, attention problems, and problems with family, school, neighborhood, and peers. Problems are attributed in large part to lack of social competence and information processing issues. Caregiver difficulties include ineffective disciplinary and communication techniques[26] as well as poor caregiver involvement due to mental illness, incarceration, substance abuse, long work hours, and so forth.[26] Furthermore, antisocial behavior is often transgenerational and can go back 2 generations.[25] Treatment approaches are often systemic, family focused, and designed to empower the child and caregivers with resources and skills to improve family relationships, overall communication, and problem-solving techniques. Ultimately the goal is to effect positive, lasting behavioral change through improved, prosocial skill development and related activities.[26]

The intersection of media violence effects and risk factors for aggressive behavior in youths provides a unique opportunity for clinicians, children, and their caregivers to discuss social cognitions, which can help the clinician better diagnose information processing issues. It can also provide a window to understand attachment and parenting style, including transactional issues between the caregiver and child.

INTERVENTIONS

Mental health providers implicitly or explicitly have a viewpoint on violent media effects and must be prepared to consider this bias, along with the direct and indirect role of violence in all media accessed by patients. Research has found clinicians' personal habits and viewpoints impact the time allocated to a given issue in a clinical interview, assessment, and treatment plan. For example, pediatricians who watch more TV spend less time talking about media with their patients.[27]

When treating youths with conduct, aggression, and antisocial behavior, it is important to take a holistic approach to treatment. The case formulation should reflect a developmental and ecological model.[28] Research recommendations are based on clinical points from evidenced-based psychotherapies for behaviorally disordered children and youths[26] as well as an integrative, cognitive-behavioral model that can be implemented by all practitioners.[28]

During the interview, pay close attention to how the child and family describe and respond to interpersonal situations (home, school, peers, teachers, and so forth). Focus on the cognitive process: How does the child perceive, code, and experience the world? Questions for the practitioner and caregiver to consider are as follows: What are the types of media the child is using? What is the child's level of maturity and intelligence regarding social cognitions? Who are the primary caregivers and role models in the child's life?[28] Can the child distinguish fantasy from reality? Does the child seem to have misattributions of other's behavioral motivations, feelings, and expectations?[28] If the violence is real, can the child describe right from wrong? Can the child discuss the consequences of the violence? Does the child identify with the perpetrator or the victim? Does the exposure desensitize the youth? Does the exposure provoke internalizing symptoms? Are externalizing symptoms of aggression or violence present? Is the behavior culturally normative? That is, does the child live in a violent neighborhood or has the child lived in a war zone?[29]

Exposure to media violence can desensitize some youths, terrorize others, but also entertain, educate, and inform. The choice of media content is a form of self-expression and provides a glimpse into a youngsters' inner world and viewpoint. Children with behavioral disorders often struggle to open up with adults and can be wary of judgment. As engagement and motivation are critical to obtaining important information, and associated with better treatment outcomes,[30] exploring favorite digital media can help establish a therapeutic alliance and jump start the interview.

DIGITAL MEDIA QUESTIONS TO EXPLORE WITH BEHAVIORALLY DISORDERED YOUTHS

- What do you watch and play, and where do you go on social media?
- Are you actively involved or are you a passive observer?
- Is there hurting of others? Is there killing? If so, what do you feel/think when you see the hurt of others?
- Do you think any of these things would happen in real life? If so, how might you react?
- Do you think your parents (or friends) know that you watch this? If so, how do you think your parents (or friends) would react if they knew what you are viewing?

CLINICAL GUIDELINES FOR AN INTERVIEW WITH THE CAREGIVER

Clinicians should consider the large disconnect between what parents report and what children report regarding parental monitoring of media.[14] Parents think media violence is a problem but typically do not think this problem impacts their child. Only 13% of parents have a media plan for the home.[31] Parents ignore media rating systems and assume their child is engaging with age-appropriate material.[32] The interview should motivate caregivers to establish a family media plan. When appropriate, children can help in the development of such a plan. Explain to caregivers that in order for the child to change behavior, the child's environment must cease sustaining the behaviors[31]:

- Are you concerned about your child's media habits?
- How well do you understand what media your child is using? Can you describe what he or she watches, plays, and does on social media?
- Where are media and video games located in the household?
- Do you coview media/coplay video games with your child? If so, how do you feel about the content? Have you had a discussion with your child about the content of his or her media activity?
- What type of media do you enjoy? What type of media do other family members use? How much time do you/other family members spend involved with media? Do you see your media habits as an influence on your family? Are you willing to alter these habits?

CLINICAL GUIDELINES FOR CAREGIVER INTERVENTION

Treatments for disordered conduct in youths are often family focused, as an ineffective caregiver discipline style can contribute to the child's problematic behaviors. Caregivers' change is crucial for effective treatment outcomes. Behavior modifications caregivers can address include emotional regulation, prosocial activity engagement, and modeling improved problem-solving skills. Encourage caregivers to seek counseling if they are unable to make changes without professional help.

Media usage discussions can serve as a positive initiator for change in communication style. The introduction of rules, and predictive routines, should be done using clear commands, devoid of coercion and punitive associations. Use positive discipline techniques, such as monitoring and ignoring and walking away.[33] At the same time, in other areas, permit and support autonomous behavior.[34] Whenever necessary, model and role play with caregivers to demonstrate effective interactions:

- Develop a family media plan with input from the entire household. If possible, replace violent media/video games with strategy, nonviolent sports and role-playing games.
- Caregivers should coplay with the child and actively discuss the video game; if using other problematic media sites, interact with the child around the content of the site; together, discuss the child's experience of the site, for example:
  - Is this realistic?
  - What is motivating the characters to use violence? Additionally, what might be some of the motivations of the media producers and other developers of violent media?[35]
  - Did the characters use good problem-solving skills? What might be an alternative, peaceful, solution?
  - What are the consequences of violence in the show/game? What might the consequences look like in reality? Discuss any differences.
- Reduce media exposure gradually, thereby balancing the child's attachment to the media, its potential toxicity, and the potential disturbance incurred by reducing access or exposure. Introduce prosocial activities whenever possible.

GUIDELINES FOR WHEN CHILD/ADOLESCENT PATIENTS ARE UNRECEPTIVE TO INTERVENTIONS

In addition to the aforementioned guidelines, encourage the caregiver to pay attention to verbal and nonverbal cues before the child's problematic behavior.[32] Use this information as a signal to change the interpersonal dynamic. Consider being more playful, affectionate, changing tone or topic, and using humor. When parents are too busy or emotionally spent to address the latter, attending and ignoring techniques may prove beneficial. Kazdin's[33] Parent Management Training for child and adolescent conduct problems coaches caregivers to ignore undesirable behavior, and attend to a positive, opposite behavior. Thus, when a child knowingly defies the family media plan, caregivers should ignore this. Do not engage in a power struggle. At another time, when the child follows the media plan, or another established household rule, caregivers should attend to the positive behavior, using positive reinforcement and praise. Consider developing point/token charts for behaviors. Another technique parents can use to address demanding child behavior is the walking away technique.[33] Caregivers should get comfortable walking away when the child is demanding something, such as wanting to watch/play violent media. Stand by the initial parenting decision; when the child eventually calms down, attend to the child. Reinforce for the child what about the calm behavior that is desirable. Clinicians have reported significant behavioral improvement in as little as 5 to 10 minutes of caregiver coaching, per treatment session for the youths.[28]

FOR THE CHILD/ADOLESCENT

- Do not enter into a confrontation over this issue; however, do not condone expansion.
- Focus on supporting positive behavior change, rather than dwelling on maladaptive behaviors. Use praise, warmth, physical affection (pat on the back), and reward/incentive systems.

- With persistence and patience, continue to introduce alternative activities with small rewards and recognition for participation in alternatives.
- Violent media is meeting a need. Is there a healthier way to match this need for peer acceptance, peer relations, or competency at a task/sport?
- Consider the impact media violence is having on the function, achievements, and developmental milestones of the child. If the impact of this exposure is negligible or there are more pressing clinical issues, then follow and monitor its evolution and influence.
- If personal bias is part of the problem, challenge caregivers to reflect on personal beliefs about media violence.

Other treatment issues for clinicians to consider are the impact of public debates about media and cultural norms. Public policy debates about societal violence, gun control, and censorship, including lay interpretation of academic findings, can alarm parents and induce exaggerated concern. Highly aroused caregivers can hinder the intake of clinical concerns, such as family history and other risk factors. Lastly, cultural norms and biases are internalized and typically unconscious.[36]

SUMMARY

Child and adolescent aggression and disordered conduct is a common and challenging clinical presentation. Research indicates that media violence effects can exacerbate risk factors. Therefore, the youths' exposure to media violence is a persisting challenge for individual families, mental health professionals, and society as a whole.

As content and means to access media, including digital violence, are rapidly changing, it is ever more difficult for caregivers to be completely knowledgeable about what their children access. Caregivers and clinicians should consider this ever-evolving challenge. Even though this exposure can have novel, intense, and toxic influence, the basic principles of child raising and child and adolescent treatment are adaptable and can be proactively applied. A family focused approach to change offers the best outcomes.

Over time, clinically useful tools, such as ratings scales and tracking of children's digital footprints, would allow practitioners to assess exposure to media violence and point out when this exposure becomes problematic. Implementation of open-ended questions about exposure to media violence should be incorporated in clinical interviews. Clinical assessments of children and adolescents would include questions about exposure and involvement with media violence and social media along with questions about family, school, and peers.

Research focused on all aspects of exposure to violent media, not just the assumed negative impacts, would help guide mental health professionals to a more balanced intervention process that not only considers the alleviation of symptoms but also offers recognition of the full range of children's needs, scaffolding, and expansion for what is going well in the children's and families' lives. Thus, mental health professionals should consider all biopsychosocial and ecological factors, develop comprehensive and individualized treatment plans, and lean toward caution when the punitive risks outweigh the benefits.

REFERENCES

1. Sanders NK, editor. Epic of Gilgamesh. London: Penguin Books; 1972.
2. Ferguson CJ. Does media violence predict societal violence? It depends on what you look at and when. J Commun 2015;65:E1–22.

3. Surgeon General's Scientific Advisory Committee on Television and Social Behavior. Television and growing up: the impact of televised violence. Rockville (MD): National Institute of Mental Health; 1972. p. 139.
4. Bushman BJ, Newman K, Calvert SL, et al. Youth violence: what we know and what we need to know. Am Psychol 2016;71(1):17–39. Citing Bushman BJ, Huesmann LR. Aggression. In: Frick TS, Gilbert DT, Lindzey, editors. Handbook of social psychology. 5th edition. New York: Wiley; 2010. p. 833–63.
5. Rideout VJ, Foehr UG, Roberts DF. Generation M^2: media in the lives of 8- to 18-year-olds. Menlo Park (CA): Henry J Kaiser Family Foundation; 2010. p. 1–79.
6. Huesmann LR. The impact of electronic media violence: scientific theory and research. J Adolesc Health 2007;41(6 Suppl 1):S6–13, p.S6.
7. Boyd RW, Swanson WS. The evolution of virtual violence: how mobile screens provide windows to real violence. Pediatrics 2016;138(2) [pii:e20161358].
8. Pecora N, Murray JP, Wartella E. Children and television: 50 years of research. Mahwah (NJ): Lawrence Erlbaum; 2007.
9. Gerbner G, Signorielli N. Violence profile 1967 through 1988-89: enduring patterns. The Annenberg School for Communication. Philadelphia: University of Pennsylvania; 1990.
10. Bandura A, Walters RH. Social learning and personality development. New York: Holt, Rinehart & Winston; 1963.
11. Pearl D, Bouthilet L, Lazar JB. Television and behavior: ten years of scientific progress and implications for the eighties, vol. 1. Bethesda (MD): US Dept. of Health and Human Services, Public Health Service, Alcohol, Drug Abuse, and Mental Health Administration, National Institute of Mental Health; 1982.
12. Anderson CA, Berkowitz L, Donnerstein E, et al. The influence of media violence on youth. Psychol Sci Public Interest 2003;4(3):81–110.
13. Bushman BJ, Huesmann R. Short-term and long-term effects of violent media on aggression in children and adults. Arch Pediatr Adolesc Med 2006;160:348–52.
14. Anderson CA, Gentile DA. Media violence, aggression, and public policy. In: Borgida E, Fiske S, editors. Beyond common sense: psychological science in the courtroom. Malden (MA): Blackwell; 2008. p. 281–300. B1.
15. Murray JP. Media violence: the effects are both real and strong. Am Behav Sci 2008;51(8):1212–30.
16. Freeman JL. Media violence and its effect on aggression: assessing the scientific evidence. Toronto: University of Toronto Press, ebook; 2013.
17. Daly LA, Perez LM. Exposure to media violence and other correlates of aggressive behavior in preschool children. 2009 Early Childhood Research and Practice. Available at: http://files.eric.ed.gov/fulltext/EJ868537.pdf. Accessed August 1, 2017.
18. Hopf WH, Huber GL, Weiß RH. Media violence and youth violence: a 2-year longitudinal study. J Media Psychol 2008;20(3):79–96.
19. Pagani LS, Fitzpatrick C, Barnett TA, et al. Prospective associations between early childhood television exposure and academic, psychosocial, and physical well-being by middle childhood. Arch Pediatr Adolesc Med 2010;164(5):425–31.
20. Fitzpatrick C, Barnett T, Pagani LS. Early exposure to media violence and later child adjustment. J Dev Behav Pediatr 2012;33(4):291–7.
21. Crick NR, Dodge KA. A review and reformulation of social information processing mechanisms in children's social adjustment. Psychol Bull 1994;115:74–101.
22. Davies D. Child development: a practitioner's guide. New York: The Guilford Press; 2004.
23. Gentile DA. Catharsis and media violence: a conceptual analysis. Societies 2013; 3:491–510.

24. Huston AC, Zillman D, Bryant J. Media influence, public policy and the family. In: Zillmann D, Bryant J, Huston AC, editors. Media, children, and the family: social scientific, psychodynamic, and clinical perspectives. Mahwah (NJ): Lawrence, Erlbaum Associates, Inc; 1994. p. 3–18.
25. Kazdin AE. Conduct disorders in childhood and adolescence. Thousand Oaks (CA): Sage Publication, Inc; 1995.
26. Weisz JR, Kazdin AE. Evidence-based psychotherapies for children and adolescents. New York: The Guilford Press; 2017.
27. Council on Communications and Media. Policy statement: children, adolescents and the media. Pediatrics 2013;132:958–61.
28. Boxer P, Frick PJ. Treating conduct problems, aggression, and antisocial behavior in children and adolescents: an integrated view. In: Steele RG, Elkin ED, Roberts M, editors. Handbook of evidence-based therapies for children and adolescents: bridging science and practice. New York: Springer-Verlag, NY, Inc; 2008. p. 241–59.
29. American Psychiatric Association. Diagnostic and statistical manual of mental disorders. 5th edition. Washington, DC: American Psychiatric Association; 2013.
30. Kazdin AE, Marciano PL, Whitley MK. The therapeutic alliance in cognitive-behavioral treatment of children referred for oppositional, aggressive, and antisocial behavior. J Consult Clin Psychol 2005;73(4):726–30.
31. Gentile DA, Nathanson AI, Rasmussen EE, et al. Do you see what I see? Parent reports of parental monitoring of media. Fam Relat 2012;61:470–87.
32. Patterson GR, Reid JB, Eddy JM. A brief history of the Oregon model. Antisocial behavior in children and adolescents: a developmental analysis and model for intervention. Washington, DC: American Psychological Association; 2002. p. 3–21.
33. Kazdin AE. Parent management training and problem-solving skills training for child and adolescent conduct problems. In: Weisz JR, Kazdin AE, editors. Evidence-based psychotherapies for children and adolescents. New York: The Guilford Press; 2017. p. 142–58.
34. Zisser-Nathenson AR, Herschell AD, Eyberg SM. Parent-child interaction therapy in the treatment of disruptive behavior disorders. In: Weisz JR, Kazdin AE, editors. Evidence-based psychotherapies for children and adolescents. New York: The Guilford Press; 2017. p. 103–21.
35. Lomonaco C, Kim T, Ottaviano L. Fact sheet: media violence. Riverside (CA): Southern California Academic Center of Excellence on Youth Violence Prevention, University of California; 2010.
36. Introduction to DSM V. Diagnostic and statistical manual of mental disorders. 5th edition. Washington, DC: American Psychiatric Association; 2013.

Electronic Screen Media Use in Youth With Autism Spectrum Disorder

McLeod Frampton Gwynette, MD[a],*, Shawn S. Sidhu, MD[b],
Tolga Atilla Ceranoglu, MD[c]

KEYWORDS

- Autism spectrum disorder • Electronic media • Social media • Screen time
- Internet addiction • Technology-aided interventions • Family media interventions
- Healthy media use

KEY POINTS

- Extended screen time has a multitude of harmful effects on typically developing youth and those with autism spectrum disorder, including but not limited to physiologic, cognitive, social, emotional, and legal/safety effects.
- Youth with autism spectrum disorder may be even more at risk than typically developing peers for many of these harmful effects.
- Several technology-aided interventions have emerged to help youth with autism spectrum disorder across multiple domains, including social skills, behaviors, communication, academic learning, and adaptive functioning.
- Parents of youth with autism spectrum disorder may benefit from several recommendations and resources from the American Academy of Pediatrics and the American Academy of Child and Adolescent Psychiatry.

INTRODUCTION

Electronic screen media (ESM) play an increasingly prominent role in the lives of children and teenagers. Many typically-developing (TD) youth use media not only for entertainment, but also as a primary form of communication, learning, information gathering, social support, and self-expression.

Disclosure Statement: Dr M.F. Gwynette has nothing to disclose. Dr S.S. Sidhu has received an honorarium for writing CME questions for the American Psychiatric Association journal, FOCUS. Dr T.A. Ceranoglu has nothing to disclose.
[a] Department of Psychiatry, Medical University of South Carolina, Project Rex, MUSC Autism Spectrum Foundation, 67 President Street, Charleston, SC 29425, USA; [b] Department of Psychiatry, University of New Mexico, 2400 Tucker Avenue NE, MSC 095 030, Albuquerque, NM 87111, USA; [c] Department of Psychiatry, Massachusetts General Hospital, Shriners Hospital for Children, Charlestown Health Care Center, 73 High Street, Charlestown, Boston, MA 02129, USA
* Corresponding author.
E-mail address: gwynette@musc.edu

Child Adolesc Psychiatric Clin N Am 27 (2018) 203–219
https://doi.org/10.1016/j.chc.2017.11.013
1056-4993/18/© 2017 Elsevier Inc. All rights reserved.

Special care must be given to those with autism spectrum disorder (ASD) in the new media environment. The core features of ASD place many individuals at risk for over-use and improper use of ESM, which could result in harmful consequences.

At the same time, the compelling nature of ESM might provide motivation for some youth with ASD to engage in technology-aided interventions (TAI) resulting in improved outcomes. This article discusses these interventions, along with some po-tential family-oriented interventions.

SCOPE OF MEDIA USE IN YOUTH WITH AUTISM SPECTRUM DISORDER

Youth with ASD watch more television than TD matched peers,[1] and spend approx-imately 4.5 hours a day on screen time with 2 or less hours dedicated to nonscreen activities.[2] Youth with ASD spend most of their free time on screens compared with 18% of TD peers, and youth with ASD play video games an average of 1 hour more per day than TD peers[3] and tend to have a preference for video games over television.[4]

The difficulty for youth with ASD in disengaging from ESM is further elaborated in parental responses to the Problem Video Game Playing questionnaire. Parents of boys and girls with ASD report snapping, yelling, or getting angry if someone interrupts them while playing video games, and thinking life would be boring without video games more than parents of gender-matched TD peers.[2] The parents of ASD boys re-ported their child playing video games longer than they intended to and saying, "just a few more minutes," and the parents of ASD girls reported that their child plays video games too much, both significantly more than gender-matched TD peers.

Potentially more important than ESM use patterns in youth with ASD is that most do not seem to be using ESM for social purposes. More than half of youth with ASD have never played with a friend over electronic media, and only 15% of youth with ASD engage friends in this manner on a weekly basis.[2] A total of 64% of children with ASD use media in a nonsocial way, such as playing video games alone or with strangers, or surfing gaming Web sites. Most do not use any form of online communi-cation via e-mail, instant messaging, chat rooms, or social networks. Although only 13% reported using media for social purposes, youth with ASD who identified as girls, Hispanic, and having higher cognitive skills did use media for social purposes signif-icantly more than matched youth with ASD.[3]

THE UNIQUE INTERPLAY BETWEEN AUTISM SPECTRUM DISORDER SYMPTOMS AND MEDIA

In the last two decades, the prevalence rate of ASD has risen two-fold and now stands at 1 in 68 children. ASD awareness has correspondingly soared through increased media coverage, culminating in the recent introduction of a new character with Autism (Julia) on PBS' Sesame Street television series.

Simultaneous to this spike in ASD prevalence, access to ESM overall has increased exponentially, doubling over a 2-year period between 2011 and 2013.[5] Children with ASD, who already have a strong predilection for ESM,[6] currently receive unprece-dented daily exposure to ESM beginning in infancy.[4,7] Research is currently underway in infants, toddlers, and children to determine if exposure to ESM can increase the risk for a child developing ASD, but published literature is still in its early development and no firm conclusions can be drawn.[8]

The exact cause of autism, although currently unknown, is almost certainly a com-plex interaction between genetic, environmental, and epigenetic factors. Research has implicated upwards of 1000 associated genes[9,10] and ASD has a high rate of heritability and genetic loading. Both youth with ASD and their parents have an increased likelihood of being proficient at technology compared with TD peers. This, combined with a predilection for technology, potentially increases their risk for excessive ESM usage. The higher prevalence of ASD in technology epicenters, such as Silicon Valley and Eindhoven, Netherlands, may be a window into the future regarding the interplay between genetics and environment in the areas of ASD and technology.

Youth with ASD seem to have a unique relationship with technology. Family members often report that loved ones with ASD possess technological "splinter" skills that far exceed those expected for their chronologic age and other areas of development. Challenges to appropriate use of ESM arise if youth with ASD outpace their parents and providers in their technological capabilities. For example, it may be difficult for parents to successfully monitor social media usage or World Wide Web browsing history if their child is particularly skilled and able to conceal such information.

Individuals with ASD also perform better on certain tasks using ESM compared with traditional materials, while generally being more attentive and motivated.[11] Youth with ASD can improve their social skills using a wide array of ESM modalities, including video games[12] and a variety of software applications and hardware. TAI can help improve executive function skills in youth with ASD, a common area of impairment, albeit not part of the Diagnostic and Statistical Manual–Fifth Edition criteria or unique to ASD.[13] Repetitive and disruptive behaviors also seem responsive to TAI. Furthermore, ESM has made a significant impact on the education of youth with ASD in the last several decades, aiding in language development and academic learning.[14] However, response to ESM may be limited, because some youth with ASD struggle to process and organize information from multimedia interventions.[15] See **Table 1** for additional details on the benefits and potential risks of technology use in youth with ASD.

SEQUELAE OF UNHEALTHY AND IMPROPER ELECTRONIC AND SOCIAL MEDIA USE IN YOUTH WITH AUTISM SPECTRUM DISORDER AND FAMILIES

Unhealthy and improper use of ESM is associated with several negative outcomes, many of which could disproportionately impact youth with ASD and their families in a detrimental way.

Table 1
Overview of potential risks and benefits of electronic screen media in youth with ASD

Potential Benefits	Autism Symptoms, Deficits	Potential Risks
• Can help with social skills, joint attention • Can promote language development	Social and communication deficits	• Tendency is to use technology nonsocially • Cyberbullying • Increased social isolation
• Can reduce repetitive behaviors • ASD patients have an affinity for technology	Restricted, repetitive interests, behaviors, and activities	• Difficulty detaching from device • Risk of Internet addiction
• May learn more efficiently using technology • Can be used to build executive functioning skills	Cognitive and executive functioning	• Possible increased risk for attention-deficit/hyperactivity disorder • May interfere with sleep

Physiologic

Obesity

The positive correlation between ESM use and body mass index has been well established in the medical literature for TD youth. Youth with ASD who are heavy media users may be especially at risk for obesity. Youth with ASD are more likely to be overweight or obese than TD peers.[1] Barriers to physical activity in youth with ASD are many and such barriers have been positively correlated to screen time.[16]

Sleep

Children with ASD are also more likely to experience sleep difficulties than matched TD peers, such as shorter total sleep time, longer sleep latency, and decreased sleep efficiency.[17] The suppression of melatonin levels associated with nighttime tablet use could serve to worsen these sleep difficulties.[18]

Bedroom access to a television or computer is more strongly associated with sleep disturbances in youth with ASD than those with attention-deficit/hyperactivity disorder (ADHD) or TD control subjects, and this effect was mediated by the number of hours spent playing video games.[19] Another study found that youth with ASD who use media within 30 minutes of bedtime have significantly greater sleep-onset delays and shorter overall sleep duration compared with youth with ASD without bedtime media.[20] The access to media in the bedroom of these youth did not seem to have any impact on sleep as it did in the aforementioned study.

Internet addiction

Preliminary data from Japan suggest the prevalence of Internet addiction may be higher in youth with ASD, especially those with comorbid ADHD.[21] This makes sense given the tendency for youth with ASD to use more ESM, having more difficulty separating from ESM, and being prone to restricted interests and repetitive behaviors. Internet addiction has widely been associated with several negative neurobiologic correlates.

Social

As ESM continues to emerge, a few studies have examined its potential impact on social skills, communication, and peer relationships in TD youth. These studies are highly applicable in ASD.

One study found that 11-year-olds who spent 5 days at an outdoor education camp without any access to media perform significantly better at reading facial expressions and interpreting nonverbal cues than control subjects who had stayed at home and used media without restriction.[22] Another study found electronic media use correlated to lower friendship trust, disrupted communication, increased rate of peer conflict, and feeling alienated.[23] Although using forms of messaging were positively associated with quality relationships, chat rooms and video games predicted decreased quality of such relationships. Lastly, Valkenburg and Peter[24] found that those who communicate online with existing friends show that technology positively impacts the closeness of their real-world friendships. However, the same was not true for those who talked with strangers or played independently.

Cognitive

Increased screen time is correlated with decreased grade point average (**Fig. 1**), increased time spent on homework, inattention, impulsivity, off-task behavior, social isolation, difficulty making friends, decreased activities, social-emotional difficulties, mood volatility issues, and sleep-onset latency issues in TD youth.[25] Many of these are known areas of difficulty for youth with ASD.

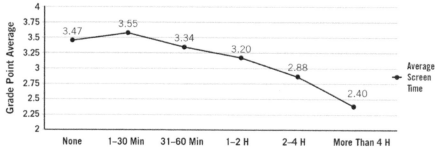

Fig. 1. Grade point averages by screen time per day for children in secondary school. (*From* Pressman RM, Owens JA, Evans AS, et al. Examining the interface of family and personal traits, media, and academic imperatives using the learning habit study. Am J Fam Ther 2014;42(5):356; with permission.)

Emotional

Although youth with ASDs are more likely to be bullied than their TD peers,[26] literature on cyberbullying in ASD is limited. Cyberbullying is associated with negative social, academic, and health consequences.

According to the American Academy of Pediatrics, ESM use patterns are an important harbinger of mood disturbances.[27] Extremes of Internet use and passive social media use are correlated to increased depression and decreased life satisfaction. These data remain highly limited.

Legal/Safety

Youth with ASD may especially be at risk for impulsivity that is coupled with social naivety, judgment difficulties, and an incomplete understanding of the ramifications for their actions. Inappropriate communications of a sexual or violent nature could result in a host of potential legal ramifications for youth with ASD. Such youth are also at increased risk of exploitation from others in the form of abuse or financial exploitation.

TECHNOLOGY-AIDED INTERVENTIONS FOR YOUTH WITH AUTISM SPECTRUM DISORDER

Children with ASD can potentially learn more efficiently from computers than from in-person teachers[14] and technology has been used to assist children with ASD for more than 40 years, beginning with early augmentative and assistive communication devices to promote language development. Since the introduction of the iPhone in 2007, there has been a massive shift away from desktop applications and toward mobile devices, along with a simultaneous explosion in publications on TAI for youth with ASD (**Fig. 2**). Results of these interventions seem promising overall, and a recent published meta-analysis confirmed the overall effectiveness of technology-based training.[28–39]

Youth with ASD use a vast array of overlapping technologies and platforms comprising various permutations of Internet-connected hardware and software, including applications or "apps" (**Fig. 3**). Autism researchers are actively studying individual aspects of the information in **Fig. 3**, but typically only after the technology has been in broad use among youth with and without ASD. Furthermore, the authors know of no published studies using interventions incorporating multiple elements of the **Fig. 3**, which may be more representative of actual day-to-day use. For example, it

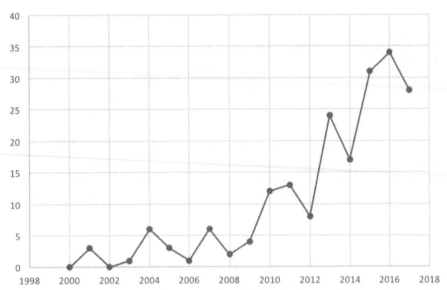

Fig. 2. Number of relevant articles returned on PubMed using search terms "Technology Treatment Autism" or "Technology Intervention Autism" for the years 2000 through 2017. Note that the number of articles for 2017 is projected based on publications through the first half of 2017.

would be valuable to research how artificial intelligence implemented through a digital assistant, such as Apple's Siri, across desktop, mobile, and wearable devices may be able to improve functioning in youth with ASD. The authors summarize research findings in key areas next.

iPad/Tablet

iPad and tablet technology for patients with ASD has evidence supporting efficacy in many areas, most significantly for enhancing and developing language, targeting social deficits and problem behaviors, and improving academic and adaptive functioning (**Fig. 4**).

Social Media/Web Sites

Social networking sites (SNS), such as Facebook, Instagram, Twitter, and Snapchat, are now ubiquitous, and represent a significant opportunity for clinicians to study social media usage in youth with ASD and potentially intervene. There is evidence supporting the use of SNS for nonanxious youth with ASD to build friendships.[40] Furthermore, parents benefit from support and information about ASD treatment they receive from other parents on SNS.[41,42] YouTube can be used for delivery and as a data gathering tool by clinicians implementing the picture exchange communication system, an intervention that provides alternative communication strategies and tools for individuals with severe language delay.[43] Overall, data in SNS and ASD are still emerging.

Importantly, youth with ASD are particularly vulnerable to bullying across physical settings and may be at risk for cyberbullying, because they struggle to detect or appreciate the subtleties of nonverbal communication while online.[22] It is therefore important for parents and clinicians to keep in mind that youth with ASD are often

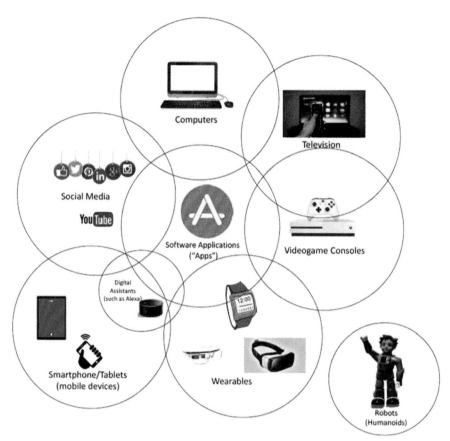

Fig. 3. Overview of technologies used by youth with ASD. The use of technology by youth with ASD involves extensive overlap between various hardware and software platforms, nearly all of which are connected to the Internet. Robot technology is on the rise and is likely to enter everyday use within some, or even throughout all, of the circles soon (see section on future directions). (Xox *Courtesy of* Microsoft, Redmond, Washington; with permission.)

less mature relative to their chronologic age or physical development and their autism symptoms do not "disappear" once they go online.[44] In clinical practice, many parents express fears about their children being victimized by peers or overage individuals while online. It is therefore strongly recommended that parents provide close supervision when their child uses social media.

Video Games

Youth with ASD spend more time playing video games compared with their TD peers. Although video games are primarily used recreationally, they can be used to improve vocabulary, communication, empathy, and social skills. Notably, the use of video games by youth with ASD, similar to TD youth, has not been shown to result in increased aggression, even when playing violent games.[45] However, playing video games can worsen sleep problems in boys.[19] In addition, video games can be more addictive and more overused for boys with ASD compared with boys with ADHD. See Mazurek and Wenstrup[2] and Ferguson and colleagues[46] for a detailed review on the use of gaming by youth with ASD.

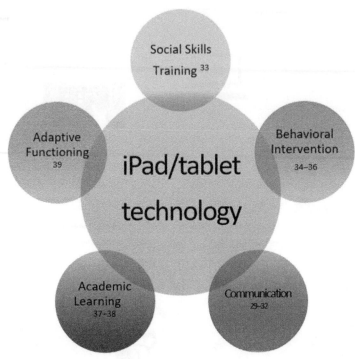

Fig. 4. The use of iPad/tablet technology for patients with ASD and corresponding references.

Desktop Computer Software

Among numerous desktop-based interventions, TeachTown is a standout software program. Implemented in multiple US school districts, TeachTown has evidence indicating its ability to improve independent living skills, enhance community skills and safety, and improve executive functioning skills.[47]

Online Games

Several online role-player games, such as World of Warcraft and Minecraft, can provide youth an opportunity to practice social skills and develop friendships. Autcraft is a customized Minecraft server environment created by individuals with ASD and designed to minimize bullying and the destruction of other people's creations (**Fig. 5**). The site aims to allow users to feel safe and confident online (see Autcraft. com and YouTube video posted by the founder of Autcraft for additional details).

Wearable Technology

Wearable technology is beneficial in multiple ways for youth with ASD including the following[48–51]:

- Assessing movements in high-risk neonates
- Monitoring autonomic response to behavioral interventions
- Monitoring to prevent elopement and wandering behaviors
- Monitoring self-regulation and intervening when needed
- Aiding in the physiologic detection of anxiety
- Characterizing the response to social cues through eye-tracking

A recent pilot study using the Apple Watch demonstrated that visual scene cues can be successfully provided in a real-time manner to supplement language in youth with ASD.

Multiple scientific teams are currently developing software for the Google Glass wearable platform designed to aid in real-time conversations outside the clinical setting. Preliminary data indicate that the use of Glass as an intervention for youth with ASD may be feasible, acceptable, and possibly effective.[52,53]

Virtual reality seems promising for the enhancement of social skills and treatment of social anxiety in youth with ASD[54–58] and for job training in young adults. Virtual reality has also been shown to be helpful for the acquisition of driving skills in adolescents with ASD,[59] a finding with major implications relevant to overall adaptive functioning and independent living skills.

FUTURE DIRECTIONS

Autism combines in myriad ways with the fast-moving and ubiquitous technological advancements of the day. Within the flurry of activity and innovation in the area of ASD and TAI, there are several key trends that are likely to continue. First, development of interventions based on mobile platforms has grown exponentially in the last 10 years and will likely be the foundation of future innovation. Mobile and wearable devices can now recognize where the user is, how they are moving, and what they are doing, all while gathering information about their surroundings. Artificial intelligence can assist youth with ASD in conversational skills and will be integrated within virtual reality platforms. This will likely result in the development of devices that can help youth with ASD navigate through the surrounding environment and interact with people and more effectively than ever.

Second, robot technology seems to be on the verge of broader implementation for the treatment of core deficits in youth with ASD,[60–62] including social/communication symptoms and repetitive behaviors. Reasons for this trend include the affinity of youth with ASD for robot technology and the rapid development of robots that seem human or "humanoid" and therefore enhance engagement (**Fig. 6**).

Third, social media posting will likely evolve more toward video posts rather than still images. Such applications as Snapchat, Facebook Live, Twitter Periscope, and the video chat application House Party help users feel like they are "actually there" with

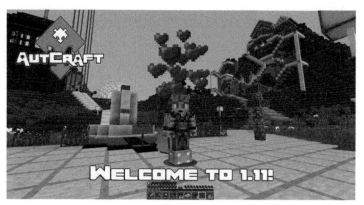

Fig. 5. Screenshot from Autcraft.com. (*Courtesy of* Autcraft, Timmins, Canada; with permission.)

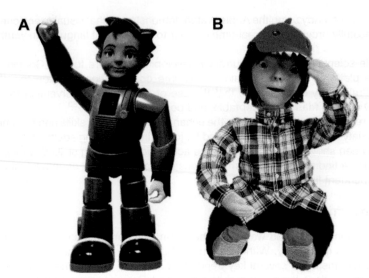

Fig. 6. (*A*) Milo and (*B*) KASPAR. Examples of robots designed for use in teaching social/communication skills to youth with ASD. (*Courtesy of* [*A*] RoboKind, Dallas, Texas; with permission; and [*B*] Zuyd University of Applied Sciences, Heerlen, Netherlands; with permission.)

each other in real time. This is an exciting possibility, but as noted in several tragic events recorded using social media, the posting of live video will continue to generate logical ethical concerns and discussion.

Fourth, emerging technology has the potential to blur the lines between fantasy and reality for youth with ASD. Products in development, such as Gatebox (see gatebox.com) will soon provide users with a holographic friend/companion based on their favorite fantasy character. These friend/companions will be programmed to keep in contact with the user throughout the day using friendly text messages until the user arrives home. This technology has the potential to provide individuals with ASD much sought-after unconditional companionship. However, the ramifications of bringing such a fantasy character into the user's real life are currently unclear.

One challenge ASD research faces is the rapid adoption and use of technology before the validation of its use as evidence-based. Odom and colleagues[63] points out that the excitement and ubiquity of technology resulted in the "unbridled adoption of applications and equipment with little regard for, or knowledge about, the efficacy of such approaches, or their potential collateral effects," including use of technology in the classroom for children in kindergarten.[22] Psychiatrist are likely to work with many families who implement technological interventions for their children without gathering input from said psychiatrist. Although technology is undoubtedly exciting as a possible treatment modality for youth with ASD, ethical issues and healthy debate concerning its risks and benefits will certainly arise. Taking a nonjudgmental approach when working with parents who may lean heavily on ESM to manage or soothe their child's behavior may be beneficial for many psychiatrists. Furthermore, each individual child represents an "N = 1," so supporting parents' implementation of "whatever works" may be useful.

Providers can play a leadership role in the dissemination of evidence-based information about technology and ASD. For example, multiple academic institutions have well-developed Web sites containing information for parents and families about treatment options and the latest development in the field. However, the demand for evidence-based information currently far outstrips the supply. With upwards of 3000 scientific articles published on ASD yearly, perhaps the next role for technology in its relationship with ASD is to serve as a fulcrum for disseminating evidence-based information to families, providers, and stakeholders in a unified way.

RECOMMENDATIONS FOR FAMILIES
The Complex Interplay Between Electronic and Social Media Use in Autism Spectrum Disorder and Family Dynamics

Many parents of youth with ASD find the management of electronic media to be a source of distress in the family.[64] Approximately half of such families have identified rules on media use, and even those who endorse having rules admit that such rules are ineffective.[65] **Table 2** outlines and categorizes risk factors that lead to negative outcomes.[25,27,65]

General Recommendations for Families

Great care should be taken in educating youth with ASD and their families in the clinical and school settings such that there is an adequate understanding of the potential consequences for inappropriate and unhealthy use of ESM. The American Academy of Pediatrics Media and Communication Toolkit[27] includes a user-friendly platform called the Family Media Plan that allows families to easily create and print a plan that works for them. The American Academy of Child and Adolescent Psychiatry also has several informative resources for families in the Facts for Families Guide. Some of these recommendations are summarized in **Table 3**.

Adaptations for Youth With Autism Spectrum Disorder

Youth with ASD may especially struggle with healthy and proper ESM use given the core symptoms of their condition. Restricted interests and repetitive behaviors, social and pragmatic communication difficulties, developmental delay, and difficulty with transitions can all create unique challenges for families. Thus, we have adapted some of the recommendations for families of youth with ASD (**Fig. 7**).

Taking an Electronic Screen Media History

Because ESM can be such an integral part of their lives, obtaining a detailed history on ESM usage is helpful during the work-up and management of patients with ASD. The authors list suggested items to gather during the clinical interview in **Table 4**.

Table 2
Risk factors potentially leading to negative outcomes for youth with ASD using electronic screen media

Home/Parent Factors	Child Factors	Negative Outcomes
• Inconsistent parenting	• Temperament	• Increased child screen time
• Parental coercion and spanking	• Externalizing behaviors	• Decreased executive functioning in child
• Exposure to inappropriate media	• Self-regulation and social-emotional problems	• Decreased verbal and nonverbal parent-child interaction
• Heavy parental use	• Difficulty disengaging	• Poorer family functioning
• Constant media background noise	• Resistance to limit setting	• Decreased child play/development
• Screen as pacifier	• ASD-related barriers	

Abbreviation: ASD, autism spectrum disorder.

Table 3
Summary of recommendations from American Academy of Child and Adolescent Psychiatry Facts for Families guide on use of electronic screen media in children and adolescents and the American Academy of Pediatrics Media and Communication Toolkit for Families Recommendations

0–18 mo	18–24 mo	2–5 y	6–12 y	Adolescents
• Avoid screens completely • Hands-on activities with human engagement facilitate normal cognitive, motor, language, and social-emotional development • Most time should be spent in hands-on activities without media in the child's environment	• Most time should be spent in hands-on activities without media • Very brief intervals • Focus on high-quality educational programming • Parents watch with children and explain content	• Most time should be spent in hands-on activities without media • <1 h per day • Still emphasize educational and age-appropriate programming • Parent still watch with children and explain content	• Consistent time limits • Limit types of media • Monitor sleep, physical activity, and behavioral health effects • Screen-free zones: bedroom, dinner table • Screen-free times: meals, bedtime, family interaction	• <2 h per day • Media-free zones and times • Ongoing education and communication • Parental supervision and limit setting • Parental modeling of healthy use • Limit media use when doing homework

Data from American Academy of Child and Adolescent Psychiatry Facts for Families: Children and screen time. Available at: https://www.aacap.org/AACAP/Families_and_Youth/Facts_for_Families/FFF-Guide/Children-And-Watching-TV-054.aspx. Accessed November 10, 2017; and AAP Council on Communications and Media. Media use in school-aged children and adolescents. Pediatrics 2016;138(5):[pii:e20162592].

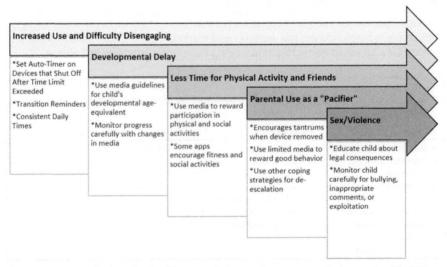

Fig. 7. Recommendations for healthy use of electronic screen media in youth with ASD.

Table 4 Taking an electronic screen media history	
Quantitative	**Qualitative**
Hours per weekday	Activity (eg, offline games, online games, social media, email, YouTube, school work)
Hours per weekend day	Type of games (if applicable): individual, online, role-player
Length of time between last use of ESM and going to bed	Emotional reaction of the child to parents setting limits on ESM

Final Recommendations

Electronic screen media presents as an opportunity for youth with ASD to improve their symptoms and as an activity with significant inherent risks. Although parents may feel unable to fully understand their child's ESM activities, active engagement can enable parents to learn about their child's usage and help navigate through the complex world of technology. Given their vulnerability secondary to a high affinity for technology and accompanying social deficits, youth with ASD will no doubt benefit from the active involvement of parents to monitor ESM usage and set appropriate limits. By gathering history on ESM usage during the clinical interview and incorporating this information into a comprehensive treatment plan, psychiatrists can better relate to their patients and potentially optimize outcomes and quality of life for youth with ASD and their families.

ACKNOWLEDGMENTS

The authors thank Ben Kinsella and Christina Whalen for their contributions to this article. They also thank several individuals who allowed them to share their impressive work as a part of this article.

REFERENCES

1. Healy S, Haegele JA, Grenier M, et al. Physical activity, screen-time behavior, and obesity among 13-year olds in Ireland with and without autism spectrum disorder. J Autism Dev Disord 2017;47(1):49–57.
2. Mazurek MO, Wenstrup C. Television, video game and social media use among children with ASD and typically developing siblings. J Autism Dev Disord 2013; 43(6):1258–71.
3. Mazurek MO, Shattuck PT, Wagner M, et al. Prevalence and correlates of screen-based media use among youths with autism spectrum disorders. J Autism Dev Disord 2012;42(8):1757–67.
4. Kuo MH, Orsmond GI, Coster WJ, et al. Media use among adolescents with autism spectrum disorder. Autism 2014;18(8):914–23.
5. Common Sense Media. Zero to eight: children's media use in America. 2013. Available at: http://www.commonsensemedia.org/research/zero-to-eight-childrens-media-use-in-america-2013. Accessed July 1, 2017.
6. Shane HC, Albert PD. Electronic screen media for persons with autism spectrum disorders: results of a survey. J Autism Dev Disord 2008;38(8):1499–508.
7. Heffler KF, Oestreicher LM. Causation model of autism: audiovisual brain specialization in infancy competes with social brain networks. Med Hypotheses 2016;91: 114–22.

8. Cheng S, Maeda T, Yoichi S, et al. Early television exposure and children's behavioral and social outcomes at age 30 months. J Epidemiol 2010;20(Suppl 2): S482–9.

9. Geschwind DH. Genetics of autism spectrum disorders. Trends Cogn Sci 2011; 15(9):409–16.

10. Murdoch JD, State MW. Recent developments in the genetics of autism spectrum disorders. Curr Opin Genet Dev 2013;23(3):310–5.

11. Whalen C, Liden L, Ingersoll B, et al. Behavioral improvements associated with computer-assisted instruction for children with developmental disabilities. J Speech Lang Pathol Appl Behav Anal 2006;1(1):11–26.

12. Wilkinson N, Ang RP, Goh DH. Online video game therapy for mental health concerns: a review. Int J Soc Psychiatry 2008;54(4):370–82.

13. Rajendran G, Mitchell P. Computer mediated interaction in Asperger's syndrome: the bubble dialogue program. Comput Educ 2000;35(3):189–207.

14. Moore M, Calvert S. Brief report: vocabulary acquisition for children with autism: teacher or computer instruction. J Autism Dev Disord 2000;30(4):359–62.

15. Grynszpan O, Martin J-C, Nadel J. Multimedia interfaces for users with high functioning autism: an empirical investigation. Int J Hum Comput Stud 2008;66(8): 628–39.

16. Must A, Phillips S, Curtin C, et al. Barriers to physical activity in children with autism spectrum disorders: relationship to physical activity and screen time. J Phys Act Health 2015;12(4):529–34.

17. Elrod MG, Hood BS. Sleep differences among children with autism spectrum disorders and typically developing peers: a meta-analysis. J Dev Behav Pediatr 2015;36(3):166–77.

18. Wood B, Rea MS, Plitnick B, et al. Light level and duration of exposure determine the impact of self-luminous tablets on melatonin suppression. Appl Ergon 2013; 44(2):237–40.

19. Engelhardt CR, Mazurek MO, Sohl K. Media use and sleep among boys with autism spectrum disorder, ADHD, or typical development. Pediatrics 2013; 132(6):1081–9.

20. Mazurek MO, Engelhardt CR, Hilgard J, et al. Bedtime electronic media use and sleep in children with autism spectrum disorder. J Dev Behav Pediatr 2016;37(7): 525–31.

21. So R, Makino K, Fujiwara M, et al. The prevalence of Internet addiction among a Japanese adolescent psychiatric clinic sample with autism spectrum disorder and/or attention-deficit hyperactivity disorder: a cross-sectional study. J Autism Dev Disord 2017;47(7):2217–24.

22. Uhls YT, Michikyan M, Morris J, et al. Five days at outdoor education camp without screens improves preteen skills with nonverbal emotion cues. Comput Hum Behav 2014;39:387–92.

23. Blais JJ, Craig WM, Pepler D, et al. Adolescents online: the importance of Internet activity choices to salient relationships. J Youth Adolesc 2008;37(5):522–36.

24. Valkenburg PM, Peter J. Preadolescents' and adolescents' online communication and their closeness to friends. Dev Psychol 2007;43(2):267–77.

25. Pressman RM, Owens JA, Evans AS, et al. Examining the interface of family and personal traits, media, and academic imperatives using the learning habit study. Am J Fam Ther 2014;42(5):347–63.

26. Maiano C, Normand CL, Salvas MC, et al. Prevalence of school bullying among youth with autism spectrum disorders: a systematic review and meta analysis. Autism Res 2016;9(6):601–15.

27. American Academy of Pediatrics Media Toolkit. Web. Available at: https://www.aap.org/en-us/advocacy-and-policy/aap-health-initiatives/pages/media-and-children.aspx. Accessed 01 Jul 2017.
28. Grynszpan O, Weiss PL, Perez-Diaz F, et al. Innovative technology-based interventions for autism spectrum disorders: a meta-analysis. Autism 2014;18(4):346–61.
29. Agius MM, Vance M. A Comparison of PECS and iPad to teach requesting to preschoolers with autistic spectrum disorders. Augment Altern Commun 2016;32(1):58–68.
30. Flores M, Musgrove K, Renner S, et al. A comparison of communication using the Apple iPad and a picture-based system. Augment Altern Commun 2012;28(2):74–84.
31. Gevarter C, O'Reilly MF, Kuhn M, et al. Assessing the acquisition of requesting a variety of preferred items using different speech generating device formats for children with autism spectrum disorder. Assist Technol 2017;29(3):153–60.
32. Irwin J, Preston J, Brancazio L, et al. Development of an audiovisual speech perception app for children with autism spectrum disorders. Clin Linguist Phon 2015;29(1):76–83.
33. Fletcher-Watson S, Petrou A, Scott-Barrett J, et al. A trial of an iPad intervention targeting social communication skills in children with autism. Autism 2016;20(7):771–82.
34. Granich J, Dass A, Busacca M, et al. Randomised controlled trial of an iPad based early intervention for autism: TOBY playpad study protocol. BMC Pediatr 2016;16(1):167.
35. Murdock LC, Ganz J, Crittendon J. Use of an iPad play story to increase play dialogue of preschoolers with autism spectrum disorders. J Autism Dev Disord 2013;43(9):2174–89.
36. Jeffries T, Crosland K, Miltenberger R. Evaluating a tablet application and differential reinforcement to increase eye contact in children with autism. J Appl Behav Anal 2016;49(1):182–7.
37. Allen ML, Hartley C, Cain K. iPads and the use of "apps" by children with autism spectrum disorder: do they promote learning? Front Psychol 2016;7:1305.
38. Stephenson J. Using the choiceboard creator app on an iPad(c) to teach choice making to a student with severe disabilities. Augment Altern Commun 2016;32(1):49–57.
39. Burckley E, Tincani M, Guld Fisher A. An iPad-based picture and video activity schedule increases community shopping skills of a young adult with autism spectrum disorder and intellectual disability. Dev Neurorehabil 2015;18(2):131–6.
40. van Schalkwyk GI, Marin CE, Ortiz M, et al. Social media use, friendship quality, and the moderating role of anxiety in adolescents with autism spectrum disorder. J Autism Dev Disord 2017;47(9):2805–13.
41. Mohd Roffeei SH, Abdullah N, Basar SK. Seeking social support on Facebook for children with autism spectrum disorders (ASDs). Int J Med Inform 2015;84(5):375–85.
42. Tangherlini TR, Roychowdhury V, Glenn B, et al. "Mommy Blogs" and the vaccination exemption narrative: results from a machine-learning approach for story aggregation on parenting social media sites. JMIR Public Health Surveill 2016;2(2):e166.
43. Jurgens A, Anderson A, Moore DW. Parent-implemented picture exchange communication system (PECS) training: an analysis of YouTube videos. Dev Neurorehabil 2012;15(5):351–60.

44. Gwynette MF, Morriss D, Warren N, et al. Social skills training for adolescents with autism spectrum disorder using Facebook (project rex connect): a survey study. JMIR Ment Health 2017;4(1):e4.

45. Engelhardt CR, Mazurek MO. Video game access, parental rules, and problem behavior: a study of boys with autism spectrum disorder. Autism 2014;18(5): 529–37.

46. Ferguson MB, Anderson-Hanley PC, Mazurek MO, et al. Game interventions for autism spectrum disorder. Games Health J 2012;1(4):248–53.

47. Whalen C, Moss D, Ilan AB, et al. Efficacy of TeachTown: basics computer-assisted intervention for the intensive comprehensive autism program in Los Angeles Unified School District. Autism 2010;14(3):179–97.

48. Billeci L, Tonacci A, Tartarisco G, et al. An integrated approach for the monitoring of brain and autonomic response of children with autism spectrum disorders during treatment by wearable technologies. Front Neurosci 2016;10:276.

49. Di Palma S, Tonacci A, Narzisi A, et al. Monitoring of autonomic response to sociocognitive tasks during treatment in children with autism spectrum disorders by wearable technologies: a feasibility study. Comput Biol Med 2017;85:143–52.

50. Kushki A, Khan A, Brian J, et al. Kalman filtering framework for physiological detection of anxiety-related arousal in children with autism spectrum disorder. IEEE Trans Biomed Eng 2015;62(3):990–1000.

51. Singleton G, Warren S, Piersel W. Clinical overview of the need for technologies for around-the-clock monitoring of the health status of severely disabled autistic children. Conf Proc IEEE Eng Med Biol Soc 2014;2014:789–91.

52. Kinsella BG, Kushki A, Chow S. Evaluating the usability of a social skills training app for children with ASD. Paper presented at: International Meeting for Autism Research. Baltimore (MD), May 13, 2016.

53. Liu R, Salisbury JP, Vahabzadeh A, et al. Feasibility of an autism-focused augmented reality smartglasses system for social communication and behavioral coaching. Front Pediatr 2017;5:145.

54. Bekele E, Crittendon J, Zheng Z, et al. Assessing the utility of a virtual environment for enhancing facial affect recognition in adolescents with autism. J Autism Dev Disord 2014;44(7):1641–50.

55. Kuriakose S, Lahiri U. Design of a physiology-sensitive VR-based social communication platform for children with autism. IEEE Trans Neural Syst Rehabil Eng 2017;25(8):1180–91.

56. Lahiri U, Bekele E, Dohrmann E, et al. A physiologically informed virtual reality based social communication system for individuals with autism. J Autism Dev Disord 2015;45(4):919–31.

57. Maskey M, Lowry J, Rodgers J, et al. Reducing specific phobia/fear in young people with autism spectrum disorders (ASDs) through a virtual reality environment intervention. PLoS One 2014;9(7):e100374.

58. Zhen B, Blackwell AF, Coulouris G. Using augmented reality to elicit pretend play for children with autism. IEEE Trans Vis Comput Graph 2015;21(5):598–610.

59. Cox DJ, Brown T, Ross V, et al. Can youth with autism spectrum disorder use virtual reality driving simulation training to evaluate and improve driving performance? An exploratory study. J Autism Dev Disord 2017;47(8):2544–55.

60. Alcorn AM, TT, Babović Dimitrijevic S, et al. Robots teaching autistic children to mind read: a feasibility study of child-robot interaction during emotion-recognition training. Paper presented at: International Meeting for Autism Research. San Francisco (CA), May 12, 2017.

61. Huijnen C, Lexis MAS, Jansens R, et al. How to implement robots in interventions for children with autism? A co-creation study involving people with autism, parents professionals. J Autism Dev Disord 2017;47(10):3079–96.
62. Robokind. Available at: http://www.robots4autism.com. Accessed July 22, 2017.
63. Odom SL, Thompson JL, Hedges S, et al. Technology-aided interventions and instruction for adolescents with autism spectrum disorder. J Autism Dev Disord 2015;45(12):3805–19.
64. Nally B, Houlton B, Ralph S. Researches in brief: the management of television and video by parents of children with autism. Autism 2000;4(3):331–7.
65. Mazurek MO, Engelhardt CR. Video game use in boys with autism spectrum disorder, ADHD, or typical development. Pediatrics 2013;132(2):260–6.

Adolescent Eating Disorder Risk and the Online World

Jennifer S. Saul, MD[a],*, Rachel F. Rodgers, PhD[b]

KEYWORDS

- Internet • Online • Eating disorders • Body image

KEY POINTS

- Internet and social media are important to consider as contexts contributing to the promotion and maintenance of eating disorders.
- The online space contains high levels of appearance pressures, but also hosts extreme content, promoting eating disorder behaviors that may be harmful.
- Clinicians should explore their patients' use of Internet and broaden their knowledge of useful online resources that may be helpful to clients or their families.

The media has been proposed to constitute an important source of sociocultural appearance pressures, and the detrimental effects of exposure to unrealistic and unrepresentative body types, and messages regarding the importance of achieving a thin and toned appearance have been highlighted.[1] The pressure to achieve such unrealistic ideals is increased by the fact that the bodies portrayed in the media are highly unrepresentative of the general population and are accompanied by a discourse that exaggerates the extent to which body weight and shape are controllable through diet and exercise, as well as a food environment that is conducive to overeating.[2] The reciprocal relationships between media use and eating disorder risk have been well documented over the past 2 decades in relation to traditional forms of media, primarily print and television content.[1] However, over the past years, the proportion of media content that is viewed online rather than via these traditional types of media has increased, particularly among youth who are at the highest risk of eating disorders.[3]

In recent years, Internet usage has increased exponentially, with 93% of teenagers now possessing Internet access at home.[4] Youth are the highest Internet and social media users, with up to 89% of 18 to 29 year olds using a social network site, largely through their mobile phones.[5] In response to this, an emerging body of literature has started to document the relationships between Internet and social media use and eating disorder risk.

Disclosure Statement: None.
[a] Child & Adolescent Psychiatry Consulting, LLC 2001 S Central Avenue, Marshfield, Suite A, WI 54449, USA; [b] Department of Applied Psychology, Northeastern University, 404 iNV, 360 Huntington Avenue, Boston, MA 02115, USA
* Corresponding author.
E-mail address: saul.jenna@gmail.com

Child Adolesc Psychiatric Clin N Am 27 (2018) 221–228
https://doi.org/10.1016/j.chc.2017.11.011
1056-4993/18/© 2017 Elsevier Inc. All rights reserved.

childpsych.theclinics.com

GENERAL INTERNET USE AND EATING DISORDER RISK
Internet and Social Media in the Context of Eating Disorders

Many theoretic frameworks have been used to ground investigations of the relationship between sociocultural influences, such as traditional media and eating disorders, including sociocultural theory, social learning theory, self-objectification theory, social identity theory, and uses and gratifications theory. These theories focus on examining the ways that media serves to increase the exposure to harmful appearance ideal, reinforces the centrality and importance of appearance, and models unhealthy appearance-altering behaviors and practices. Social identity theory additionally highlights how the salience of appearance or eating-related behaviors as a condition for group membership may serve to promote eating disorders.

Online forms of media, including social media, have attributes that make them particularly relevant to eating disorders. The first is their highly visual nature. Most online content comprises images rather than text, which makes it saturated in appearance-related content. Furthermore, youth may use types of social media that are particularly picture oriented and that encourage them to spend time curating the images of themselves that appear online, and examining images of their peers or celebrities. The second is its capacity to tailor itself to a person's interests, building on previous content through targeted advertising, search histories, and so forth, leading to an online environment that becomes increasingly person specific the more time that is spent online. For example, a large number of Web sites will have advertisements that are selectively produced based on a person's past search history, meaning that someone who has looked for dieting or weight loss–related content will be likely to view advertisements for weight-loss products.[6] Similarly, a content analysis of advertisements on popular Web sites targeting teenagers highlighted the high proportion of cosmetic and beauty products being promoted.[7] The third aspect is the interactive nature of the online world. In this way, and particularly with social media, the online world combines aspects of traditional media influence as related to eating disorders but also interpersonal influences, including peer relationships, teasing, and such. Finally, the Internet provides the opportunity for access to a wider variety of social groups than the offline world, particularly for youth. Furthermore, through facilitating the coming together of people with marginal interests, the Internet provides a space for groups with attitudes and opinions that are on the more extreme ends of the spectrum. One example of this is pro–eating disorder communities, which is discussed in greater detail later.

Two of the broader characteristics of the Internet that are also relevant are the lack of capacity to moderate Internet content as well as its principal use for commercial purposes. One illustration of the consequences of this is the proliferation of weight-loss products, applications (apps), and methods being sold on the Internet. Most of these products or apps are not empirically based or supported,[8,9] making it unclear whether they can be helpful in any way. Furthermore, for individuals at risk of eating disorders, such products or mobile apps may promote behaviors such as calorie counting that can precipitate or maintain eating disorder behaviors.

In this way, the Internet presents many relevant aspects to the development and maintenance of eating disorders. Given this, the relationship between eating disorders and Internet and social media has received increased research attention. In later discussion, the authors provide a synthetic review of the empirical studies examining this relationship. Overall, the literature provides support for such a relationship with small effect sizes. It is important to remember, however, that social media use occurs in addition to exposure to traditional media and its detrimental effects on body image (**Box 1**).

Box 1
Internet characteristics relevant to eating disorders

- Highly visual: Little text, mostly images, with some of the most-popular apps being entirely photograph based

- User-influenced: Content tailored to each user based on previous online activity and interest. Capacity to become an increasingly appearance and diet–saturated environment

- Interactive medium that combines media influences and peer feedback

- Capacity to bring together individuals with marginal interests and facilitate the normalization behaviors such as eating disorder symptoms

- Lack of moderation and supervision

- Presence of commercial interests, including the diet, beauty, and fitness industries

---

Empirical Evidence

Many correlational and experimental studies have provided support for the relationship between Internet use and higher levels of disordered eating, and eating disorder symptoms, in addition to a small number of longitudinal studies. Earlier studies focused on identifying a relationship between general Internet use and eating disorder symptoms and provided evidence for this association in samples of adults,[10,11] undergraduates,[12] and adolescents.[13,14] Furthermore, in one of the few existing longitudinal studies, Facebook use was a prospective predictor of increased eating disorder symptoms.[15] More recently, however, it has emerged that engagement in online platforms that promote engagement in photograph-based activities are most related to eating disorder risk factors. Among female adolescents, those who used appearance-related forms of Internet and social media displayed the highest levels of eating disorder risk factors.[16] Similarly, among female adolescents, those who spent more time editing their images for social media reported higher levels of body dissatisfaction and dieting.[17,18] Among young women, use of the photograph features specifically on Facebook was found to be associated with drive for thinness and body image concerns, whereas general Facebook use was not.[19] Among adolescent girls, selfie taking and a preoccupation with curating an online self is correlated with risk for developing eating disorders.[17]

In this way, involvement with photograph-related activities on the Internet seems to be particularly related to eating disorder risk. Although the mechanisms accounting for this still warrant further investigation, it is likely that appearance comparisons play an important role. Support for this comes from studies identifying appearance comparison as a mediating factor in the relationships between Facebook exposure and body image concerns.[20] In addition to social comparison, however, the feedback received from peers on social media may play an important role. For example, undergraduates who received negative feedback on their online profiles reported higher levels of eating disorder abnormality.[21] Thus, there is emerging evidence that receiving negative feedback on social media may increase eating disorder symptoms.

Much of the content on the Internet serves to promote individuals, brands, and products. To date, little research has investigated how targeted advertising to individuals with existing body image and eating concerns might maintain or exacerbate eating disorder symptoms. Very recent research has provided initial evidence that apps and programs promoted in the context of fitness and weight loss are indeed unhelpful to individuals at risk of eating disorders. Among college students who reported using fitness tracking apps, calorie counting and fitness tracking were associated with eating disorder behaviors.[22]

In sum, greater Internet and social media use has been shown to be associated with eating disorder behaviors, particularly greater use of photograph-based apps and among individuals who are most invested in their online self-presentation.

EATING DISORDER–SPECIFIC CONTENT

In addition to examining the relationship between Internet and social media use and eating disorder risk, research attention has been directed toward understanding the ways in which content specific to eating disorders exists online, and how it is related to the eating disorder outcomes.

Pro–Eating Disorder Content

As described above, one of the ways in which the Internet is relevant to eating disorders is through the coming together of individuals with minority beliefs. One such example is pro–eating disorder content and communities that use the Internet as a means of expressing their belief in the fact that eating disorders are a life choice as opposed to a form of mental illness, and seek to support individuals in the maintenance and often concealment of their eating disorder.[23] The typical content includes pictures of very thin individuals, "thinspirations" (sometimes digitally modified so as to appear even more emaciated).[24] They also frequently present advice or "tips" for maintaining disordered eating symptoms, including extremely unhealthy weight-loss methods or techniques for concealing symptoms from family and friends.[24] Furthermore, they often include some means of interactive communication (notice board, blog, or instant messaging) through which members communicate and provide each other with encouragement and support.

Content analyses of the interactions on pro–eating disorder Web sites have highlighted the importance of shared deception and concealment for fear of stigma or imposed treatment and the way in which this reinforces the separation between the group of members and the outside world.[25]

A small body of research has provided support for the relationship between use of pro–eating disorder Web sites and eating disorder symptoms.[26,27] For example, in interviews by Schroeder[28] with women undergoing eating disorder treatment, participants reported that the tips and tricks on pro–eating disorder Web sites had worsened their eating disorder symptoms by prompting feelings of being "triggered" to act on eating disorder–related urges (eg, obsessions about nutritional information) and by teaching inappropriate, hazardous compensatory behaviors. In addition, a systematic review and meta-analysis of the findings of experimental studies investigating the effects of exposure to pro–eating disorder content found a consistent small to moderate size effect on eating disorder symptoms. Evidence points to the fact that such Web sites and online content are harmful and may constitute a serious barrier to treatment.[29]

Despite the focus on maintaining eating disorder symptoms of these communities, however, many studies have also found that the possibility of receiving social support was one of the main motivations for individuals to participate in these online communities.[23,30] Individuals suffering from eating disorders are known to experience a lack of social support in their interpersonal environment and report shame and stigma.[22,31] Given this, the Internet provides a safe space where their behaviors and attitudes will be received without judgment and where they can encounter others with similar experiences.

Given the evidence for the harmfulness of pro–eating disorder online content, efforts to limit the presence of such content have increased. Social media platforms such as

Pinterest and Tumblr have banned such groups from forming, and legislation has emerged at the international level banning pro–eating disorder Web sites.[29] Professional organizations such as ANAD (Anorexia Nervosa and Associated Disorders) have been involved in advocating for the removal of pro–eating disorder online content; however, unfortunately monitoring the online space is difficult.

Pro-Recovery, Information, and Support Networks

Although the Internet does allow for individuals endorsing pro–eating disorder positions to come together, it also facilitates the creation of support groups. Several online pro-recovery groups for eating disorders do exist and have been shown to provide both information and emotional support.[32] Furthermore, online groups may fulfill needs, which face-to-face groups have more difficulty meeting, such as being available late at night, and may fill an important gap in available resources.[33] The creation of more supportive online content around treatment seeking is an important need, and clinicians should investigate innovative ways of using the Internet as a means of providing outreach and support.

RESOURCES AND FUTURE DIRECTIONS

The evidence for the ways in which the Internet and social media may serve to promote and maintain eating disorder abnormality is increasing. However, the Internet also provides a means of providing access to information and resources regarding eating disorders. For example, using the Internet has been shown to be a successful means of disseminating mental health first aid for eating disorders.[34] Similarly, The Reach out And Recover Web site provides a useful screening tool for parents or friends who are concerned about a loved one's eating behaviors. In addition, it provides a printout summary and recommendations for referral that can be provided to a general practitioner (http://www.reachoutandrecover.com.au). Clinicians should investigate their client's use of Internet and social media and be able to direct them and their families to accurate and helpful online resources.

In addition, given the evidence for the lack of social support for individuals with eating disorders, strengthening the offline relationships of individuals who suffer from eating disorders may help satisfy their need for social support and, in turn, inhibit their desire to visit pro–eating disorder Web sites. Furthermore, increasing the number of social support resources online for individuals with eating disorders could also be a promising direction. In response to the documented effects of engagement in photograph-based online activities on eating disorder risk, programs targeting media literacy around social media have started to emerge and revealed promise among adolescents.[35] More research in this direction is warranted. Longitudinal studies examining social media use by younger children and subsequent development of eating disorders are indicated.

More broadly, it might also be helpful for clinicians to encourage clients to consider their relationship to social media and the Internet, and their reliance on it. It has been suggested that the constant solicitations of social media might also increase stress and anxiety.[36] In the context of eating disorders, it might also increase the frequency of appearance comparisons and other unhelpful behaviors. Therefore, some clients may also benefit from considering the value of limiting their time online. In the case of youth, parental mediation of Internet use has been shown to be helpful and increase positive Internet use.[37] Parents should be advised to monitor their children's online activities with specific attention to their children's choices of posted photographs and the extent to which they have been edited (**Box 2**).

Box 2
Key findings and future directions concerning the Internet and eating disorders

Key findings

- Greater Internet and social media use, particularly photograph-based apps, has been shown to be associated with eating disorder behaviors
- Individuals who are most invested in their online self-presentation may be most vulnerable
- Pro–eating disorder Web sites advocate for eating disorders as a lifestyle rather than a disorder
- Exposure to pro–eating disorder Web sites has been shown to be detrimental and increase eating disorder symptoms
- Pro-recovery content is rarer

Directions

- Clients' Internet and social media use should be taken into account as an influence for recovery or maintenance of eating disorder symptoms
- Clinicians should investigate innovative ways of using the Internet as a means of providing outreach and support
- Clinicians should learn to direct clients and their families to accurate and helpful online resources
- Clinicians should encourage clients to consider their relationship to social media, and in the case of minors, encourage parental mediation of online content

---

SUMMARY

The Internet has created a more visual and interactive media, such that youth are more likely to view images of a thin ideal and compare it to their own.

Social media has also given youth access to a much wider group of people and interests than they otherwise encounter, in a way that can support and promote eating disordered behaviors.

Professional organizations have advocated for the removal of pro–eating disorder online content, and several sites have taken action; still, monitoring the online space is difficult. The creation of more supportive online content around treatment seeking is an important need, and the effectiveness of such interventions should be measured. Clinicians should explore their patients' use of Internet and social media and consider its impact on treatment. In addition, clinicians should broaden their knowledge of useful online resources that may be helpful to clients or their families.

REFERENCES

1. Levine MP, Murnen SK. "Everybody knows that mass media are/are not [pick one] a cause of eating disorders": a critical review of evidence for a causal link between media, negative body image, and disordered eating in females. J Soc Clin Psychol 2009;28:9–42.
2. Rodgers RF. The role of the "Healthy Weight" discourse in body image and eating concerns: an extension of sociocultural theory. Eat Behav 2016;22:194–8.
3. Swanson SA, Crow SJ, Le Grange D, et al. Prevalence and correlates of eating disorders in adolescents: results from the national comorbidity survey replication adolescent supplement. Arch Gen Psychiatry 2011;68:714–23.

4. Madden M, Zickuhr K. 65% of online adult users use social networking sites. Washington, DC: Pew Internet and American Life Project Report. 2011.
5. Rodgers RF, Melioli T. The relationship between body image concerns, eating disorders and internet use, part I: a review of empirical support. Adolesc Res Rev 2016;1:95–119.
6. Yu J, Cude B. 'Hello, Mrs Sarah Jones! We recommend this product!' Consumers' perceptions about personalized advertising: comparisons across advertisements delivered via three different types of media. Int J Consum Stud 2009;33:503–14.
7. Slater A, Tiggemann M, Hawkins K, et al. Just one click: a content analysis of advertisements on teen web sites. J Adolesc Health 2012;50:339–45.
8. Pagoto S, Schneider K, Jojic M, et al. Evidence-based strategies in weight-loss mobile apps. Am J Prev Med 2013;45:576–82.
9. Breton ER, Fuemmeler BF, Abroms LC. Weight loss—there is an app for that! But does it adhere to evidence-informed practices? Transl Behav Med 2011;1:523–9.
10. Peat CM, Von Holle A, Watson H, et al. The association between internet and television access and disordered eating in a Chinese sample. Int J Eat Disord 2015;48:663–9.
11. Melioli T, Rodgers RF, Rodriges M, et al. The role of body image in the relationship between Internet use and bulimic symptoms: three theoretical frameworks. CyberPsychol Behav Soc Netw 2015;18:682–6.
12. Bair CE, Kelly NR, Serdar KL, et al. Does the Internet function like magazines? An exploration of image-focused media, eating pathology, and body dissatisfaction. Eat Behav 2012;13:398–401.
13. Tiggemann M, Slater A. NetGirls: the Internet, Facebook, and body image concern in adolescent girls. Int J Eat Disord 2013;46(6):630–3.
14. Tiggemann M, Slater A. NetTweens: the internet and body image concerns in pre-teenage girls. J Early Adolesc 2014;34(5):606–20.
15. Mabe AG, Forney KJ, Keel PK. Do you "like" my photo? Facebook use maintains eating disorder risk. Int J Eat Disord 2014;47(5):516–23.
16. Tiggemann M, Miller J. The internet and adolescent girls' weight satisfaction and drive for thinness. Sex Roles 2010;63:79–90.
17. McLean SA, Paxton SJ, Wertheim EH, et al. Photoshopping the selfie: self photo editing and photo investment are associated with body dissatisfaction in adolescent girls. Int J Eat Disord 2015;48:1132–40.
18. McLean SA, Paxton SJ, Wertheim EH, et al. Selfies and social media: relationships between self-image editing and photo-investment and body dissatisfaction and dietary restraint. J Eat Disord 2015;3:O21.
19. Meier EP, Gray J. Facebook photo activity associated with body image disturbance in adolescent girls. Cyberpsychol Behav Soc Netw 2014;17(4):199–206.
20. Fardouly J, Diedrichs PC, Vartanian LR, et al. Social comparisons on social media: the impact of Facebook on young women's body image concerns and mood. Body Image 2015;13:38–45.
21. Hummel AC, Smith AR. Ask and you shall receive: desire and receipt of feedback via Facebook predicts disordered eating concerns. Int J Eat Disord 2015;48:436–42.
22. Simpson CC, Mazzeo SE. Calorie counting and fitness tracking technology: associations with eating disorder symptomatology. Eat Behav 2017;26:89–92.
23. Rodgers RF, Skowron S, Chabrol H. Disordered eating and group membership among members of a pro-anorexic online community. Eur Eat Disord Rev 2012;20:9–12.

24. Borzekowski DLG, Schenk S, Wilson JL, et al. e-Ana and e-Mia: a content analysis of pro–eating disorder web sites. Am J Public Health 2010;100:1526.
25. Sharpe H, Musiat P, Knapton O, et al. Pro-eating disorder websites: facts, fictions and fixes. J Public Ment Health 2011;10:34–44.
26. Custers K, Van den Bulck J. Viewership of pro-anorexia websites in seventh, ninth and eleventh graders. Eur Eat Disord Rev 2009;17:214–9.
27. Juarez L, Soto E, Pritchard ME. Drive for muscularity and drive for thinness: the impact of pro-anorexia websites. Eat Disord 2012;20:99–112.
28. Schroeder P. Adolescent girls in recovery for eating disorders: exploring past pro-anorexia internet community experiences [Dissertation]. Dissertation Abstracts International: Section B: The Sciences and Engineering 2010;71:1354.
29. Rodgers RF, Lowy AS, Halperin DM, et al. A meta-analysis examining the influence of pro-eating disorder websites on body image and eating pathology. Eur Eat Disord Rev 2016;24:3–8.
30. Rouleau CR, von Ranson KM. Potential risks of pro-eating disorder websites. Clin Psychol Rev 2011;31:525–31.
31. Stewart MC, Schiavo RS, Herzog DB, et al. Stereotypes, prejudice and discrimination of women with anorexia nervosa. Eur Eat Disord Rev 2008;16:311–8.
32. Eichhorn KC. Soliciting and providing social support over the Internet: an investigation of online eating disorder support groups. J Comput Mediat Commun 2008;14:67–78.
33. Winzelberg A. The analysis of an electronic support group for individuals with eating disorders. Comput Human Behav 1997;13:393–407.
34. Melioli T, Rispal M, Hart LM, et al. French mental health first aid guidelines for eating disorders: an exploration of user characteristics and usefulness among college students. Early Interv Psychiatry 2016. [Epub ahead of print].
35. McLean SA, Wertheim EH, Masters J, et al. A pilot evaluation of a social media literacy intervention to reduce risk factors for eating disorders. Int J Eat Disord 2017;50(7):847–51.
36. Gazzaley A, Rosen LD. The distracted mind: ancient brains in a high-tech world. Cambridge (MA): MIT Press; 2016.
37. Elsaesser C, Russell B, Ohannessian CM, et al. Parenting in a digital age: a review of parents' role in preventing adolescent cyberbullying. Aggression and Violent Behavior 2017;35:62–72.

Youth Screen Media Habits and Sleep

Sleep-Friendly Screen Behavior Recommendations for Clinicians, Educators, and Parents

Lauren Hale, PhD[a],*, Gregory W. Kirschen, PhD[b],
Monique K. LeBourgeois, PhD[c], Michael Gradisar, PhD[d],
Michelle M. Garrison, PhD[e,f], Hawley Montgomery-Downs, PhD[g],
Howard Kirschen, MD[h], Susan M. McHale, PhD[i],
Anne-Marie Chang, PhD[j,k], Orfeu M. Buxton, PhD[j,l,m,n]

KEYWORDS

• Youth • Screen media habits • Sleep • Screen behavior recommendations

Disclosures: Authors on this paper were supported in part by the Eunice Kennedy Shriver National Institute of Child Health and Human Development (NICHD) of the National Institutes of Health (NIH) under award numbers R01HD073352 (supporting Dr L. Hale, Dr A.M. Chang, G.W. Kirschen, and Dr O.M. Buxton), R01HD087707 (supporting Dr M.K. LeBourgeois), and R01HD071937 (supporting Dr M.M. Garrison). The content is solely the responsibility of the authors and does not necessarily represent the official views of the National Institutes of Health. Outside of the current work, Dr O.M. Buxton received subcontracts from Mobile Sleep Technologies for National Science Foundation award 1622766 and NIH/National Institute on Aging (NIA) R43AG056250. Dr M. Gradisar has received consultancies from Johnson & Johnson, the Australian Psychological Society, the National Health & Medical Research Council, Access Macquarie, and Little Brown Book Company.

[a] Program in Public Health, Department of Family, Population, and Preventive Medicine, Stony Brook Medicine, HSC Level 3, Room 071, Stony Brook, NY 11794-8338, USA; [b] Medical Scientist Training Program, Stony Brook Medicine, HSC Level 3, Room 071, Stony Brook, NY 11794-8338, USA; [c] Department of Integrative Physiology, University of Colorado Boulder, Boulder, CO 80309-0354, USA; [d] Department of Psychology, Flinders University, GPO Box 2100, Adelaide 5001, South Australia; [e] Division of Child and Adolescent Psychiatry, University of Washington School of Medicine, 4333 Brooklyn Avenue NE, Seattle, WA 98195-9455, USA; [f] Department of Health Services, University of Washington School of Public Health, Seattle, WA, USA; [g] Department of Psychology, West Virginia University, PO Box 6040, 53 Campus Drive, 1124 LSB, Morgantown, WV 26506-6040, USA; [h] Child, Adolescent, Adult Psychiatry and Psychotherapy Private Practice, 366 N Broadway Street 210, Jericho, NY 11753, USA; [i] Department of Human Development and Family Studies, The Pennsylvania State University, 114 Henderson, University Park, PA 16802, USA; [j] Department of Biobehavioral Health, The Pennsylvania State University, Biobehavioral Health Building, University Park, PA 16802, USA; [k] College of Nursing, The Pennsylvania State University, Nursing Sciences Building, University Park, PA 16802, USA; [l] Division of Sleep Medicine, Harvard Medical School, 221 Longwood Avenue, Boston, MA 02115, USA; [m] Division of Sleep and Circadian Disorders, Departments of Medicine and Neurology, Sleep Health Institute, Brigham and Women's Hospital, 221 Longwood Avenue, Boston, MA 02115, USA; [n] Department of Social and Behavioral Sciences, Harvard Chan School of Public Health, 677 Huntington Avenue, Boston, MA 02115, USA
* Corresponding author.
E-mail addresses: Lauren.Hale@stonybrook.edu; Lauren.Hale@stonybrookmedicine.edu

Child Adolesc Psychiatric Clin N Am 27 (2018) 229–245
https://doi.org/10.1016/j.chc.2017.11.014
1056-4993/18/© 2017 Elsevier Inc. All rights reserved.

KEY POINTS

- Use of screen media by youth is associated with shorter total sleep time, delayed sleep onset, shorter sleep duration, later bedtime, and poorer sleep quality.
- Mechanisms underlying the relationship between screen media habits and sleep outcomes include displacement of sleep time spent, psychological stimulation from content, and (3) alerting and circadian effects of exposure to light from screens.
- Clinicians, educators, and parents should prioritize the need of youth to get sufficient sleep by maintaining regular and consistent bedtime routines.
- There is a need for more basic, translational, and clinical research examining the effects of screen media on sleep and related health and health behavior consequences.

Abbreviations

FERRET	Food, Emotions, Routine, Restrict, Environment and Timing
IVGA	Internet and video game addiction
NSF	National Sleep Foundation

INTRODUCTION

The widespread use of portable electronic devices and the normalization of screen media devices in the bedroom is accompanied by a high prevalence of insufficient sleep, affecting a majority of adolescents, and 30% of toddlers, preschoolers, and school-age children.[1–6] Three-fourths of American children and adolescents report the presence of at least 1 screen media device in their bedroom, with roughly 60% reporting regular use of these devices during the hour before bedtime.[7,8]

Parents, educators, and clinicians express concern about whether excessive use of screen media among young people affects sleep and well-being. In this article, we provide an overview of the current science on screens and sleep, with a focus on recommendations to reduce the potentially problematic influence of screen time on pediatric sleep. We then review how impaired sleep in pediatric populations may lead to a range of adverse behaviors, physical health problems, and well-being outcomes. We begin with a summary of the 2 consensus statements on child and adolescent sleep needs. Then, we summarize the range of screen habits among youth, focusing on screen habits at bedtime. Next, we review current literature on evidence of the effects of youth screen habits on sleep, and the mechanisms by which screen habits may impact sleep. We conclude with evidence-based strategies to improve sleep through sleep-friendly screen behavior recommendations and other take-home messages for families and practitioners.

SLEEP REQUIREMENTS FOR CHILDREN AND ADOLESCENTS

Two independent sleep associations—the National Sleep Foundation (NSF) and American Academy of Sleep Medicine—each convened teams of sleep researchers and other experts to establish consenuses to guide health care providers and the public about sleep duration requirements across the lifespan, based on the best available evidence. Both groups used a modified RAND/UCLA Appropriateness Method[9] to arrive at their recommendations. For the pediatric population, the NSF panel recommended that newborns (0–3 months) obtain 14 to 17 hours of sleep daily, infants (4–11 months) obtain 12 to 15 hours, toddlers (1–2 years) obtain 11 to 14 hours, pre-schoolers (3–5 years) obtain 10 to 13 hours, school-aged children (6–13 years) obtain 9 to 11 hours, and teenagers (14–17 years) obtain 8 to 10 hours.[10] The American Academy of Sleep Medicine recommendations were identical to those of the NSF, except the former suggested that infants aged 4 to 12 months obtain 12 to 16 hours of sleep per day (including naps) and children aged 6 to 12 obtain 9 to 12 hours.[11]

Consequences of Insufficient Sleep for Cognitive, Psychological, and Physical Well-Being

Sleep problems in early life predict a greater likelihood of later development of psychopathology in childhood and adolescence.[12] In a large study (N = 32,662), short sleep duration (≤10 hours per night by maternal report) and nocturnal awakenings (≥3 per night) in toddlers were associated with the development of behavioral and emotional problems at age 5.[13] Sleep problems at age 4 have been found to predict a greater incidence of behavioral and emotional problems emerging by mid-adolescence.[14] In experimental studies, toddler napping seems to be important for self-regulation. A challenging puzzle task after 5 days of regular napping (compared with not napping) elicited fewer perseverative behaviors, and less negative self-appraisals.[15] Imposing sleep restriction on healthy teens rapidly degrades mood and emotion regulation,[16] as with adults. A large cross-sectional study of adolescents identified associations between short sleep duration and emotional problems, peer conflict, and suicidal ideation.[17] In a metaanalysis of longitudinal and intervention studies, adolescent sleep problems seem to precede the emergence of depression.[18] Although more work on the modifiable aspects of sleep duration, sleep quality, and regularity of sleep timing are needed, the current literature suggests that each of these factors is important for psychological health. These relationships may be bidirectional, because sleep and psychological problems influence one another throughout development,[19] suggesting a resonance phenomenon or a vicious cycle that may be exacerbated by excessive screen media habits. Williams and colleagues[20] have proposed a developmental cascade model, supported by longitudinal data on children, to explain the reciprocal interactions of sleep and emotion and attention self-regulation.

Beyond emotional and behavioral problems, a metaanalysis of cross-sectional studies revealed that short sleep duration was reliably associated with weight gain, adiposity, and obesity risk in both children and adults.[4] Infants obtaining less than 12 hours of sleep per day, measured by maternal report, were more likely to be overweight at age 3 and have higher levels of adiposity.[21] In a longitudinal study of children age 1 to 7 years, sleep duration was associated with greater increases in body mass index, fat mass, and waist-to-hip ratio.[22] In a controlled, laboratory-based experimental study, 3-year-old children exposed to acute sleep restriction (skipping a nap and bedtime delayed by approximately 2.3 hours) consumed greater amounts of carbohydrate and fat and more total calories,[23] which may explain the increased risk of obesity caused by insufficient sleep. A recent review identified sleep as among the socioeconomic, family, environmental, and behavioral factors contributing to childhood obesity.[24]

In a longitudinal study of children in the third grade, bedtimes after 8 PM were associated with a greater odds of increased adiposity measured in the sixth grade. As with children, insufficient sleep in adolescence has been shown to promote dietary behaviors that lead to obesity,[25] with additional effects mediated via decreased physical activity and neuroendocrine changes that bolster fat storage. More evidence is needed, particularly in interventions that counteract the effects of screen media consumption leading to insufficient quantity or inadequate quality sleep, that in turn influence weight gain in childhood. However, the "weight" of available evidence suggests that obesity may be a sleep loss-related outcome of excessive screen media consumption.

WHAT ARE THE BEDTIME SCREEN HABITS OF INFANTS, CHILDREN, AND ADOLESCENTS?

Although the scientific and clinical communities continue to express concern regarding the negative impacts of screen media on sleep, electronics in the bedroom and screen time use around bedtime remain common among youth.[26–28] A large-scale, nationally representative sample of American parents in 2013[26] revealed that about one-third of young children (36%) had televisions in their bedrooms, including 16% of children under 2 years of age, 37% of 2- to 4-year-olds, and 45% of 5- to 8-year-olds. Additionally, among parents of infants and young children who allowed a bedroom television, 22% did so to help their child fall asleep, 14% did so to get their child to fall asleep in his or her own room, and 4% did so because their child slept in a family room containing a television.[26] The presence of a television in the bedroom varies by cultural, socioeconomic, and structural factors. Data from a 2016 nationally representative study of more than 2600 US youth indicated that 47% of tweens and 57% of teens have televisions in their bedrooms.[27] Media devices in the bedroom were more common in lower income youth (68% vs 37%). The authors speculated that the higher rate of media in the bedrooms of lower income tweens and teens may be the result of more frequent room sharing, sleeping in a multipurposed room, or differing family preferences. Parent-reported data from the 2014 *Sleep in America* poll by the NSF revealed that 75% of youth keep at least 1 type of electronic device in their bedroom. The poll also found that the 28% of school-aged children and 57% of teenagers who leave an electronic device on in their bedroom after bedtime obtained less total sleep and had lower sleep quality.[7]

About 50% of parents endorse the belief that watching television helps their infant, toddler, or preschooler "wind down" in the evening.[28] Likewise, multiple studies documented that adolescents report using media at bedtime to "help" them fall asleep.[29] There is a current programming trend toward developing calming shows and apps aimed at helping children relax before bedtime and transition to sleep. To our knowledge, no published research exists on the effectiveness of such content. Such evidence should be a minimum requirement for these approaches to be recommended.

Importantly, over the past decade, the landscape of screen media devices has changed markedly, dramatically altering children and adolescents engage with their environment. Data from large national US samples in 2011 and 2013 show an increase in ownership of tablet devices in young children (age 0–8) from 8% to 40% and an increase in access to mobile "smart" devices at home from 52% to 75%.[26] Another report indicated that, from 2011 to 2013, the percentage of children under 2 years of age who had used a mobile device increased from 10% to 38%.[26]

SCREEN MEDIA, ESPECIALLY NEAR BEDTIME, IS ADVERSELY ASSOCIATED WITH SLEEP TIME AND QUANTITY

In relation to a growing interest in the association between screen time and sleep patterns, data from more than 60 associated studies have been examined in 2 systematic literature reviews[3,30] and 2 related metaanalyses.[31,32] In the time since those articles were published, at least a dozen more studies have surfaced (eg, see[6,8,33–42]), from a wide range of cultural contexts including Thailand,[37] Saudi Arabia,[40] and Norway.[8]

The vast majority of these studies indicate that the extent of screen time among children and adolescents is associated with delayed bedtime and shorter total sleep time.[43–45] Several studies also found associations between screen time and reduced sleep quality,[46,47] longer sleep onset latency,[48] and increased daytime tiredness.[49,50] One recent study found that electronic media use accounted for 30% of all variance in adolescent sleep efficiency, as measured by actigraphy.[34] Most studies examined total daily screen time as a predictor, but even greater effects on sleep have been documented in evening media use in the bedroom (ie, in the 1–2 hours before bedtime[51,52]) and in use of violent media at any time.[53,54]

One metaanalysis investigated the association between portable screen-based media devices and sleep outcomes.[32] Merging results from 20 studies and more than 125,000 youth, the authors consistently found that bedtime media usage is associated with insufficient sleep duration (odds ratio, 2.17; $P < .001$), poor sleep quality (odds ratio, 1.46; $P < .01$), and excessive daytime sleepiness (odds ratio, 2.72; $P < .01$). This metaanalysis found that the mere presence of a portable screen-based media device in the bedroom has adverse associations with sleep outcomes. In 1 study of 600 preschoolers, those with a television in their bedroom watched twice as much evening television (about 28 minutes vs 13 minutes, respectively) and watched more shows with violent, scary, or "mature" content (29% vs 13%).[53] Most related studies focused on typically developing children, but results of studies on children with attention deficit hyperactivity disorder and autism spectrum disorders show similar patterns. One such study found that exposure to violent programming within 30 minutes before bedtime was associated with longer sleep latency and shorter sleep duration.[54]

Negative associations with sleep have been found with use of a range of screen media devices, including televisions, computers, video games, and mobile devices such as smartphones and tablets.[29,48,51,52,55–64] However, there are mixed results regarding whether the type, size, or interactivity level of the screen affects sleep outcomes. In a study of 2048 children in grades 4 and 7, having either a television or small screen device near where they sleep—as well as more daily screen time—was associated with obtaining less sleep.[6] The increase in interactive media options may increase the impact of media use on sleep; some studies have found that interactive screen media use (eg, video games and mobile devices) may have a greater impact on sleep than passive use, such as watching television.[6,45,65–70] One recent metaanalysis found no association between television watching and sleep duration,[31] but did find that computer use is associated with a shorter total sleep duration. Another study shows that use of interactive screen media increases the odds of nighttime awakenings and daytime tiredness,[41] but other studies examining the effects of video game use on sleep have shown more modest effects.[67,71] One study compared 1 hour of bedtime tablet use with 3 different lighting profiles and found minimal differences in the impact on sleep and next-day functioning.[72] However, longer durations of bright screen use (between 1.5 and 5.0 hours) have been shown to increase alertness before sleep.[73–76]

MECHANISMS THROUGH WHICH SCREENS AFFECT SLEEP

Because many of the existing studies are observational and cross-sectional, causality is difficult to discern. Several potential mechanisms, along with supporting evidence, are briefly discussed, including time displacement, psychological stimulation from content, and the alerting and circadian effects of light.

Time Displacement of Sleep

Screen media use can lead to behavioral bedtime delay, as children or adolescents postpone bedtime to prolong screen entertainment.[65,77,78] Using a screen-based device displaces time that would otherwise have been spent sleeping. This time displacement mechanism is particularly powerful when screens are used at night, when sleep is most likely the activity being directly offset.

Psychological Stimulation from Media Content Disrupting Sleep

Research has found mixed results regarding the effect of screen media use on psychological, emotional, and/or physiologic arousal, but this relationship likely mediates some effect of screen media use on sleep.[79–82] Video games, particularly violent games, are often thrilling for enthusiasts, typically simulating life-or-death experiences requiring players' full attention to succeed. Violent video game play before bed increase arousal compared with nonviolent gameplay. However, arousal is a likely mediator of sleep problems even in nonviolent media use.[46] In another controlled experiment, playing an "exciting" video game was associated with increased heart rate, slightly delayed sleep-onset, and decreased REM sleep, further suggesting that the effect of screen use on sleep is mediated via arousal.[60]

Effects of Light-Emitting Screens on Child and Adolescent Sleep

Exposure to the light emitted by screens in the evening hours before and/or during bedtime is another likely mechanism by which use of screen media negatively impacts sleep. Screen-based light may affect sleep via several pathways:

1. Increasing arousal and reducing sleepiness at bedtime,
2. Disrupting sleep architecture as assessed by polysomnographic recording, and
3. Delaying the circadian rhythm and subsequently postponing sleep-onset, which results in shortened sleep duration unless wake time is also delayed.

Studies of young adults demonstrated that evening use of light-emitting devices increases alertness and decreases sleepiness before bedtime, as determined by cognitive performance, self-reported scales, and waking electroencephalographic measures.[73,75,83] These studies also showed that this light suppresses blood levels of the sleep-promoting hormone melatonin, which normally increases in the hours before bedtime.[73,75,76,83] Similar results were found in an experimental study of adolescents, in which exposure to LED screens before bedtime decreased self-reported sleepiness and melatonin levels.[74] Exposure to nonscreen artificial light in the evening also increases alertness (quelling underlying sleep drive) and suppresses melatonin levels, delaying sleep onset. The light emitted from screen media devices includes greater short-wavelength light in the blue light range, which has been shown to induce stronger melatonin-suppressing responses.[84] In fact, in the aforementioned study of adolescents,[74] both subjective alertness and melatonin suppression were significantly attenuated when study participants wore glasses that filtered out short-wavelength light.

Few studies have directly measured the effects of light from screens on polysomnographic measures of sleep.[72,74,75] One such study in young adults found that exposure to light-emitting devices before bedtime caused a phase delay of melatonin release and modestly increased the time to fall asleep and reduced the duration of REM sleep.[75] It is impossible to determine whether longer sleep latency or reduced REM sleep duration was due to decreased sleepiness before bedtime, suppression of melatonin, a phase delay of the circadian clock, or a combination of these factors. Other published reports, including a study of adolescents,[72] found no significant changes on subsequent polysomnography with evening exposure to light-emitting devices.[72,74]

Although limited research documents the effects of light from digital media on sleep, the results are particularly applicable to youth, who may be more sensitive to light than adults.[85] One study[86] found that the magnitude of melatonin suppression induced by moderately bright indoor light levels in the evening was twice as much in primary school children as in adults. This difference could be related to pupil diameter, which is significantly larger in children than adults. Another study[87] found that children showed significantly greater melatonin suppression compared with adolescents in response to varying degrees of evening light exposure. Taken together, these results suggest that the light from screen media use around bedtime adversely affects sleep, particularly in younger children. Furthermore, these findings indicate the need for further research on the effect of screen media devices on sleep, especially in youth.

INTERNET AND VIDEO GAME ADDICTION AND SLEEP

There is growing concern that technology habits can become uncontrollable and excessive to the point of interference with normal daily functioning. For example, the *Diagnostic and Statistical Manual of Mental Disorders*, 5th edition, recognizes 1 type of technology addiction, Internet gaming disorder, as a "condition for further study."[88] More broadly, the concept of Internet and video game addiction (IVGA), has gained traction in the psychological and psychiatric communities, due in part to the disorder's deleterious effects on sleep. IVGA is classified as an inability of Internet users to limit excessive Internet use, with ensuing psychosocial dysfunction.[89] A recent systematic literature review and other studies show a particularly strong association between use of massively multiplayer online role-playing games and poor sleep quality.[90–92] IVGA has been associated with subjective insomnia and insufficient sleep among afflicted adolescents.[90] Existing literature on this association remains limited and causality is unproven, but there seems to be a strong association between IVGA and sleep problems.

MODERATING FACTORS

New evidence suggests some young people are particularly susceptible to the ill effects of screen media on sleep quality. As early as 2009, researchers documented individual differences in teenagers' heart rate variability when playing violent video games.[82] A subsequent study[46] demonstrated that adolescents' level of gaming experience moderated the effect between their video game use, heart rate variability, and sleep. Inexperienced gamers reported poorer sleep after playing a violent video game, in contrast with experienced gamers, who reported poorer sleep after a nonviolent video game. Physiologic trait differences can also amplify technology exposure effects by directly delaying bedtimes.[52] An experimental laboratory study by Reynolds and colleagues[78] revealed that adolescents who perceived fewer consequences from risk taking were more likely to end daily video gaming sessions at a later time, thus delaying sleep onset, compared with their peers. Smith and colleagues[93] found that adolescents who self-reported higher trait flow (the ability to easily immerse oneself into an activity) were also more likely to delay bedtime via extended periods of evening gaming. Their follow-up laboratory study replicated this effect, but only for video games that were both challenging and enjoyable (ie, when game difficulty was set to "hard" instead of "easy"). Similarly, poor self-control in combination with unstructured television viewing has been associated with delayed bedtimes in adults, a finding supported in a follow-up study.[94] This emerging research suggests that identifying predisposing individual traits and characteristics of the technology use helps to discern youth whose technology habits are most likely to delay sleep onset.

INTERVENTIONS, POLICIES, AND STRATEGIES DESIGNED TO IMPROVE CHILD AND ADOLESCENT SLEEP

The American Academy of Pediatrics issued a Statement of Endorsement in support of the American Academy of Sleep Medicine guidelines, which recommends that screen-based devices not be allowed in children's bedrooms and be turned off 30 minutes before bedtime.[95] These are commonly suggested approaches, but modifying media content may be another effective means of protecting sleep. A randomized trial found that a harm reduction intervention that attempted to change the media exposure of preschool children away from violent and toward educational and prosocial content, significantly decreased odds of sleep problems across follow-up at 6, 12, and 18 months, compared with controls.[96]

Experimental studies seeking to evaluate interventions to improve sleep outcomes in children and adolescents are sparse, and have typically incorporated multifaceted sleep hygiene programs that address multiple elements in addition to screen media before bed. Nevertheless, existing literature suggests that limiting screen time during the 30 to 60 minutes before bedtime may yield modest benefits in terms of "lights out time" as well as sleep quality and duration. A 1-week program, consisting of classes teaching sleep physiology, biological significance, and the consequences of sleep deprivation, resulted in more regular bedtimes and shorter sleep onset latency among 58 adolescents (mean, 16 years of age), but no benefit on sleep quality or daytime sleepiness.[97] Another investigation assessed the usefulness of the FERRET (Food, Emotions, Routine, Restrict, Environment and Timing) sleep hygiene program among 22 adolescents (mean, 13 years of age). FERRET instructed adolescents to comply with 3 rules for each of the domains of the acronym (eg, restrict—no electronic media at least 30 minutes before bed, no exercise 3 hours before bed, no other activities in bed except for sleep).[98] This program significantly improved scores on the Adolescent Sleep Hygiene Scale, Pittsburgh Sleep Quality Index, and Sleep Disturbance Scale for Children, although objective sleep duration did not change significantly. A targeted intervention of mobile phone restriction in the hour before bed among 63 adolescents (mean, 16 years of age) resulted in "lights out" 17 minutes earlier and a total sleep time increase of 19 minutes per night.[99] However, the authors reported a low 26% recruitment rate, highlighting the difficulty of implementing such a regimented screen-limiting schedule in teens. In another study, limiting screen media around bedtime for healthy adolescents with good sleep did not significantly impact sleep outcomes. In a study of high school athletes (mean, 17 years of age) whose baseline consisted of sufficient sleep (eg, total sleep time, 7:49 weekdays, 9:11 weekends), a strict "no electronic media" rule after 10:00 PM resulted in no benefit in terms of total sleep time, sleep quality, or daytime functioning.[100] In sum, limited existing research suggests that sleep hygiene interventions may be practically challenging to achieve but yield benefits to those children and adolescents with insufficient sleep. Larger, multisite studies are urgently needed given the increasing intrusion of evening screen media use in of the lives of modern youth, including gaming, social media, and homework.

CLINICIAN'S PERSPECTIVE

Clinicians can help families to improve their sleep health and screen media habits by encouraging parenting marked by high levels of warmth and support, as well as limits that are clearly communicated, consistently applied appropriate to the child's behavior and context, and allow for developmentally appropriate autonomy (ie, an authoritative parenting style[101,102]; **Box 1**). All parents should begin instilling family bedtime routines and healthy sleep habits early in life, and adjust these routines as youth mature (**Box 2**). If the youth health behaviors and habits become part of the child's own daily routine, she or he will be better able to take charge of her or his own sleep health behaviors when this becomes appropriate in later years. For younger children, these routines mean establishing household rules related to screens and

---

Box 1
Sleep-friendly screen behavior recommendations for clinicians and educators

- Talk with families about the importance of adequate sleep.

- Recommend building healthy sleep habits starting as young as possible.

- Teach families about the negative effects of evening use of light-emitting screens on sleep.

- Encourage regular bedtimes that allow adequate time for sleep, and regular bedtime routines in the hour before bed, consisting of calming activities and avoidance of screen media.

- Advise families to restrict all screen devices from bedrooms, including TVs, video games, computers, tablets, and cell phones. Encourage parents to be good role models by following these rules themselves.

- Consider insufficient sleep as a contributing factor for youth exhibiting mood, academic, or behavioral problems.

- Inspire children of all ages to develop autonomy and self-regulatory skills to maintain healthy screen media habits.

Adapted from Lemola S, Perkinson-Gloor N, Brand S, et al. Adolescents' electronic media use at night, sleep disturbance, and depressive symptoms in the smartphone age. J Youth Adolesc 2015;44(2):405–18; and Mindell JA, Owens JA. A clinical guide to pediatric sleep: diagnosis and management of sleep problems, 2nd edition. Philadelphia: Lippincott Williams & Wilkins; 2015; with permission.

---

sleep early on. For older children and adolescents, they involve open conversations about the core reasons for behaviors. This proactive and engaged parenting style promotes cooperation and parent–child shared goals for children's health and well-being, and aims to help children develop self-regulation skills, and eventually increasing autonomy to govern their own behavior.

Examples from health psychology provide accessible guidance. A teen with a healthy diet does not typically result from the rigid imposition of a such a diet after a lifetime of unhealthy foods, but with a healthy and balanced eating habits instilled from a young age. A healthy "screen media diet" may be a resonant and useful concept for many children, parents, educators, and clinicians. It is difficult for parents who smoke to mandate a no smoking policy. Role modeling and a health risk prevention approach is far more likely to be effective than a secondary prevention approach (eg, smoking cessation). Successful parenting ideally starts early and sets appropriate norms and boundaries while maintaining parental warmth, rather than holding off on setting boundaries until a problem develops requiring discipline. Encouraging the development of age-appropriate autonomy will help teenagers to develop a sense of responsibility for maintaining a healthy lifestyle.

For teenagers presenting with excessive screen time, a few clinical pearls may help families to follow the recommendations laid out in **Boxes 1** and **2**. First, one must always focus on the chief complaint, that is, what brought the patient to seek help in the first place. In cases of excessive nighttime screen media use, children and adolescents are often seen in the clinician's office for poor academic performance or lack of concentration in school. Upon taking a careful history, the clinician often discovers a significant lack of sleep, often attributable to patients staying up late while using mobile devices, computers, or video games. Clinicians must discover the underlying factors (eg, social or family stress) that drive the patient to use the screens in the late hours. Addressing such factors directly may be essential to motivating families to achieve healthier screen habits.

Box 2
Sleep-friendly screen behavior recommendations for parents

- Establish screen media habits for your children that enable healthy sleep.[3,7,111]
  o Plan a bedtime that allows for adequate sleep.
  o Avoid screen media in the hour before bedtime and at nighttime.
  o Replace evening screen time with calm activities for your children (reading, coloring, conversation, etc).
  o Keep all screen devices (televisions, video games, computers, tablets, and smartphones) out of bedrooms.
  o Avoid passive background media: Children may be affected by screen media even when they are not actively engaged.
  o Content matters: Avoid violent and/or scary media, which can negatively affect your children's sleep.
  o Family rules and routines are most effective when applied to all children in the household.
- Establish other healthy sleep practices for your child and yourself.[112–114]
  o Set and abide by regular bedtimes every day, including weekends, allowing the child sufficient sleep duration for his or her age.[10]
  o Bedtime should follow a predictable routine (eg, brush teeth, read a story, lights out).
  o Bedrooms should be cool (65°F–70°F), comfortable, dark, and quiet.
  o Avoid evening intake of chocolate or beverages that interfere with sleep (soda, tea, coffee, energy drinks).
  o Include physical exercise into the daily routine, and spend time outdoors during sunlight hours when possible.
- Be a healthy sleep role model by prioritizing your own sleep.
  o Improve your own sleep-related behaviors (eg, reduce screen time before bedtime, establish a regular bedtime)[113] to improve your health and well-being.[115]
  o Turn off electronic media devices in the evening throughout the household and charge all mobile devices in a central location outside bedrooms.
  o Parents who are overtired are less well able to parent effectively, including being proactive in orchestrating child routines and dealing effectively and calmly with daily hassles that are part of everyday life.
- Parent your child with clear communication, awareness, and fair, consistent, developmentally appropriate rules.[116]
  o Talk with your child or teen early and often about the importance of adequate sleep for optimal health.
  o Be aware of how much time your child or teen spends engaging in screen media, including before and after bedtime.[75]
  o Pay attention to your child or teen's mood and behavior at home, and discuss concerns you may have. Mood impairment is often caused by inadequate sleep.
  o Establish and enforce appropriate media and sleep rules for your children as early in their lives as possible; consistently point out after-effects of failing to follow those rules (eg, being tired and cranky the next day after playing games too late) to develop your child's understanding of the effects of inadequate sleep.
  o Work with teens to jointly develop healthy sleep routines that also allow them to meet obligations (eg, homework or sports) and are consistent with these guidelines.
  Developing autonomy and ability to self-regulate is important for teens, as is consistency.

The clinician should then work with families to reduce evening and nighttime screen media use via structural and behavioral modifications to improve sleep health (see **Box 2**). Many adolescents are reluctant to change their health behaviors,[103] yet providing them with education about the positive benefits of sufficient sleep as well as the negative consequences of poor sleep can help to motivate such change.[104–108] For example, pointing out that a change in sleep habits may improve concentration, daytime alertness, and academic performance may motivate youth to modify nighttime habits. Discussing the negative repercussions of inadequate sleep on qualities that are important to the patient, such as body weight or athletic performance, may likewise motivate the patient to reduce nighttime screen media use and establish other healthy bedtime habits. Perhaps most important, parents and children should remove screen-based devices from the bedroom to ensure that they are not used at night.

Changing bedtime screen media use habits in our young patients is challenging. However, several tools and strategies increase our chances of success, with the goal of promoting healthy sleep habits that children and adolescents will continue to follow throughout their lives.

RECOMMENDATIONS FOR CLINICIANS, EDUCATORS, AND PARENTS

Based on our current understanding of clinical practice and sleep health research, we have developed sleep-friendly screen behavior recommendations for clinicians and educators (see **Box 1**) and for parents (see **Box 2**) to help minimize the adverse effects of screen-based media on the sleep of children and adolescents.

FUTURE DIRECTIONS

Research indicates that screen-based media represents a threat to the sleep quality of youth, many of whom already have insufficient sleep. However, very few studies demonstrate easy-to-implement and effective interventions. Future research should develop, implement, and evaluate sustainable interventions that minimize the adverse effects of evening screen use on sleep. For example, a means of reducing fear of missing out from social media and other screen-based activities may significantly improve the sleep of adolescents.[109,110] There is a clear need for more basic, translational, and clinical research into the effects of screen-based media on sleep and related health consequences among children and adolescents, to educate and motivate parents, clinicians, teachers, and youth to foster healthy sleep habits.

ACKNOWLEDGMENTS

The authors are grateful to Guest Editor, Paul Weigle, MD, for his careful review and constructive feedback on this article.

REFERENCES

1. National Sleep Foundation (NSF). Children and sleep. 2004. Available at: https://sleepfoundation.org/sites/default/files/FINAL%20SOF%202004.pdf. Accessed June 10, 2017.
2. National Sleep Foundation (NSF). Sleep in America poll: teens and sleep. 2006. Available at: https://sleepfoundation.org/sites/default/files/2006_summary_of_findings.pdf. Accessed June 10, 2017.
3. Hale L, Guan S. Screen time and sleep among school-aged children and adolescents: a systematic literature review. Sleep Med Rev 2015;21:50–8.
4. Cappuccio FP, Taggart FM, Kandala NB, et al. Meta-analysis of short sleep duration and obesity in children and adults. Sleep 2008;31:619–26.
5. Beebe DW. Cognitive, behavioral, and functional consequences of inadequate sleep in children and adolescents. Pediatr Clin North Am 2011;58:649–65.
6. Falbe J, Davison KK, Franckle RL, et al. Sleep duration, restfulness, and screens in the sleep environment. Pediatrics 2015;135:e367–75.
7. Buxton OM, Chang AM, Spilsbury JC, et al. Sleep in the modern family: protective family routines for child and adolescent sleep. Sleep Health 2015;1:15–27.

8. Hysing M, Pallesen S, Stormark KM, et al. Sleep and use of electronic devices in adolescence: results from a large population-based study. BMJ Open 2015;5: e006748.
9. Finch KB, Bernstein SJ, Aguilar MD, et al. The RAND/UCLA appropriateness method user's manual. Santa Monica (CA): RAND; 2001.
10. Hirshkowitz M, Whiton K, Albert SM, et al. National Sleep Foundation's sleep time duration recommendations: methodology and results summary. Sleep Health 2015;1:40–3.
11. Paruthi S, Brooks LJ, D'Ambrosio C, et al. Consensus statement of the American Academy of Sleep Medicine on the recommended amount of sleep for healthy children: methodology and discussion. J Clin Sleep Med 2016;12:1549–61.
12. Sadeh A, Tikotzky L, Kahn M. Sleep in infancy and childhood: implications for emotional and behavioral difficulties in adolescence and beyond. Curr Opin Psychiatry 2014;27:453–9.
13. Sivertsen B, Harvey AG, Reichborn-Kjennerud T, et al. Later emotional and behavioral problems associated with sleep problems in toddlers: a longitudinal study. JAMA Pediatr 2015;169:575–82.
14. Gregory AM, O'Connor TG. Sleep problems in childhood: a longitudinal study of developmental change and association with behavioral problems. J Am Acad Child Adolesc Psychiatry 2002;41:964–71.
15. Miller AL, Seifer R, Crossin R, et al. Toddler's self-regulation strategies in a challenge context are nap-dependent. J Sleep Res 2015;24:279–87.
16. Baum KT, Desai A, Field J, et al. Sleep restriction worsens mood and emotion regulation in adolescents. J Child Psychol Psychiatry 2014;55:180–90.
17. Sarchiapone M, Mandelli L, Carli V, et al. Hours of sleep in adolescents and its association with anxiety, emotional concerns, and suicidal ideation. Sleep Med 2014;15:248–54.
18. Lovato N, Gradisar M. A meta-analysis and model of the relationship between sleep and depression in adolescents: recommendations for future research and clinical practice. Sleep Med Rev 2014;18:521–9.
19. Tesler N, Gerstenberg M, Huber R. Developmental changes in sleep and their relationships to psychiatric illnesses. Curr Opin Psychiatry 2013;26:572–9.
20. Williams KE, Berthelsen D, Walker S, et al. A developmental cascade model of behavioral sleep problems and emotional and attentional self-regulation across early childhood. Behav Sleep Med 2017;15:1–21.
21. Taveras EM, Rifas-Shiman SL, Oken E, et al. Short sleep duration in infancy and risk of childhood overweight. Arch Pediatr Adolesc Med 2008;162:305–11.
22. Taveras EM, Gillman MW, Pena MM, et al. Chronic sleep curtailment and adiposity. Pediatrics 2014;133:1013–22.
23. Mullins EN, Miller AL, Cherian SS, et al. Acute sleep restriction increases dietary intake in preschool-age children. J Sleep Res 2017;26:48–54.
24. Woo Baidal JA, Locks LM, Cheng ER, et al. Risk factors for childhood obesity in the first 1,000 days: a systematic review. Am J Prev Med 2016;50:761–79.
25. Franckle RL, Falbe J, Gortmaker S, et al. Insufficient sleep among elementary and middle school students is linked with elevated soda consumption and other unhealthy dietary behaviors. Prev Med 2015;74:36–41.
26. Zero to eight: children's media use in America 2013. San Francisco (CA): Common Sense Media Inc.; 2013.
27. The common sense census: media use by tweens and teens. San Francisco (CA): Common Sense Media Inc.; 2015.

28. Rideout V, Hamel E. The media family: electronic media in the lives of infants, toddlers, preschoolers and their parents. Menlo Park (CA): Henry J. Kaiser Family Foundation; 2006.

29. Eggermont S, Van den Bulck J. Nodding off or switching off? The use of popular media as a sleep aid in secondary-school children. J Paediatr Child Health 2006;42:428–33.

30. Cain N, Gradisar M. Electronic media use and sleep in school-aged children and adolescents: a review. Sleep Med 2010;11:735–42.

31. Bartel KA, Gradisar M, Williamson P. Protective and risk factors for adolescent sleep: a meta-analytic review. Sleep Med Rev 2015;21:72–85.

32. Carter B, Rees P, Hale L, et al. Association between portable screen-based media device access or use and sleep outcomes: a systematic review and meta-analysis. JAMA Pediatr 2016;170:1202–8.

33. Harbard E, Allen NB, Trinder J, et al. What's keeping teenagers up? prebedtime behaviors and actigraphy-assessed sleep over school and vacation. J Adolesc Health 2016;58:426–32.

34. Fobian AD, Avis K, Schwebel DC. Impact of media use on adolescent sleep efficiency. J Dev Behav Pediatr 2016;37:9–14.

35. Muller D, Signal L, Elder D, et al. Environmental and behavioural factors associated with school children's sleep in Aotearoa/New Zealand. J Paediatr Child Health 2017;53:68–74.

36. Exelmans L, Van den Bulck J. Sleep quality is negatively related to video gaming volume in adults. J Sleep Res 2015;24:189–96.

37. Vijakkhana N, Wilaisakditipakorn T, Ruedeekhajorn K, et al. Evening media exposure reduces night-time sleep. Acta Paediatr 2015;104:306–12.

38. Sijtsma A, Koller M, Sauer PJ, et al. Television, sleep, outdoor play and BMI in young children: the GECKO Drenthe cohort. Eur J Pediatr 2015;174:631–9.

39. Chaput JP, Leduc G, Boyer C, et al. Electronic screens in children's bedrooms and adiposity, physical activity and sleep: do the number and type of electronic devices matter? Can J Public Health 2014;105:e273–9.

40. Al-Hazzaa HM, Al-Sobayel HI, Abahussain NA, et al. Association of dietary habits with levels of physical activity and screen time among adolescents living in Saudi Arabia. J Hum Nutr Diet 2014;27(Suppl 2):204–13.

41. Jiang X, Hardy LL, Baur LA, et al. Sleep duration, schedule and quality among urban Chinese children and adolescents: associations with routine after-school activities. PLoS One 2015;10:e0115326.

42. Yland J, Guan S, Emanuele E, et al. Interactive vs passive screen time and night-time sleep duration among school-aged children. Sleep Health 2015;1:191–6.

43. King DL, Delfabbro PH, Zwaans T, et al. Sleep interference effects of pathological electronic media use during adolescence. Int J Ment Health 2013;1.

44. Nuutinen T, Ray C, Roos E. Do computer use, TV viewing, and the presence of the media in the bedroom predict school-aged children's sleep habits in a longitudinal study? BMC Public Health 2013;13:684.

45. Oka Y, Suzuki S, Inoue Y. Bedtime activities, sleep environment, and sleep/wake patterns of Japanese elementary school children. Behav Sleep Med 2008;6:220–33.

46. Ivarsson M, Anderson M, Akerstedt T, et al. The effect of violent and nonviolent video games on heart rate variability, sleep, and emotions in adolescents with different violent gaming habits. Psychosom Med 2013;75:390–6.

47. Munezawa T, Kaneita Y, Osaki Y, et al. The association between use of mobile phones after lights out and sleep disturbances among Japanese adolescents: a nationwide cross-sectional survey. Sleep 2011;34:1013–20.

48. Alexandru G, Michikazu S, Shimako H, et al. Epidemiological aspects of self-reported sleep onset latency in Japanese junior high school children. J Sleep Res 2006;15:266–75.
49. Wallenius M, Punamäki RL, Rimpelä A. Digital game playing and direct and indirect aggression in early adolescence: the roles of age, social intelligence, and parent-child communication. J Youth Adolescence 2007;36:325–36.
50. Lemola S, Brand S, Vogler N, et al. Habitual computer game playing at night is related to depressive symptoms. Personality Individ Differ 2011;51:117–22.
51. Owens J, Maxim R, McGuinn M, et al. Television-viewing habits and sleep disturbance in school children. Pediatrics 1999;104:e27.
52. Van den Bulck J. Television viewing, computer game playing, and Internet use and self-reported time to bed and time out of bed in secondary-school children. Sleep 2004;27:101–4.
53. Garrison MM, Liekweg K, Christakis DA. Media use and child sleep: the impact of content, timing, and environment. Pediatrics 2011;128:29–35.
54. Mazurek MO, Engelhardt CR, Hilgard J, et al. Bedtime electronic media use and sleep in children with autism spectrum disorder. J Dev Behav Pediatr 2016;37:525–31.
55. Johnson JG, Cohen P, Kasen S, et al. Association between television viewing and sleep problems during adolescence and early adulthood. Arch Pediatr Adolesc Med 2004;158:562–8.
56. Li S, Jin X, Wu S, et al. The impact of media use on sleep patterns and sleep disorders among school-aged children in China. Sleep 2007;30:361–7.
57. Thompson DA, Christakis DA. The association between television viewing and irregular sleep schedules among children less than 3 years of age. Pediatrics 2005;116:851–6.
58. Adam EK, Snell EK, Pendry P. Sleep timing and quantity in ecological and family context: a nationally representative time-diary study. J Fam Psychol 2007;21:4–19.
59. Dworak M, Schierl T, Bruns T, et al. Impact of singular excessive computer game and television exposure on sleep patterns and memory performance of school-aged children. Pediatrics 2007;120:978–85.
60. Higuchi S, Motohashi Y, Liu Y, et al. Effects of playing a computer game using a bright display on presleep physiological variables, sleep latency, slow wave sleep and REM sleep. J Sleep Res 2005;14:267–73.
61. Yen CF, Ko CH, Yen JY, et al. The multidimensional correlates associated with short nocturnal sleep duration and subjective insomnia among Taiwanese adolescents. Sleep 2008;31:1515–25.
62. Choi K, Son H, Park M, et al. Internet overuse and excessive daytime sleepiness in adolescents. Psychiatry Clin Neurosci 2009;63:455–62.
63. Punamaki RL, Wallenius M, Nygard CH, et al. Use of information and communication technology (ICT) and perceived health in adolescence: the role of sleeping habits and waking-time tiredness. J Adolesc 2007;30:569–85.
64. Mesquita G, Reimao R. Nightly use of computer by adolescents: its effect on quality of sleep. Arq Neuropsiquiatr 2007;65:428–32.
65. Arora T, Broglia E, Thomas GN, et al. Associations between specific technologies and adolescent sleep quantity, sleep quality, and parasomnias. Sleep Med 2014;15:240–7.
66. Arora T, Hussain S, Hubert Lam KB, et al. Exploring the complex pathways among specific types of technology, self-reported sleep duration and body mass index in UK adolescents. Int J Obes (Lond) 2013;37:1254–60.

67. Weaver E, Gradisar M, Dohnt H, et al. The effect of presleep video-game playing on adolescent sleep. J Clin Sleep Med 2010;6:184–9.
68. Lemola S, Perkinson-Gloor N, Brand S, et al. Adolescents' electronic media use at night, sleep disturbance, and depressive symptoms in the smartphone age. J Youth Adolesc 2015;44:405–18.
69. Chahal H, Fung C, Kuhle S, et al. Availability and night-time use of electronic entertainment and communication devices are associated with short sleep duration and obesity among Canadian children. Pediatr Obes 2013;8:42–51.
70. Gradisar M, Wolfson AR, Harvey AG, et al. The sleep and technology use of Americans: findings from the National Sleep Foundation's 2011 Sleep in America poll. J Clin Sleep Med 2013;9:1291–9.
71. King DL, Gradisar M, Drummond A, et al. The impact of prolonged violent video-gaming on adolescent sleep: an experimental study. J Sleep Res 2013;22:137–43.
72. Heath M, Sutherland C, Bartel K, et al. Does one hour of bright or short-wavelength filtered tablet screenlight have a meaningful effect on adolescents' pre-bedtime alertness, sleep, and daytime functioning? Chronobiol Int 2014;31: 496–505.
73. Cajochen C, Frey S, Anders D, et al. Evening exposure to a light-emitting diodes (LED)-backlit computer screen affects circadian physiology and cognitive performance. J Appl Physiol (1985) 2011;110:1432–8.
74. van der Lely S, Frey S, Garbazza C, et al. Blue blocker glasses as a countermeasure for alerting effects of evening light-emitting diode screen exposure in male teenagers. J Adolesc Health 2015;56:113–9.
75. Chang AM, Aeschbach D, Duffy JF, et al. Evening use of light-emitting eReaders negatively affects sleep, circadian timing, and next-morning alertness. Proc Natl Acad Sci U S A 2015;112:1232–7.
76. Wood B, Rea MS, Plitnick B, et al. Light level and duration of exposure determine the impact of self-luminous tablets on melatonin suppression. Appl Ergon 2013;44:237–40.
77. Bruni O, Sette S, Fontanesi L, et al. Technology use and sleep quality in preadolescence and adolescence. J Clin Sleep Med 2015;11:1433–41.
78. Reynolds CM, Gradisar M, Kar K, et al. Adolescents who perceive fewer consequences of risk-taking choose to switch off games later at night. Acta Paediatr 2015;104:e222–7.
79. van der Vijgh B, Beun RJ, Van Rood M, et al. Meta-analysis of digital game and study characteristics eliciting physiological stress responses. Psychophysiology 2015;52:1080–98.
80. Barlett CP, Rodeheffer C. Effects of realism on extended violent and nonviolent video game play on aggressive thoughts, feelings, and physiological arousal. Aggress Behav 2009;35:213–24.
81. Lin TC. Effects of gender and game type on autonomic nervous system physiological parameters in long-hour online game players. Cyberpsychol Behav Soc Netw 2013;16:820–7.
82. Ivarsson M, Anderson M, Akerstedt T, et al. Playing a violent television game affects heart rate variability. Acta Paediatr 2009;98:166–72.
83. Higuchi S, Motohashi Y, Liu Y, et al. Effects of VDT tasks with a bright display at night on melatonin, core temperature, heart rate, and sleepiness. J Appl Physiol (1985) 2003;94:1773–6.
84. Lockley SW, Brainard GC, Czeisler CA. High sensitivity of the human circadian melatonin rhythm to resetting by short wavelength light. J Clin Endocrinol Metab 2003;88:4502–5.

85. Turner PL, Mainster MA. Circadian photoreception: ageing and the eye's important role in systemic health. Br J Ophthalmol 2008;92:1439–44.

86. Higuchi S, Nagafuchi Y, Lee SI, et al. Influence of light at night on melatonin suppression in children. J Clin Endocrinol Metab 2014;99:3298–303.

87. Crowley SJ, Cain SW, Burns AC, et al. Increased sensitivity of the circadian system to light in early/mid-puberty. J Clin Endocrinol Metab 2015;100:4067–73.

88. Association Psychiatric Association. Diagnostic and statistical manual of mental disorders (5th edition). Washington, DC: American Psychiatric Publishing; 2013.

89. Goldsmith TD, Shapira NA. Problematic internet use. In: Hollander E, Stein DJ, editors. Clinical manual of impulse-control disorders. 1st edition. Washington, DC: American Psychiatric Publishing; 2005. p. 291–308.

90. Lam LT. Internet gaming addiction, problematic use of the internet, and sleep problems: a systematic review. Curr Psychiatry Rep 2014;16:444.

91. Achab S, Nicolier M, Mauny F, et al. Massively multiplayer online role-playing games: comparing characteristics of addict vs non-addict online recruited gamers in a French adult population. BMC Psychiatry 2011;11:144.

92. Rehbein F, Kleimann M, Mossle T. Prevalence and risk factors of video game dependency in adolescence: results of a German nationwide survey. Cyberpsychol Behav Soc Netw 2010;13:269–77.

93. Smith LJ, Gradisar M, King DL, et al. Intrinsic and extrinsic predictors of video-gaming behaviour and adolescent bedtimes: the relationship between flow states, self-perceived risk-taking, device accessibility, parental regulation of media and bedtime. Sleep Med 2017;30:64–70.

94. Exelmans, L, VD, BJ. Ego depletion both increases and decreases time to bed: a dual pathway model. Presented at the 23rd Congress of the European Sleep Research Society, Bologna (Italy), September 13–16, 2016.

95. American Academy of Pediatrics Supports Childhood Sleep Guidelines. American Academy of Pediatrics (2016).

96. Garrison MM, Christakis DA. The impact of a healthy media use intervention on sleep in preschool children. Pediatrics 2012;130:492–9.

97. de Sousa IC, Araujo JF, de Azevedo CVM, et al. The effect of a sleep hygiene education program on the sleep–wake cycle of Brazilian adolescent students. Sleep Biol Rhythms 2007;5:251–8.

98. Tan E, Healey D, Gray AR, et al. Sleep hygiene intervention for youth aged 10 to 18 years with problematic sleep: a before-after pilot study. BMC Pediatr 2012; 12:189.

99. Bartel K, Gradisar M. An adolescent's worst nightmare? Altering pre-bedtime phone use to achieve better sleep health. J Sleep Res 2016;25:141.

100. Harris A, Gundersen H, Mørk-Andreassen P, et al. Restricted use of electronic media, sleep, performance, and mood in high school athletes—a randomized trial. Sleep Health 2015;1:314–21.

101. Klein HA, Ballantine J. For parents particularly: raising competent kids: the authoritative parenting style. Child Education 2012;79(1):46–7.

102. Grusec JE. A history of research on parenting strategies and children's internalization of values. In: Grusec JE, Kuczynski L, editors. Parenting and children's internalization of values. Hoboken (NJ): Wiley; 1997. p. 3–22.

103. Gayes LA, Steele RG. A meta-analysis of motivational interviewing interventions for pediatric health behavior change. J Consult Clin Psychol 2014;82:521–35.

104. Prochaska JO, DiClemente CC. Stages and processes of self-change of smoking: toward an integrative model of change. J Consult Clin Psychol 1983;51: 390–5.

105. Cain N, Gradisar M, Moseley L. A motivational school-based intervention for adolescent sleep problems. Sleep Med 2011;12:246–51.
106. Bonnar D, Gradisar M, Moseley L, et al. Evaluation of novel school-based interventions for adolescent sleep problems: does parental involvement and bright light improve outcomes? Sleep Health 2015;1:66–74.
107. Cassoff J, Knauper B, Michaelsen S, et al. School-based sleep promotion programs: effectiveness, feasibility and insights for future research. Sleep Med Rev 2013;17:207–14.
108. Gradisar M, Smits MG, Bjorvatn B. Assessment and treatment of delayed sleep phase disorder in adolescents: recent innovations and cautions. Sleep Med Clin 2014;9:199–210.
109. Beyens I, Frison E, Eggermont S. "I don't want to miss a thing": adolescents' fear of missing out and its relationship to adolescents' social needs, Facebook use, and Facebook related stress. Comput Hum Behav 2016;64:1–8.
110. Elhai JD, Levine JC, Dvorak RD, et al. Fear of missing out, need for touch, anxiety and depression are related to problematic smartphone use. Comput Hum Behav 2016;63:509–16.
111. National Sleep Foundation (NSF). Electronics in the bedroom: Why it's necessary to turn off before you tuck in. 2017. Available at: https://sleepfoundation.org/ask-the-expert/electronics-the-bedroom. Accessed June 10, 2017.
112. Mindell J, Owens J. A clinical guide to pediatric sleep: diagnosis and management of sleep problems. Philadelphia: Lippincott Williams & Wilkins; 2015.
113. National Sleep Foundation (NSF). Back to school sleep tips. 2017. Available at: http://sleepfoundation.org/sleep-news/back-school-sleep-tips-0. Accessed June 10, 2017.
114. National Sleep Foundation (NSF). Healthy sleep tips. 2017. Available at: https://sleepfoundation.org/sleep-tools-tips/healthy-sleep-tips. Accessed June 10, 2017.
115. Watson NF, Badr MS, Belenky G, et al. Recommended amount of sleep for a healthy adult: a joint consensus statement of the American Academy of Sleep Medicine and sleep research society. Sleep 2015;38:843–4.
116. Positive Parenting Practices. Center for Disease Control and Prevention. 2016. Available at: http://www.cdc.gov/healthyyouth/protective/positiveparenting/monitoring.htm. Accessed June 10, 2017.

Geeks, Fandoms, and Social Engagement

Dale Peeples, MD[a],*, Jennifer Yen, MD[b], Paul Weigle, MD[c]

KEYWORDS

- Geek • Cosplay • Fanfiction • Subculture • Gamer • Social engagement • Internet

KEY POINTS

- "Geek" culture is broad and growing, and often enthusiasts are involved in many different fandoms.
- Fandoms are participatory in nature. Although often based on a media property, such as a book, comic book, or television show, fans take ownership and transform the original work.
- Fanfiction is a creative outlet in which writers build off existing creative works to explore relationships and themes from the original material.
- Cosplay, a form of costuming that often takes place at conventions, involves the crafting of a costume of a favorite character, along with light role-playing elements.

INTRODUCTION

Whereas the other articles in this journal focus on medical, psychiatric, and social impacts of the Internet and technology on children and adolescents, this article examines cultural considerations. The Internet succeeded in connecting the world. Ideas are rapidly transmitted around the globe. International trends spread virally, and receive a local makeover influenced by the existing cultural context of communities in which they take root. Like-minded individuals easily connect with one another based on interests, and overcoming limitations geography formerly placed on the establishment of communities.

Interests that are typically stigmatized now form the basis of online communities in which enthusiasts receive support and affirmation, and gain cultural capital through activities and interests that once remained hidden. This leads to increased comfort expressing these interests in public, increasing visibility of previously marginalized groups. These changes were facilitated by the second stage of development of the

No conflicts of interest to disclose (D. Peeples). Speaker Bureau for Assurex Health (J. Yen).
[a] The Medical College of Georgia at Augusta University, Department of Psychiatry & Health Behavior, 997 Street, Sebastian Way, Augusta, GA 30912, USA; [b] Baylor College of Medicine, Department of Psychiatry & Behavioral Sciences, 1977 Butler Boulevard, Houston, TX 77030, USA; [c] Natchaug Hospital, 189 Storrs Road, PO Box 260, Mansfield Center, CT 06250-0260, USA
* Corresponding author.
E-mail address: dpeeples@augusta.edu

World Wide Web, called Web 2.0, which was characterized by the change from static Web pages to dynamic, user-generated content and the growth of social media in the early 2000s.[1] Public interaction with Web sites in the 1990s was static and geared toward consumption, not interaction. The realization of Web 2.0 brought interactivity. Readers of a site began to communicate, comment, and contribute. This is the defining feature of social media, and enables organization of virtual communities.

Virtual communities form around any interest, but we focus our discussion on geek culture, and its subgenres. Geek culture thrives on the Internet, to the point that it is spilling out into the mainstream, while still retaining a measure of stigma. Superficial knowledge of geek interests leads to stereotypes and misconceptions. By better understanding cultural trends, practitioners can facilitate rapport with and understanding of our patients, decrease family discord, help patients identify overlooked strengths, and offer guidance on the developmental task of identity exploration in adolescence.

To better understand geek culture, our first step is to explore the history of youth culture studies. This research occurs largely outside of the field of psychiatry, across a multidisciplinary spectrum from sociology to anthropology, to media and consumer studies. Randomized controlled trials are few in the literature, and often the focus is on ethnographic studies. Using this approach, researchers immerse themselves in a culture, make observations, and conduct semistructured interviews with members of the group. Ethnographic studies adapt to investigate online communities by observing Internet forums and interviewing online members. Modern researchers often touch base with both virtual and real-world communities in the same study.

Our focus now shifts to geek culture writ large. Many activities and interests fall under the broad definition of geek. More prominent activities receive close examination, specifically social media use, cosplay, fanfiction, comics, and gaming. Some geek subsets experience greater stigma, such as furries and bronies, and consequently deserve further attention to facilitate understanding in the face of stereotypes. Attention is given to exploration and expression of identity, building cultural capital, as well as risks and benefits of subcultural participation.

THE HISTORY OF YOUTH STUDIES

The concept of an adolescence is relatively new to human history. Anthropology focuses on rites of passage transitioning a child into the adult world.[2] Cultural ceremonies, such as a bar mitzvah or a quinceañera, are well-known examples of communities welcoming members into the stage of young adulthood. In North America, the concept of the "teenager" as an extended phase of life came about primarily after World War II, as families had more resources to devote to children, allowing for participation in higher education and slowing the transition to independence, marriage, and work. This allowed for the formation of the teenager as an identity, separate from the broader culture of children or adults.

Taking a step back to the early 1900s, the first youth studies were conducted at the University of Chicago under Robert Park and Ernest Burgess. In keeping with the progressive nature of Chicago, the researchers sought to determine the causes of juvenile delinquency in the hopes of achieving reform.[2] To explore causes of delinquency, they mapped the neighborhoods of Chicago by culture and social groups, paying attention to social spaces that unite individuals and cultural bonds holding them together.

Delinquency remained the primary focus of youth studies until the 1960s, when a shift toward examination of subcultures began. The postwar era allowed for the formation of the "teenager" identity, and social scientists began to take interest in this new subculture.[3] It should be noted that the use of the term "subculture" draws some criticism due to pejorative connotations, especially given youth studies' initial focus on delinquency.[4] Different fields favor different terminology, but subculture, countercul-ture, fandom, affinity group, neo-tribes, and lifestyle may be used somewhat inter-changeably. Using the terminology of the time, most youth studies during the 1960s and 1970s focused on music-affiliated youth subcultures. A British perspective moved to the forefront of the field, driven by the Center for Contemporary Cultural Studies at the University of Birmingham.[4]

The Birmingham formulation of youth studies uses a Marxist lens, viewing youth cul-tures as an outgrowth of class struggles. Disempowered working-class youth adopt styles, music, and rituals to resolve social contradictions they experience.[4] Teddy boys, mods, rockers, hippies, skinheads, punks, Goths, and ravers have all been the subject of study over the decades. During this period, researchers trivialized or ignored female-driven subcultures.[2]

Since the 1990s, the Marxist conceptualization draws more criticism, as has the term "subculture." Various new fields of study explore youth cultures, multiplying the number of terms used to describe their social connections created by a shared in-terest. Some argue that music is no longer as much of a driving force in defining youth cultures.[5] The Internet is culpable for this change, as music is now typically consumed in personalized, streaming fashion. Radio and traditional media hold less influence in defining universal musical preferences. The personalized music consumption makes it harder for music subcultures to gain broad mass appeal as they did in the 1960s through the 1980s.

Subculture studies now focus on areas of shared interest outside of music. Life-styles, affinity groups, neo-tribes, and fandoms are a variety of terms used to describe communities bonded over similar pursuits.[4] The Internet serves to concentrate these groups, connecting individuals from across the globe.

THE GEEK

Historically, "geek" is a term of derision, but like other slurs, it has been reappropri-ated, and is now used with pride for self-identification. The name has roots in carnival side shows, but took on its current meaning around the 1950s, describing a socially awkward individual. Beginning in the 1980s, computer technology moved out of lab-oratories and into everyday lives in the forms of personal computers and video-game systems.[5] Geek interests became more relevant to the public, ushering in a gradual acceptance of the value of the geek. With the rise in popularity of the superhero movie genre and video gaming in the early 2000s geek culture has greater social relevance and recognition, drawing more into the fold. With this growth, practitioners are likely to encounter individuals identifying as geeks, but our knowledge and attitudes regarding this group are often dated.

A defining trait of the geek is obsessive interest and knowledge in a given field.[5] As the term geek sheds stigma, it can attach to areas of interests previously outside of the geek domain. For instance, a "sports geek" may be hyperfocused on team statistics, fantasy sports, or wear flamboyant dress and face paint at a game. This discussion focuses on more traditional geek pursuits. Broadly speaking, these interests fall into science and technology fields, and obscure media, such as genre literature, comic books, and gaming.

Examining activities at multigenre conventions (or "cons") gives examples of geek pursuits (**Table 1**) and is a method used in the literature to assess engagement with geek interests.[6] Cons feature a wide variety of activities. These include meeting celeb-rities for autographs, attending panel discussions by the creators or fans of particular media properties, watching movies, listening to live music, and shopping. At larger

Table 1 Geek interests	
Anime	Japanese animation. The most accepted use of the term is to describe any animation originating from Japan. Some will use it to describe animation that is Japanese inspired, but this can head to intense debate.
Comics	The world of comic entertainment moved beyond the physical comic book. In addition to electronic publishing, many comic stories are retold in cartoons, video games, television series, and movies. There are comic fans who have never bought a comic book.
Cosplay	A mix of costuming and light role playing first popularized in Japan. It has grown to become a common feature of fan conventions worldwide.
Fanfiction	Fan-created works based off existing literary properties, which are then shared among fans. One of the best-known works coming out of the fanfiction world is *Fifty Shades of Gray*, which was inspired by the *Twilight* series.
Fantasy	Entertainment focused on magical and mythical elements. High fantasy tends to involve clear acts of magic and fantastical beasts and epic battles of good and evil. Low fantasy involves tales that could almost be set in real history, with a very light imprint from magic, and characters that are often morally gray. *The Lord of the Rings* is an example of high fantasy, whereas *A Game of Thrones* fits in as low fantasy.
Flik	The folk music of conventions. Songs often have a parody quality, and use lyrics referencing sci-fi and fantasy.
Horror	Representations in literature, television, and movies. Zombies and post-apocalyptic representations tend to be popular.
Manga	Japanese comic books. Genres geared toward boys, girls, men, and women exist. Manga is read from right to left, and top to bottom, reversing the typical left to right pattern found in Western comics.
Paranormal	Interest in spirts and paranormal investigation. This can include fictional representations, like the *X-Files*, or how to conduct paranormal investigations, like those on reality TV.
Science	Robotics, rocketry, space exploration, the Internet, and hacking lend themselves to discussion at geek conventions.
Sci-Fi	Science fiction. The fandom around science fiction is the oldest of the geek genres, and established conventions and fanzines that were the primary social outlets for geeks before the Internet. *Star Wars*, *Star Trek*, and *Doctor Who* remain some of the most beloved franchises.
Tabletop games	A wide collection of gaming styles that are typically played among a small group of friends, and often have complex game mechanics. Role-playing games, like Dungeons & Dragons, are perhaps the most well-known subgenre of tabletop gaming.
Video games	Any form of electronic gaming ranging from apps on smart phones to well-known console games to multiplayer games on a personal computer. In addition to gaming consoles like the PlayStation 4, Xbox One, and Nintendo Switch, PC gaming is very popular, with Steam serving as one of the largest distribution platforms.
YA Lit	Young adult literature. Fiction geared toward younger readers, thus carrying some social stigma for adult fans. The *Harry Potter* series, and *Hunger Games* are well-known examples.

cons, groups of similar interests sort into tracks. Broad topics, like science, genre literature, sci-fi, gaming, theater, and anime, are broken into subcategories, or tracks. For instance, gaming is divided into tracks for tabletop gaming, video gaming, and LAN (local area network) gaming. Using track listings to define interests does offer challenges, as tracks change from year to year and differ between cons. Tastes and culture are constantly evolving, so to determine common interests in the geek community, looking at areas of interest at conventions is a sensible approach.

Participation defines fandom.[7] Most of the world's population has some measure of exposure to sci-fi franchises like *Star Wars* and *Star Trek*. Watching a sci-fi movie does not make an individual a geek. Rather, passion that drives an individual to engage with a film, to discuss it with friends, and to create something of their own around it makes that individual a geek. Consumption consists of sitting down and watching a film. Engagement entails discussing it with friends, writing stories about further events in the movie's world, or making costumes representative of the characters. As traditional geek interests were relatively obscure, sharing such passion was very difficult before the advent of the Internet.

Geek interests carry social stigma.[7–9] In broader society, geeks are viewed as juvenile ("cosplay is just dress-up") or low-culture pursuits ("genre fiction isn't real literature"). This prompts the question of why don't geeks shift interests to more socially acceptable pastimes? Engagement may be motivated by 3 factors: the use of fantasy as an escape from real-world pressures, finding a sense of belongingness in a subgroup, and pleasure in engagement with media beyond passive consumption. A controlled study[6] of geeks found evidence for the use of fantasy as an escape but also high engagement in normal life activities, except for politics. Friendships are strong with those who share their interests, but this does not lead to a larger, more traditional social network. Geek responders report being open to experiences and valuing creativity, giving some support to motivation stemming from a drive to actively engage with media.

SOCIAL MEDIA ENGAGEMENT

Before the digital age, those who identified themselves as "geeks" were typically isolated both in their interests and from their peers.[6] After all, many geek activities (reading, writing, and gaming) were considered inherently "less social," as they were typically performed alone. Geeks' enjoyment of them could be perceived as antisocial or representing disinterest in social interactions. Even geeks living in large cities struggled to find and connect with others who participated in the same subcultures.

With the advent of the Internet, the online world quickly became inhabited by people expressing all sorts of interests, even those considered taboo or controversial. With one click of the mouse, introductions could be made and conversations started without ever meeting someone face-to-face. Users quickly embraced this new way of meeting others free from constraints of time, distance, gender, or age. As in real life, individuals with shared similarities began gathering in virtual meeting spaces to socialize. Not unexpectedly, youth were the fastest adapters of this new social media, aided by their capacity to adapt to technology with minimal effort. Social media can help adolescents to combat loneliness, establish intimacy, and maintain relationships.[10]

The World Wide Web offered geeks plagued by social difficulties opportunities to connect to others more easily. One can share as little or as much as one wishes without the fear of discrimination based on appearance, social class, or financial situation. Awkward individuals have the opportunity to review and edit their responses as many times as needed for comfort before sharing them. Significant communication issues (such as autism or social anxiety) can be hidden more effectively. A readymade commonality with other geeks diminishes fear of being judged for their love of their subculture. This is particularly true when interacting with a shared fandom, a community of fans dedicated to a specific person, book, or show.

One of the first (and arguably most popular) Web portals/service providers was AOL. Its chatrooms became popular once users realized they could congregate in virtual groups clearly segregated by interest or subculture. Anyone entering these chats could have a built-in topic of mutual interest with which to connect to others. These groups also self-delineated into smaller subsets when enough members were willing to break away. AOL chatrooms conferred the option to send an instant message to someone within the chat for a private conversation. For example, one could enter a *Star Trek* chatroom, then find oneself entering a subgroup dedicated to *The Next Generation* series as opposed to the original. During this period, technology thought-leaders took note of the popularity of instant online interactions. A subtle shift began from Web service to social media, and more and more content became geared specifically toward the geek audience. Even at the earliest stages of social media, one-fifth of American teenagers used the Internet specifically for instant messaging, where they were increasingly likely to find their close friends online.[11]

Habbo (2000) and Friendster (2002) both originated as gaming-based platforms with a social networking component, connecting those with a love of video games. Myspace (2003), Skype (2003), and Facebook (2004) all launched shortly after. By the time Tumblr (2007), Pinterest (2010), Instagram (2010), and a variety of fanfiction sites were launched, geeks around the world were using them to create and share content for their fandoms. Geek youths tend to gravitate toward platforms that enable constant, live communication. Adolescents spend a great deal of time creating and propagating material about their favorite fandoms, in the form of memes, video clips, screen captures, blogs, or vlogs.

YouTube (2005) spawned new types of entertainers, many of whom are teenagers creating geek-related content. Content often consists of as live gameplay, reactions to show episodes, and fan videos for their favorite romantic pairing (known as "One True Pairing" or OTP). Tumblr and YouTube give those same creators a voice and a chance to make fans of their own, people who admire the content they create and share their interests. Twitter offers an even more expansive reach for adolescents. Not only does it allow for the same creative freedom and social connection, it has also become the platform with which geek youth effect change. Although the idea of real-life politics might be intimidating or overwhelming for teens, they can participate in activism through Twitter.

There have been many recent examples of how a passionate group of geeks enacted change in their fandoms. For example, after *Timeless*, a science fiction television program, was announced as canceled by NBC, fans came together to complain on Twitter for 2 days later until the show was renewed. Similarly, following the cancellation of Netflix's *Sense8*, a show with a diverse cast and bold social commentary fan response brought about a 2-hour special farewell episode. Fans of Freeform's *Stitchers*, a smart show filled with pop culture references and geek characters, successfully petitioned the network for a third season, and are actively pursuing a fourth. Although geek youth sometimes feel powerless to effect change in societal issues, they learn valuable skills by participating in these movements as practice for social activism.

Although the Internet has reduced the social isolation and encouraged communication for many, it comes with it its own unique problems. Within geek culture, fandoms have fought with each other and even among themselves. The anonymity of social media enables some users to spout vitriol or eschew civil behavior with little fear of consequences. This phenomenon is likely why online interactions are associated with higher frequencies of verbally aggressive behaviors than traditional communication.[12] These behaviors may manifest in cyberbullying, also called "trolling" or "flaming"; often targeting individuals who are prominent fixtures within those fandoms. Social media platforms are unable to monitor every message posted by their users, contributing to the belief that there are no true consequences for these misbehaviors. This idea can be dangerous when youths apply those same aggressive attitudes within their real-life interactions.

COSPLAY

Cosplay is a form of costumed role-playing developed through shared eastern and western influences. The name was coined in 1983 when a Japanese reporter, Nobuyuki Takahashi, described his attendance at the 1983 World Science Fiction Convention in Los Angeles.[13,14] Costuming at sci-fi conventions in the United States has documentation going back to the 1930s, but became more commonplace in the late 1960s after *Star Trek* and *Batman* appeared on national television. In Japan, interest in anime and manga provided the inspiration for a committed approach to costuming, which led to the international spread of cosplay.

Cosplay is a loosely defined activity. Traditional mainstream costuming takes place under a variety of circumstances, such as on Halloween or at the theater. Cosplay involves not only donning a costume but also an element of role-playing, distinguishing it from traditional costuming.[13,15] Acting and role-playing elements are limited in cosplay, often merely affecting the mannerisms of a reference character, or perhaps a few lines of dialogue. Generally, this serves to provide interaction with a fellow fan right before posing for a photograph. Cosplay competitions and masquerades sometimes take place at cons. In these events, registered attendees go on stage in costume, and perform signature poses of their characters. Short acting skits may be incorporated into cosplay.

Like most geek pursuits, cosplay activity is split between in-person experiences at cons, and online interactions.[13] Online activities typically begin with research and discussion. An individual selects a character to portray, and researches images to plan details of the prospective costume. Cosplayers often use the Internet to locate base materials for costumes, or to contact artisans specializing in prop or costume production. Some fans purchase completed costumes. However, cultural capital is gained based on both quality of the costume, and the amount of labor a fan invested in it.[13,16] Sharing the steps that went into crafting a costume is a common discussion.

Online communication often helps a cosplayer navigate challenging details of costume construction.[15] Formal costuming organizations offer detailed instructions for costume parts and make recommendations on source materials. One such example is the 501st Legion, a worldwide organization whose members portray imperial forces from of the *Star Wars* franchise. Most costuming groups limit membership to those age 18 and older, partly due to liability issues. However, ancillary groups exist for children, such as the Galactic Academy of *Star Wars* fans. Costume specifications are often publicly available, so it is not necessary to be a member to get help and advice about costuming. Some cosplayers record construction of costumes and upload videos to YouTube to share details of costume design. This has an altruistic element and enhances their status in the community. High-speed Internet connections enable more sharing of costuming knowledge through video and images. The ability to easily share crafting techniques granted by the Internet enhances the level of craft cosplayers can display.

Cosplayers often share images of completed costumes in social media or online cosplay communities. Cosplayers are frequently photographed at conventions, and many also do photoshoots in a setting complementary to their character. For a select few, this modeling cosplay can become a profession of sorts.[16] Professional cosplayers attend cons, selling photos and signing autographs. Some of the most successful cosplay models can transition to a traditional modeling career, publish books, or create television shows such as *Heroes of Cosplay*. Cosplayers report being motivated by the positive feedback they receive from peers. Posting photos and videos online is an easy way to attract an audience.

Aside from online activities, most cosplay engagement takes place at cons. With the rise in popularity of manga and anime in the United States in the 1990s, cons reflected more Japanese influences. Cosplay gradually became an integral part of the con experience. It is common for cosplayers to switch out multiple costumes over the course of the convention. Friends may dress as a group of affiliated heroes or the cast of a television show. Cosplayers show off in designated photo areas, or stroll the convention floor while posing for other fans. Attendees often change out of costume to more comfortable, casual dress for part of the day while shopping, eating, or listening to panel discussions (**Fig. 1**).

Studies have reported mixed findings regarding the demographics of cosplayers. Teens and young adults are the most numerous participants, but prevalence varies from genre to genre. Steampunk is a form of cosplay that blends sci-fi and Victorian-era dress. It has a bimodal distribution, with a peak in the 16-year-old to 24-year-old range as well as the 46-year-old to 54-year-old age group.[17] Stereotypically, cosplay is viewed as a feminine pursuit, in contrast to the larger world of geek culture.[16] However, reported numbers on gender vary, likely due to the nature of particular cons attended.

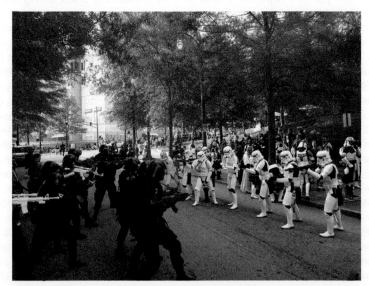

Fig. 1. Dragon Con 2014: Cobra Troopers versus Stormtroopers. Unsurprisingly, no one was hit. (*Courtesy of* D. Peeples, MD, Augusta, GA.)

Motivations to cosplay include the exploration of identity and connecting with a personal hero or interest. Others enjoy the creative element of costume design or performance.[16] The inclusive atmosphere facilitates meeting others who share interests, another motivation to cosplay. Some participants enjoy being treated like a minor celebrity, with strangers giving complements and taking pictures.[18]

Many cosplayers' families are supportive of the hobby.[18] In Japan, where cosplay has a longer period of cultural acceptance, reports[19] suggest that parents who grew up around cosplay are more supportive of their children's interest. In cultures characterized by less familiarity with cosplay, parents are typically warier. Parental concerns include engagement in a frivolous hobby, and donning a sexualized costume.[19]

Parents often object to revealing costumes, and may have concerns over costumes that cross traditional gender boundaries. Crossplay is a subset of cosplay in which costume inspiration is drawn from a character of another gender. This can occur in 1 of 2 ways. An individual may or may not transform the costume to fit their identified gender. For instance, a boy created a Wonder Woman costume adopted to masculine tastes. He follows her color scheme, and includes her hallmark objects, like the lasso of truth and the bracelets of submission. Otherwise, he tailors the costume to resemble traditional male clothing. With the presence of several key items, other fans recognize the homage to Wonder Woman. Conversely, he might decide to appear exactly as his favorite representation of Wonder Woman, donning a skirt, wig, and makeup, in addition to the lasso and bracelets.

Crossplay is common in the United States, and typically goes unremarked at cons. However, it is generally more acceptable for women than men to engage in crossplay.[16,18] Reports[8,16] list a variety of reasons individuals crossplay. Some are mundane, such as friends doing a group cosplay that requires one to fill a cross-gender role. Sometimes crossplay is done for humor, particularly when little to no effort is made to fit gender norms, such as a man with a beard crossplaying Supergirl. Some individuals crossplay to consciously challenge gender norms and expectations. Women sometimes crossplay to avoid the male gaze, as female superhero costumes are typically relatively revealing. Source material may come into play. For example, Kawaii or "cute" style in manga represents characters in a childlike depiction, in which gender is less defining. Similarly, manga has a history of stories featuring gender reversals, leading fans to incorporate those elements in a costume.[14]

Cosplayers generally express satisfaction with the hobby. However, 2 types of complaint are infrequently voiced in the community. Some cosplayers feel pressure to stick to characters that appear like them in terms of age, ethnicity, and body habitus.[15] The appeal of cosplay is to connect with a beloved fictional character, but cosplayers often bear little resemblance to their favorite characters. Transformative cosplay involves making a reference character fit one's physical characteristics, including ethnicity, gender, and body type. Unfortunately, online "trolls" are quick to criticize those who cosplay across ethnicity. Another complaint arises regarding the treatment of (typically female) cosplayers wearing erotic or revealing costumes. Inappropriate comments, contact, and unwanted photography sometimes occur.[16,20] Often cons feature signs indicating "cosplay is not consent" to remind attendees that it is polite to ask before taking a photograph, and it is never acceptable to touch someone without their permission.

Observational research suggests that even at conventions attended predominantly by costumed men, women are photographed more. Asking permission before taking pictures appears to be the exception, as a cosplayer often strikes a pose after talking to one photographer, quickly attracting several more. Child cosplayers are frequently photographed without parental permission.[20] Although cons take place in public settings, children and parents are often unaware that they may lose control over their child's image if attending a con in costume (**Fig. 2**).

COMIC BOOKS

The history of comic books, or comics, has interesting overlaps with that of psychiatry that, to this day, informs how we interpret the impact of media on children. The comic book genre is arguably the geek interest with the most visible impact on pop culture, since the rise of superhero blockbuster movies in the early 2000s. Understanding the history of comic books helps to understand its fans, and controversies that exist within their community.

Comics first achieved popularity in the United States during the 1930s, and featured a wide variety of genres aimed at both adults and children. Horror, mystery, romance, and westerns were well represented, as well as superheroes. During the Second World War, comics were distributed to soldiers as a cheap and easily sharable form of entertainment. Comic sales grew to more than 100 million copies a month by the early 1950s. Romance comics topped sales, reflecting a broad market composed of a fairly even age and gender distribution.[9,21]

The comics backlash began shortly after their appearance and grew through the 1950s. Civic groups alleged comic books promoted fantasy and immorality, leading to the moral decay of children. Crime comic books were thought to directly cause delinquency. Fears circulated that poor print type would cause vision problems for children and contribute to illiteracy by diluting text with pictures.

Local municipalities passed ordinances against the distribution of comics, and public opinion turned against comics, causing adult readership to decline. Dr Fredric Wertham, a prominent psychiatrist, became the most famous critic of comic books. He alleged that depictions of criminal activity encouraged criminal behavior in readers, and denounced purported homoerotic themes hidden in superhero comics. This

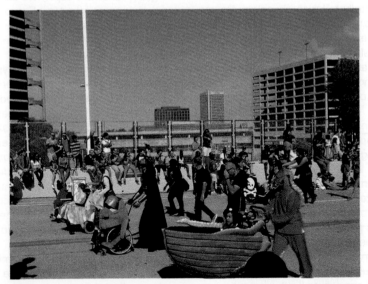

Fig. 2. Dragon Con 2016: children and families participating in the Dragon Con parade. (*Courtesy of* D. Peeples, MD, Augusta, GA.)

was based on his own case reports, described in articles and famously in his book *Seduction of the Innocent* (1954). This led to his testimony advocating comic book regulations at a Senate Subcommittee on Juvenile Delinquency.[9,21]

After the committee hearing, the comic book industry agreed to self-censor by creating the Comics Code Authority. Comics completely ceased depictions of the planning and execution of crime, graphic violence, drug use, and sexually suggestive material. Readership plummeted, multiple publishers closed, and genres withered. One of the few types to survive were superhero stories. The social stigma regarding comics became firmly entrenched in American culture. Interestingly, this was not the case across the globe. In Europe and Japan, the comic book genre continued to appeal to a broad readership via a variety of genres. This fact informs contemporary American comic culture, following the globalized market facilitated by the Internet.

A group of adolescent and young adult male individuals who grew up reading comics began to form a community in the 1960s. Cons and fanzines provided the new group's social connection. Fanzines are publications produced by enthusiasts to discuss comics and share art and related stories. Market forces led to the rise of comic book stores in the late 1970s.[9] These shops became a physical location for collectors to meet and interact on a regular basis, helping solidify comics culture. The collection of comic books provided the only source for knowledge of comic lore, which served as social capital among fans. Combined with market forces, this fact led to a boom in comic collecting, which ended in a crash during the 1990s.

The market faced collapse and major publishers were in financial trouble. To improve sales, many comic books skirted the Comics Code, to again tell "mature" stories. The "graphic novel" format, featuring a collection of self-contained stories printed on higher-quality paper stock, gained acceptance from libraries and literary critics, eroding the juvenile reputation attached to comics over the prior 50 years.[9]

In the late 1990s an influx of Japanese comics, called "manga" contributed to the survival of comics (**Table 2** for manga terminology). The popularity of Japanese anime shows such as *Pokémon* and *Sailor Moon* created a new audience for comics. The expansion of Internet access enabled enthusiasts to learn more about Japanese entertainment. Japan already had a rich history of marketing comics to all ages and genders, so with some translation, publishers had a large back-catalogue of material to market in the United States.

This shift has changed the demographics of comic collectors. In the 1970s and 1980s, approximately 90% of collectors were male.[9] Recent estimates indicate a much more equal gender split.[22] Mainstream comic books traditionally underrepresented or poorly represented women and minorities, alienating potential readers.

Table 2 **Manga terminology**	
Chibi	Little or cute. A stylistic approach rendering characters in a childlike fashion.
Kawaii	Cute, but not as infantile a representation as Chibi style. Still reliant on large eyes/pupils, large heads, and simplified design.
Josei	Manga marketed toward teenage and young adult women.
Otaku	A Japanese geek. The term has negative connotations in Japan, but is generally acceptable among Western fans.
Seinen	Manga marketed toward teenage and young adult men.
Shonen	Manga marketed toward young boys.
Shojo	Manga marketed toward young girls.

The Internet facilitates communication between the audience and creators in a way that is much more immediate and efficient than the traditional "letters to the editor" column in the back of a comic book. Publishers received increasingly negative feedback regarding the marginalization of women and minorities in comic books, resulting in the medium becoming more inclusive and balanced.

However, reactionary elements in the comic book community bemoan these changes online. Women readers report discomfort engaging with the comic book–collecting community at stores.[22] Female collectors are wary of being regarded by male storeowners or patrons as a neophyte or outsider, lacking the cultural capital to successfully navigate the social scene. Comic book stores host social events including board and card games events, serving as a local gateway into geek culture. Thus, female fans often feel excluded from an active local social network. Instead, most female fans report using the Internet for social interactions related to comic books. Recent sales data suggest that as much as 40% of comic book sales (both digital and print) are now made online.[23] The cultural capital of the physical comic book collection and the importance of the comic book store is declining, as the stories and lore of comics are now readily available online. The advent of Internet fan sites continued the traditions of fanzines while eliminating obstacles of production and distribution.

Around the same time that broadband Internet access become widespread in the United States, comic-based movies became popular. Every summer, one can now expect the release of 3 or more blockbusters based on comic franchises. Comic book stories also have successfully transitioned to television series, live-action as well as cartoon, and video games. These stories draw from classic comic book storylines. Currently there is a subclass of "comic book fans" who never actually read comics.

Comic book history shows how cultural biases shaped the medium. Public outcry denouncing comic books in the 1950s was based more in fear and personal opinion than in science. In a cultural reversal, public libraries now add comic books to curricula encouraging children to read. This serves as a reminder, when psychiatrists advise families or the media about the effects of media exposure on children, we need to look at the best available evidence and avoid getting caught up in the latest moral panic.

FANFICTION

When it comes to geeks, they often express their love for their fandom through writing fanfiction. Fanfiction, or fanfic, are works of fiction created by fans of a specific book, television show, or movie.[24] It has risen in popularity over the past few decades, but has been around for more than 70 years. The original use of the term in 1939 was in a derogatory manner (as with many things associated with geeks) when referencing amateur science fiction.[25] By 1944, it took on the current definition, but fanfiction did not gain traction until the *Star Trek* fandom began publishing in the fanzines of the 1960s. Interestingly, women dominated the fanfiction sector as early as the 1970s, something that was not seen in any other arena of fandom. This led one scholar to note it as a departure from the traditionally male activity in literary science fiction starting from the 1930s. She postulated it was the result of the need of the female audience for fictional narratives that expand the boundary of the official source products.[26]

Either way, fanfiction's appeal has always stemmed from an individual's ability to delve into the backgrounds, outside lives, and potential futures of their favorite characters through the process of writing.[27] It offers a chance for a regular fan to participate in molding and directing the journey of the characters. What started out as an expressive outlet turned into a vast network of geeks who both create and consume such works. Readers can filter through a selection of written stories by authors of varying degrees of talent and skill. In some cases, coauthors have collaborated on the same story arc or as chains in a linked anthology. A plethora of different themes, topics, and pairings can be found, and, in some cases, brand new characters can be brought to life that are just as, if not more, engaging than the ones already in existence.

There are many types of fanfiction, and stories are categorized under general headings or tags based on the themes, fandoms, characters and pairings, reader ratings, and keywords. For example, a story can be based on a popular television show, focused on a specific OTP, with mature language and content, and involve death or angst. They are gathered under a limited number of Web sites and servers dedicated to collecting and cataloging them for consumption. Some of these include the aptly titled Fanfiction.net, AOX3 (Archive of Our Own), A Teaspoon and An Open Mind, Quotev, Kindle World, and Wattpad, among others. These Web sites are designed to allow for easy searching by the reader through tags, and offer the ability to save favorite works or subscribe to an author for future works.

One of the reasons why fanfiction has grown in popularity within the geek community is the unrestrictive nature of the activity. Authors of all ages (although typically age restricted to 13 or older) may post their works and share them with other fans of the series. The Web sites offer the ability to let the writer know that the work has been lauded, and they can interact directly with their readers through the comments sections. With a diverse audience, the authors can produce works on topics or themes that might be otherwise considered socially inappropriate or risqué without fear of isolation or retaliation. Similarly, the readers are able to find someone who is willing to produce material along the lines of their interests. In fact, it is not unusual to find dedicated fans of the authors themselves who wait with bated breath for the next installment. It is a place where artists hone their craft, and where people come together to bond over their shared fandoms.

Recently, the popularity of the *Fifty Shades* series by E.L. James has catapulted fanfiction into the mainstream, as it is widely known that these books were originally created as fiction based on the *Twilight* series, by author Stephanie Meyer. If examined closely for parallels, a reader who is familiar with both sets of works can easily spot the similarities, while also recognizing the much more taboo themes of BDSM (bondage and discipline, dominance and submission, and sadism and masochism) represented in James' books. It is the popularity of the author's fanfiction that originally prompted her to stop writing short stories based on her favorite books and transition into an original project of her own. Now undoubtedly there is fanfiction based on James' characters, written by would-be authors who hope for the same eventual success.

Due to its popularity with geeks and geek youth, psychologists have begun researching fanfiction, looking into the motivations and perceived benefits of writing these stories. Some studies have suggested that fanfiction offers both writers and readers a way to fulfill practical and emotional needs.[28] Many writers have disclosed that they use the characters as a vehicle to work through their own issues or challenges in a less threatening manner. Readers in turn may connect with the difficulties of one character and use the shared experience to learn how to cope. It is research into the latter that has led some therapists to look at fanfiction as a form of expressive therapy.[27] The written works can reveal a great deal about the inner workings of the individual, while giving the clinician a way of providing therapeutic interventions. Its use is intended as a less intimidating way to engage patients and encourage exploration of sensitive topics.

GAMING

The acts of play and gaming are core to the human experience, and central to the important task of practicing and mastering skills. Games have near-universal appeal, and most do not carry the type of social stigma attached to geek culture. Sports are a mainstream form of gaming that generally do not appeal to geeks, with the notable exception of the Harry Potter–inspired game quidditch. As part of geek culture, gaming broadly refers to tabletop gaming and video games. Role-playing games (RPGs), either tabletop or video games, typically incorporate elements of sci-fi and fantasy and are most closely associated with geek culture.

Like comics, the history of gaming informs our current perceptions. RPGs evolved from war-strategy games. The latter has a tradition dating back to antiquity, but developed in a modern form as part of military officer training in the late 1800s. Gradually, a small group of wargaming enthusiasts began meeting, primarily on college campuses. Influenced by the antiwar movement of the 1960s, some members of the gaming community broke from tabletop reenactment of historical battles, in favor of a noncompetitive experience. Incorporating fantasy elements, the seminal RPG, Dungeons & Dragons (D&D), broke off as a noncompetitive wargame in 1973.[29] In D&D, a "dungeon master" acts as a referee and narrator, guiding the actions of the other players as they take on the roles of heroes undergoing a quest. By nature, RPGs are a very social activity. The games are more of a cooperative than competitive endeavor, and fans frequently modify RPGs to suit their individual tastes. As discussed, participation and interaction with a form of entertainment, as opposed to passive consumption, is a defining feature of geek fandom. Modification of games extends beyond the tabletop, as fan-produced mods are a common feature of video games as well.

The moral panic of the 1980s concerning RPGs, specifically directed at D&D, was partially the result of coincidental timing.[29] RPGs were already associated with the antiwar and counterculture movements. RPGs typically lack the element of competition, the traditional hallmark defining mainstream board games. At the time, the threat of cults loomed large in public consciousness. The interest and dedication some fans devoted to this new pastime, and its ability to attract youth, raised concerns to outsiders that D&D too might represent a cult. The presence of taboo elements in D&D gave further credence to this concern. D&D features a pantheon of gods, characters defined by moral alignments, magic, and sorcery, along with demons and devils. Despite mainstream society's mistrust of fantasy gaming, a small study of psychiatrists found that they were more likely than others to have played a role-playing game. Attitudes toward negative impact on gaming tended to be based on the responder's age.

Video gaming encompasses a wide variety of styles, and even single-player games form communities through fandoms. Since the late 1990s, online gaming has expanded the social aspect of video games from that of a shared interest to what is often a shared activity.[30] Even before processing power allowed for advanced graphics in online gaming, college campuses saw multiplayer fantasy games spring up in computer laboratories in the mid-1970s. These were known as MUDs or multi-user dungeons. Primitive by today's standards, MUDs allowed several players to work together through a text-based fantasy adventure.

Gradually, online gaming spread from campus computer laboratories to personal computers to game consoles. Online gaming takes many forms, including first-person shooters, fighting games, and RPGs (**Table 3** for gaming terminology). Of all the video-gaming options, massive multiplayer online RPGs (MMORPGs) are among the most social. MMORPGs have a player base of approximately 50 million worldwide, and the

Table 3 Gaming terminology	
Clan	A large faction of united players in a video game.
Avatar	The player's representation in a video game. Avatar customization is an important part of role-playing games.
Casual gamer	"Casuals" is sometimes used as a term of derision by very active gamers who judge that someone has less commitment to gaming. Industry often uses the term to refer to games that have less complex gameplay, such as smartphone apps.
e-Sports	Competitive gaming. Real-time strategy games and fighting simulators are popular in e-Sport competitions, and prizes are up into the millions of dollars.
FPS	First-person shooter. Generally competitive online games, often with military settings.
Guild	A smaller group of players who regularly play together. Most commonly used in the context of a massive multiplayer online role-playing game.
Hardcore gamer	Players who devote extensive time and energy to gaming. Often they prefer real-time strategy, first-person shooters, or role-playing games.
LAN party	A local area network consists of local computers or gaming systems connected to play a multiplayer game in the physical company of friends.
MMORPG	Massive multiplayer online role-playing game. Cooperative role-playing games involving thousands of players.
NPC	Nonplayer character. These characters are not under the direct control of a gamer, but allow for interaction and storytelling.
RPG	Role-playing game. A story-driven game, often in a fantasy or sci-fi setting.
RTS	Real-time strategy game. Single or multiplayer games that rely heavily on tactics and resource management.
Sandbox	Games with a large open world for players to freely explore without the confines of specific level areas.

players spend an average of 20 hours a week engaged with these games.[31] While playing these online games, players frequently text or talk to one another. MMORPGs generally allow for solitary activities, but often bring players together in clans or guilds to participate in organized activities. Unlike other forms of gaming, when any given player is not actively playing the MMORPG, the game continues without them.[31]

Players give a variety of reasons for investing time and money in the online world. Some are "killers," who enjoy the competition. Others identify as "explorers," discovering the massive yet intricate open game worlds. "Achievers" take pride in completing in-game tasks and accomplishments, whereas "socializers" come for comradery and interaction with others. Relaxation and avoiding life stress are also reasons players game.[31]

Issues surrounding gaming and gender have created controversy among gamers in recent years. Gamers are almost equally divided between the sexes, but the hobby remains stereotyped as a male pursuit. Given limited representation and hypersexualization of female characters as pointed out by critics of the gaming industry, it is not surprising that this stereotype continues. The "#Gamergate" controversy of 2014, in which a vocal group of male gamers embarked on a harassment campaign against several female gaming journalists, exemplifies the animosity directed at some female gamers.[32]

The stereotype of the white, male, socially awkward gamer discourages women from self-identifying as gamers, as does the lack of visible female role models in the gaming industry, e-Sports, review sites, streaming sites, and the games themselves.

Women feel less comfortable using online voice chat in games, compared with men, so their presence often goes unnoticed by other players. These elements create a feedback loop reinforcing the male gamer stereotype.[32] However, culture can change quickly. Video gaming has become more and more of mainstream activity, and some level of engagement is nearly ubiquitous among youth. The gaming culture is beginning to lose some of its stereotypes, and more popular games no longer carry social stigma. With better female representation in games and greater visibility in gaming culture, it will become more comfortable for female gamers.

For decades, children have dreamed of someday making a living playing video games. This remains only a dream for most, but game-related revenue options are expanding. Online streaming and e-Sports can be financially lucrative endeavors for a small group of highly skilled players. Profits from streaming video-game play depends on ad revenue and donations from subscribers. E-Sports is a form of competitive gaming, in which players focus on mastery of a single popular game, rather than playing a variety of games. The average e-Sports player is between 15 and 25 years old, and plays 3 to 4 times a week for 2 to 4 hours at a time.[33] E-Sports games are played online or on a LAN, and typically involve teams of players training together to compete in tournaments. Achievement may be the most significant motivator for e-Sport participation, but socialization can be a large motivating factor as well.

The participatory aspect of geek culture is central to gaming. Beyond the individual or group activity of gaming itself, gamers can participate by rating or reviewing games, craft strategy guides, and livestream or upload their own gameplay footage to share. As geek interests often overlap, video-game characters are popular subjects for cosplay, as well as fanfiction.

GEEK MUSIC

Links between music and the geek community are diffuse. Music allows for easy participation as well as exploration of esoteric topics, making it a fertile medium for geek interests. Countless subgenres exist for exploration, and it is very easy to engage in creative activities in music through performance, organization of performances, photography, fanzines, and blogs. Cons offer performances of different music genres, typically in the evening. Flik, punk, Goth, and electronic dance music have crossover appeal. However, no single music genre is attractive to all geeks. Some genres, like Flik, the folk music of conventions, were birthed out of the convention scene.

Flik developed organically among convention goers forming song circles more than 30 years ago. It is an amorphous genre, as there are no clear rules for what defines Flik. However, Flik generally contains sci-fi and fantasy references in its lyrics. Some songs are original compositions, others operate like parodies, substituting lyrics in a well-known pop song. Wizard rock, or wrock, originated around 2002, and draws inspiration from the Harry Potter book series. No musical style unites wrock, only lyrical content. Wrock and other types of Flik originated at cons, but other music genres are commonly performed at con events as well.[34]

The Goth subculture is based in both music and aesthetics. Goth derived from the early 1980s post-punk music scene, and in turn influenced multiple subgenres like darkwave and industrial. Dark hair and dress are common signifiers, as is heavy makeup. Although its popularity peaked in the 1980s, Goth remains a vibrant subculture, with strong influences on the aesthetics of other subcultures such as emo. Goths' bold alternative style and countercultural attitudes toward organized religion and sexuality often make them targets for bullying and intimidation in public, in a manner similar to geeks.[35]

Goth typifies the Internet's impact on music subcultures. Despite the historical trappings of the Goth community, it has always embraced technology. Goth influenced the cyberpunk literary genre, as well as industrial music in the late 1980s and 1990s. Goth Web sites and UseNet groups were common in the early days of the Web.[36]

The Internet drastically changed the way music subcultures develop cultural capital. Some music genres blur the line between the performer and the audience, a feature of punk, and post-punk subcultures like Goth. Members once demonstrated belonging through music collections and esoteric knowledge only available through time invested in the community. With the advent of high-speed Internet, exploring the history of a music subculture, and familiarizing oneself with definitive songs requires minimal effort. New members find it easy to build up a knowledge base previously associated with social capital within the subculture.

Often new members become aware of distinct aspects of online discussions. Online communities are typically guarded toward newcomers. Within a specific group, online communication etiquette has unique traits. Members learn what topics to avoid to maintain engagement in a virtual community. Learning nuances of the community's language is important. Acronyms are a staple part of text-based communication, and subcultures develop their own terminology, with Goths often using abbreviations for band names, or to refer to in-jokes.[36]

FURRIES AND BRONIES

Furries are a fringe branch of geek who identify with anthropomorphized animals. Furry fandom is associated with cosplay because both involve wearing costumes, which furries call fursuits. However, furries are defined by aspects that have little in common with cosplay. Furries express a bond with anthropomorphic animals through drawing human-animal hybrids in a manga style, the creation and enjoyment of related fanfiction, and interaction with the community online. Highly committed furries with disposable income may create and wear a fursuit, the penultimate step in exploring their animalistic identity.[37]

As with all geek communities, furries use the Internet to supplement face-to-face communication. Online, 2 primary forums exist for socialization. The first is chatrooms and discussion boards focusing on furry interests. These facilitate the exchange of art, fanfiction, or conversation on costuming or the furry lifestyle. The second avenue furries use to come together is online gaming. Several online games offer options in which anthropomorphic avatars represent the gamer. The 2 most common for furries are Second Life and World of Warcraft. Second Life is as a sim, or simulation, game. Players go about daily activities of their choosing using a representative avatar. World of Warcraft offers a more traditional gaming approach, in which furries also can use animalistic avatars and use chat functions to connect socially. Real-life contact, as with most geek pursuits, primarily centers around the con. Furry-specific cons occur throughout the year in larger cities. Furries also attend multigenre geek cons. A fursuit can take months to craft and potentially cost thousands of dollars, so wearing one at a convention is not necessary for furry status. Animal ears and tails are common, affordable substitutes for furry costumes, and some furries choose not to dress in costume at all.

Furries are perhaps the most highly stigmatized of geek subcultures, even among other geeks. Some Furries self-identify as human-animal hybrids who find self-expression in wearing their fursuit. Other geeks, who make a greater distinction between their interests and their identity, view them as extreme. As with many communities, hardcore members are often marginalized, for fear outsiders will judge the entire community through the belief of its most extreme members. A subsection of the furry community, referred to as yiffies or plushies,[37] engage in sexual activity while wearing fursuits. Although a minority of the community, the stigma associated with yiffies is often applied to all furries.

Due to the social stigma, furries take different approaches to managing their identity in their local community. Approaches to managing public perception are threefold. Some choose to keep their life compartmentalized, and do not discuss their fandom outside of the furry community. Others express only a general connection to geek culture, focusing on interests in anime and manga to divert attention from the furry identity. A few advertise their furry identity, often promoting the playful and fun aspects of the subculture, making light of it in discussion, or going out with friends in costume to unexpected places.[37]

Although both share an interest in anthropomorphic animals, bronies are distinct from furries. The typical brony is an adolescent to young adult male individual engaging in the fandom of the television show My Little Pony: Friendship Is Magic. The cartoon debuted in 2010 and is currently on its seventh season. The program follows the adventures of anthropomorphic ponies based on a Hasbro toy line marketed to young girls. The brony subculture could almost certainly not exist if it were not for the Internet.

This latest My Little Pony reboot reimagined the ponies in a Japanese kawaii character style, characterized by a cuter, childlike design including larger eyes, dilated pupils, larger heads, and rounded lines. The series takes place in a complex world with a rich backstory, aspects appealing to geek sensibilities. Cultural references in the series are made to geek interests such as D&D, Star Trek, Star Wars, and Poltergeist.

The Internet obsession with My Little Pony began on 4chan.[38] This is a notorious discussion board formed in 2003, and initially served as an outlet for English-speakers to anonymously discuss manga and anime as well as share related images. The scope of 4chan grew with its influence, to cover multiple areas of interest. 4chan is renowned for generating Internet memes (catchphrases or images that quickly spread across the Internet), and has ties to activist groups such as Anonymous and the alt-right movement. My Little Pony discussion overwhelmed 4chan following the release of My Little Pony: Friendship Is Magic. With upward of 6000 posts a day, a specific board, Ponychan, was created to contain the discussion.

Bronies describe their admiration for the TV series as appreciation of the aesthetic design and the positive messages of friendship and acceptance. Some critics suggest that this is "neo-sincerity."[38] Bronies may indeed enjoy these elements of the show, but they do so with a sense of a postmodern irony and cynicism. They understand that mainstream society views their appreciation of My Little Pony as deviant. Bronies use irony to protect themselves from potential backlash. The name "Brony" is a portmanteau of "bro" (a hypermasculinization of brother) and the stereotypically feminine pony. Mashing up masculinity and effeminate identity signify their ironic stance in the fandom.

Bronies are 87% male, 53% younger than 20, and most live in North America. As with other geeks, brony fandom has a large participatory element, which is mainly conducted online. There bronies vigorously discuss My Little Pony, using avatars of pony characters to represent themselves on social media. Pony fanfiction is common, with "clop-fic" delving into erotic tales. Many fans generate art based off the ponies, some of which takes on sexualized tones. The sexualized content contributes to the negative views many in the broader geek community and society at large have toward bronies.

SUMMARY/DISCUSSION

The exploration of identity is vital to adolescent psychological development. Each individual has multiple facets comprising the sum of their being, with contributions from family, ethnicity, country of origin, gender, and interests. Hobbies and pastimes are fluid options for youth to experiment with as they figure out who they are. The Internet opened a staggering number of choices for youth to select from in defining themselves and presenting themselves to the world. It has removed the geographic barriers previously separating individuals with niche passions, enabling them to pursue their interests together.

Interests and tastes continue to change such that pursuits that once carried enormous social stigma can suddenly earn one social capital online. In geek fandoms, adolescents can find a sense of belonging. Through creating videos and engaging in online discussion, youth obtain new skills to create and build. They can find a receptive audience for their writing or music. They can show off artistic skills through photography, crafting, and drawing. The celebration of shared geek interests is not new to fandom; it has existed for more than 75 years in the forms of conventions and fanzines. However, the Internet has dramatically improved the individual's ability to access and participate since the early 2000s.

Geek fandoms can be wonderful for youth who find a group with whom to belong, and develop a sense of pride in their contributions to these burgeoning cultures. As clinicians who work with youth, it is helpful to have a working understanding of these mostly hidden communities. A youth's interest in cosplay or fanfiction may be met with familial skepticism and mistrust. A familiarity with such hobbies helps us to help youth participate in a safe and productive manner, and provide them precious acceptance and support that may be missing from other domains of their lives.

REFERENCES

1. Croft R. Blessed are the geeks: an ethnographic study of consumer networks in social media, 2006–2012. J Market Manag 2013;29(5–6):545–61.
2. Bucholtz M. Youth and cultural practice. Annu Rev Anthropol 2002;31:525–52.
3. Bernstein S, Chatelain E. Twenty-first century teenage monsters: representations of coming of age on the fringes of America. Studies in the Humanities 2016; 43(1/2):52–64.
4. Blackman S. Youth subcultural theory: a critical engagement with the concept, its origins and politics, from the Chicago school to postmodernism. J Youth Stud 2005;8(1):1–20.
5. McArthur J. Digital subculture: a geek meaning of style. J Commun Inq 2009; 33(1):58–70.
6. McCain J, Gentile B, Campbell W. A psychological exploration of engagement in geek culture. PLoS One 2015;10(11):e0142200.
7. Kozinets R. Utopian enterprise: articulating the meanings of Star Trek's culture of consumption. J Consum Res 2001;28(1):67–88.
8. Gn J. Queer simulation: the practice, performance and pleasure of cosplay. Continuum J Media Cult Stud 2011;25(4):583–93.
9. Lopes P. Culture and stigma: popular culture and the case of comic books. Sociological Forum 2006;3:387–414.
10. Wood MA, Bukowski MW, Lis E. The digital self: how social media serves as a setting that shapes youth's emotional experiences. Adolesc Res Rev 2016;1: 163–73.

11. Pew Internet and American Life Project. Teenage life online: the rise of the instant message generation and the Internet's impact on friendships and family relationships. 2001. Available at: http://www.pewinternet.org/2001/06/21/teenage-life-online/. Accessed July 1, 2017.

12. Hellenga K. "Social space, the final Frontier: adolescents on the Internet." The changing adolescent experience: societal trends and transition to adulthood. New York: Cambridge University Press; 2002. p. 208–47.

13. Tsai S, Chen M. From fiction to reality. Eye Magazine 2015;8:38–41.

14. Winge T. Costuming the imagination: origins of Anime and Manga cosplay. Mechademia 2006;65–76.

15. Lamerichs N. Costuming as subculture: the multiple bodies of cosplay. Scene (2044-3714) 2014;2(1/2):113–25.

16. Sergina A, Weijo H. Play at any cost: how cosplayers produce and sustain their ludic communal consumption experiences. J Consum Res 2017;44(1):139–59.

17. Danahay M. Steampunk and the performance of gender and sexuality. Neo-Victorian Studies 2016;9(1):123–50.

18. Peirson-Smith A. Fashioning the fantastical self: an examination of the cosplay dress-up phenomenon in Southeast Asia. Fashion Theory: The Journal of Dress, Body & Culture 2013;17(1):77–111.

19. Rahman O, Liu W, Cheung B. "Cosplay": imaginative self and performing identity. Fashion Theory: The Journal of Dress, Body and Culture 2012;16(3):317–41.

20. Kunkel H, Twist M, McDaniel R, et al. Consent and cosplay: considerations for individuals and families. Poster presentation at Society for the Scientific Study of Sexuality Annual Conference. Phoenix (AZ), November 19, 2016.

21. Brown J. Comic book fandom and cultural capital. J Popular Cult 1997;30(4):13–32.

22. Orme S. Femininity and fandom: the dual-stigmatisation of female comic book fans. Journal of Graphic Novels & Comics 2016;7(4):403.

23. Woo B. The Android's dungeon: comic-bookstores, cultural spaces, and the social practices of audiences. Journal of Graphic Novels and Comics 2011;2(2):125–36.

24. Prucher J, editor. Brave new words: the Oxford dictionary of science fiction. New York: Oxford University Press, Inc; 2007. p. 57.

25. Verba JM. Boldly writing: a trekker fan & zine history, 1967-1987. Minnetonka (MN): FTL Publications; 2003.

26. Bacon-Smith C. Science fiction culture. Philadelphia: University of Pennsylvania Press; 2000. p. 112–3.

27. Thomas A. Fan fiction online: engagement, critical response and affective play through writing. Aust J Lang Literacy 2006;29(3):226–39.

28. Thomas A. Blurring and breaking through the boundaries of narrative, literacy, and identity in adolescent fan fiction. In: Knobel M, Lankshear C, editors. New literacies sampler. New York: Peter Lang; 2007. p. 137–66.

29. Laycock J. Dangerous games: what the moral panic over role-playing games says about play, religion, and imagined worlds. Oakland (CA): University of California Press; 2015.

30. Cade R, Gates J. Gamers and video game culture: an introduction for counselors. The Family Journal 2017;25(1):70–5.

31. Badrinarayanan V, Sierra J, Taute H. Determinants and outcomes of online brand tribalism: exploring communities of massively multiplayer online role playing games (MMORPGs). Psychol Market 2014;31(10):853–70.

32. Paaßen B, Morgenroth T, Stratemeyer M. What is a true gamer? The male gamer stereotype and the marginalization of women in video game culture. Sex Roles 2017;76(7/8):421–35.

33. Martončik M. e-Sports: playing just for fun or playing to satisfy life goals? Comput Human Behav 2015;48:208–11.

34. Tatum M. Identity and authenticity in the Filk community. Transformative Works & Cultures 2009;3:2.

35. Hodkinson P, Garland J. Targeted harassment, subcultural identity and the embrace of difference: a case study. Br J Sociol 2016;67(3):541–61.

36. Whittaker J. Dark webs: goth subcultures in cyberspace. Gothic Studies 2007; 9(1):35–79.

37. Healy M, Beverland M. Being sub-culturally authentic and acceptable to the mainstream: civilizing practices and self-authentication. J Bus Res 2016;69(1): 224–33.

38. Robertson V. Of ponies and men: My Little Pony: Friendship is Magic and the Brony fandom. Int J Cult Stud 2014;17(1):21–37.

Media Engagement and Identity Formation Among Minority Youth

Amy Mayhew, MD, MPH[a],*, Paul Weigle, MD[b]

KEYWORDS

- Identity • Race • Ethnicity • Internet • Racism • Discrimination • Social media

KEY POINTS

- There are significant differences in how media is used by youth of different ethnic and racial groups.
- Media and social media help inform the creation of a social identity for youth.
- Youth members of different ethnic groups have varying attitudes toward racism, familiarity with members of other groups, and understanding of racially charged events portrayed in the media.
- Child mental health professionals should become familiar with issues of race on and off screen and be willing to engage with their patients and families about such matters.

INTRODUCTION

Youth in the United States currently spend an unprecedented amount of time engaged with media of all kinds: television and movies, streaming services, social media, video games, and listening to music. According to a 2015 study by Common Sense Media, 13 to 18 year olds spend an average of 8.5 hours per day of electronic media use for entertainment, excluding time spent on schoolwork, and tweens (those 8–12 years old) spend an average of 6 hours per day on entertainment media.[1] Entertainment media includes watching TV, movies, and online videos; playing games on various devices; using the Internet; and listening to music, often with more than one form of media at a time. It can be difficult to precisely define media engagement, because devices are often portable, ubiquitous, and used in short bursts throughout the day or left on in the background.[2] This level of media exposure provides a near-constant barrage of messages about peer and family relationships, gender roles, expected and

Disclosure statement: No conflicts of interest to disclose.
[a] Psychiatry, Psychiatry Access Service, Cambridge Health Alliance, Harvard Medical School, 1493 Cambridge Street, Cambridge, MA 02124, USA; [b] Natchaug Hospital, Hartford Healthcare, 189 Storrs Road, Mansfield Center, CT 06250, USA
* Corresponding author.
E-mail address: amymmayhew@gmail.com

Child Adolesc Psychiatric Clin N Am 27 (2018) 269–285
https://doi.org/10.1016/j.chc.2017.11.012
1056-4993/18/© 2017 Elsevier Inc. All rights reserved.

childpsych.theclinics.com

acceptable behaviors, social mobility, stereotypes of various sorts, and social values. Individual media usage varies, and media use patterns between racial groups differ significantly. Clinicians who work with youth should understand how they engage with media, including differences between ethnic groups, and how to maximize positive potential of media use for youth and minimize negative consequences.

The rise of the Internet and social media in our culture has led to both greater connectedness and greater fragmentation. Greater ability to find and connect with peers who share a common interest, identity, or viewpoint allows for feelings of solidarity and community. These relationships may enhance perspectives created from experiences in the nondigital world (ie, interactions with friends, family, and the larger community) or provide a valuable alternative perspective that is otherwise lacking. The common restriction of one's Internet experiences to narrow pursuits and ideas may heighten the significance of online relationships, both positive and negative. For youth who identify as a minority, due to ethnicity, race, gender identity, or sexual preference, online experiences may carry greater weight, as a venue to explore their identity within a mainstream culture that may not have varied representations of their culture or experience. For youth who do not identify as a minority, the meaning attached to exposure to minority youth presentations online may similarly carry more weight, especially for those without exposure to those peers in their daily lives. For example, someone who spends all their time playing *Grand Theft Auto*, with no real-world contact with African Americans, may be more susceptible to certain stereotypes about African Americans involving criminal behavior, greed, and dysfunctional families. Such a person who also watches "Black-ish" and "Scandal" would have exposure to different media representations and may develop a more nuanced understanding of African Americans and be less susceptible to stereotypes.

This article presents data summarizing patterns of media use by youth, with an emphasis on specific ethnic and racial populations, predominantly European Americans, African Americans, and Hispanic Americans, because these groups are most largely represented in available US data. The authors then discuss identity formation and social identity theory as they relate to online influences, benefits, and risks of online engagement specific to minority populations, and how child mental health professionals may use this information to better treat patients and their families. The relationship between online and offline realities should be kept in mind, paying particular attention to issues of online racism, cyber aggression, ethnic and racial identity, and risky online behaviors.

Nearly all modern-day children interact online, so that the question becomes not if they will do so, but when and how. According to the Pew Research Center, 92% of adolescents connect to the Internet daily and 24% of them are online "almost constantly."[3] An increasing proportion of adolescents routinely communicate with peers via digital communication: texting (88%), instant messaging (79%), social media (72%), and video chat (59%).[3] More than 20 million youth across the globe use Facebook, 7.5 million of whom are under the "required" age of 13.[4] Adolescents are both passive and active participants in the online world, sometimes perusing peer contributions without comment, other times remarking on that content by texting, tweeting, and posting. Users co-create reality online, meaning they are constantly forming and being formed by the reality in which they engage, and being reinforced by that reality, for better and worse. For example, an individual consumed by watching their peers' Facebook feed, mentally documenting all the events to which he or she was uninvited, may feel the world is passing him or her by without concern. If that person engages with a WhatsApp group of friends to provide mutual support, converse, and share daily experiences, he or she may feel more connected and understood. Parents and professionals struggle to provide youth guidance on appropriate online behavior, help them understand content, show them how to make positive use of media, and advise them on how to manage online situations when they arise. One reason for this difficulty is that adolescents are typically more engaged in the virtual world than adults, regardless of socioeconomic status, race, or ethnicity.[5]

The effects model is a popular paradigm for understanding how screen media content affects attitudes, thoughts, and behavior. Two major tasks of adolescence are exploring intimacy and developing a stable identity incorporating gender, sexual, moral, political, ethnic/racial, and religious factors. A stable identity encompasses self-definition, roles, relationships, personal values, and moral beliefs.[6] Adolescents have long looked to mass media for information about sex and identity, and the Internet is simply a new tool for this ageless task. Understanding how adolescents in general, and minority adolescents in particular, are influenced by online content can help professionals and parents guide them in navigating these worlds.

Social groups, including those defined by ethnicity and race, are social constructs; therefore, an explanation of related terminology used in this article is warranted. The authors chose to use the terms "African American," "Hispanic American" (referring to people from Latin America and the Caribbean who primarily speak Spanish), "Asian American," and "European American" to refer to different ethnic/racial groups. These categorizations represent groups defined in the studies referenced in this article, which allowed for identification with only one group. "European American" is used for "white" interchangeably. Although there are certainly "white" people that are not by family origin strictly from Europe, and those that are called "white" often have ancestors from Latin America or Africa, the purpose is to generalize to the mainstream definition despite the arbitrary nature of how individuals are categorized based on social constructs. People of non-European identified groups are called "minorities," reflecting the situation within the United States but not necessarily that of the wider world, where "minorities" are often a majority (eg, people of Asian descent are not a "minority" in Asia, or even in the world population in general). Scientific data are not completely free from subjective social conventions.

Most of the data cited did not include Asian Americans, Native Americans, and multiracial individuals as defined groups because of sample size; when those data were available, they are included.

Media Habits of Adolescents

The Kaiser Foundation survey of youth media habits, recently rebranded as the Common Sense Media Survey, provides information from 4 waves of surveys of media usage among thousands of youth from across the country in 1999, 2004, 2009, and 2015. The study found that from 2004 to 2015 there was a large increase in total media use among all youth. In 2004, youth 8 to 18 years of age spent 6:21 hours per day with media. In 2009, media time had increased to 7:38 hours, which decreased only slightly to 7:26 in 2015. Watching TV and listening to music dominate media activities. Nearly two-thirds (62%) of tweens watch TV every day, and two-thirds of teens (66%) listen to music.[2] Within these averages, there are large individual variations. On a given day, 6% of teens use no media, 17% use media 2 hours or less, 31% spend 4 to 8 hours, and 26% spend more than 8 hours. In addition, different media use patterns emerge: light users, readers, mobile game users, heavy users, social networkers, and video gamers, with each group spending differing amounts of time on various media activities. Among teens, social networkers and gamers/computer users both use media about 7 hours per day, but social networkers spend about 3 hours (3:17) on social media and 44 minutes on games, whereas gamers spend about 2.5 hours on games (2:27) and 53 minutes with social media. Heavy users spend amazingly 13:27 hours with entertainment media each day. There also is a significant difference between boys' and girls' media use patterns, with boys spending significantly more time on game consoles than girls.[1]

The increase in media consumption is likely directly related to an increase in access via technology. In 2009, 20% of youth media consumption happened via mobile devices.[2] By 2015, that number jumped to 44%.[1] Between 2004 and 2009, the proportion of 8 to 18 year olds with their own cell phone exploded from 39% to 66%. Home Internet access during that same time period increased from 74% to 84%, and laptop ownership increased from 12% to 29%.[2] For a generation defined by their engagement with social media, most tweens and teens spend more time with traditional media such as TV programs and music, and just 1:11 hours per day on social media. Forty-five percent of teens use social media "every day," but a larger proportion daily listens to music (66%) or watches TV (58%). Only 10% of teens rank social media as their favorite media-related activity.[1]

When youth pass into their teen years, media use increases by more than 3 hours per day, a change that remained constant in the 2009 and 2015 surveys. Thirteen to 18 year olds in the 2015 survey spend an average of 8:56 hours per day with electronic media, whereas 8 to 12 year olds use 5:55.[1] Teens spent 39% of media time in "passive consumption," such as reading, listening to music, or watching TV programs; 25% in "interactive consumption," such as playing games or browsing the Internet; 26% in "communication," for example, video chat or social media; 3% in "content creation," meaning creating digital art or music; and 7% in "other" forms of media.[1]

The Kaiser Foundation study grouped the youth into high media users (more than 16 hours per day, 21%), moderate users (3–16 hours, 63%), and light users (<3 hours per day, 17%). Heavy media users are twice as likely (47%) to get fair to poor grades (Cs or lower) than light media users (23%). Heavy media users are also more likely to say they often get into trouble, are often sad or unhappy, and are often bored. These relationships persisted even controlling for factors, such as age, gender, race, parent education, and single versus 2-parent households.[2]

DIFFERENCES IN MEDIA HABITS BETWEEN RACIAL AND ETHNIC GROUPS

Differences in total media use between racial and ethnic groups are significant, even when controlling for age, parent education, or single- or 2-parent families; that said, individuals from historically disadvantaged groups such as African Americans and Hispanic Americans are also more likely to have lower socioeconomic status and parent education. It is difficult to discern which variable is most strongly associated with differences in media use, but it is useful to look at the differences between groups regardless. Most 8 to 18 year olds have a computer at home, regardless of race or ethnicity. However, 92% of youth who live in a high income ($100,000+ per year) household have a laptop computer in the home compared with 54% of those in a low income (<$35,000 per year) household.[1] The increase in total media usage between 1999 and 2009 was greater among Hispanic and African American youth compared with European Americans.[2]

Total Media Use

African American and Hispanic American children and those in lower socioeconomic groups spend more time using screen media than their peers. African American tweens spend an average of 6:22 hours per day, Hispanic Americans spend 5:18 hours per day, and European American tweens spend 4:00 hours per day. African American teens average 11:10 hours of media exposure daily compared with 8:51 hours among Hispanic

Americans and 8:27 hours among European Americans. African American teens spend more time using media than their peers. Lower-income teens use screen media about 3 hours more than their higher-income peers (8:56 vs 5:55). Children from lower socio-economic groups spend more time on media than those from higher economic status, a difference of 2:45 hours (10:35 vs 7:50). According to Kaiser Family Foundation Survey, there is no significant difference in the time spent multitasking media: 44% of African American middle and high school students, 41% of Hispanics, and 37% of European Americans report using another medium "most of the time" while watching TV.[2]

Television and Video Viewing

Although there is not a difference between teens of different ethnic groups about whether they watch TV on a daily basis, there is a difference in the amount of time spent. African American teens spend more time doing so: 4:33 hours versus 3:22 hours for Hispanic Americans and 2:56 hours for European Americans. Those in a lower socioeconomic group also spend more time watching TV than their peers. Among tweens, African American tweens watch 3:40 TV daily compared with 3:14 for Hispanic Americans and 2:29 for European Americans.[1]

According to the Kaiser Family Foundation Study, African American and Hispanic youth are more likely to have TV sets in their bedrooms (84% of African Americans, 77% of Hispanic Americans, 64% of European Americans and Asian Americans). African Americans (78%) and Hispanics (67%) are also more likely to have the TV on during meal times than European Americans (58%) and Asian Americans (55%). African American children under 6 years old are twice as likely as European American children to have a TV in their bedroom, and more than twice as likely to go to sleep with the TV on.[2]

Music

Listening to music is ubiquitous among teens, with no significant differences between racial and ethnic groups in regard to participation. African American teens spend more time doing so: 2:27 compared with 2:04 for Hispanic American teens, and 1:44 for European American teens. Among tweens, those from lower income families listen to more music, as do those whose parents have less than a college education. African American tweens listened to an average of 2:11 hours per day versus 1:17 for European Americans and 1:39 for Hispanic Americans.[1]

Gaming

Seventy-one percent of European American tweens play some type of video games versus 62% of African Americans and 61% of Hispanic Americans. Those whose parents have a college education play 36 minutes less than those whose parents have a high school education or less.[1]

Computer Use

European American tweens, those from higher income families, and especially those with more highly educated parents are more likely to use a computer than those in other groups.[1]

According to the Kaiser Family Foundation Survey, Asian Americans spent the most time in recreational computer use: 2:53 per day, compared with 1:49 for Hispanics, 1:24 for African Americans, and 1:27 for European Americans. Asian American youth have more computers at home and are more likely to have the computer in their bedroom (55% compared with 39% of Hispanics, 34% of African Americans, and 32% of European Americans). There was no significant difference in the amount of time different ethnic groups spent on a computer for schoolwork.[2]

Reading

According to the Common Sense Media Survey, there was no difference between youth of various ethnicities regarding whether they read on a particular day. However, there were differences by income and education, with 45% of those who parents had a college degree reading on a given day versus 29% of those whose parents had no more than a high school education.

The variable technology habits between groups may carry significant mental health consequences. For example, one study found that African American boys suffer more adverse mental health effects of computer use than European American boys or girls of either race. The study attributed this effect to the fact that African American boys use computers for video game play the most. The study found that using computers for communication or video games did not contribute favorably to youth well-being as did using computers for other purposes.[7]

In homes where parents limit youth media use (through rules or the home environment), children spend less time with media. Parental limits include no TV allowed in the bedroom, no TV on during meals or in the background, and other restrictions. Youth are more likely to report their parents talk to them about online safety and responsibility than how much time they spend using media. Seventy-two percent of tweens and 53% of teens say their parents have talked to them about how much time they spend on media. More youth, however, indicate their parents spoke to them about what media content they are allowed to use: 66% of teens and 84% of tweens. Most report their parents know "a lot" or at least "some" of their media content, but 25% indicate their parents know "little" or "nothing" about what they do or say online and 30% say their parents know little to nothing about their social media use. Parents are more likely to set limits on content than the amount of time with media. When parents do set limits, children spend less time with media. Those youth with some rules about media use spend nearly 3 hours less with media each day. European American parents are more likely to impose controls on content; 40% for European American children versus 30% of African American children and 24% of Hispanic children.[2,8]

SOCIAL IDENTITY THEORY

To understand how youth's screen media experiences influence their individual and collective identities, it is useful to consider social identity theory. Henri Tajfel, a Polish Jewish survivor of World War II, and Turner[9] first conceptualized that social identity consists of an individual's knowledge of membership to a particular group together with the "emotional significance attached to that membership." The theory explains implications of social identity for one's perceptions and behaviors as well as relationships between individuals and groups. Social identity is related to personal identity. People can use various strategies to derive a positive personal identity, distinct from strategies that improve social identity. Social identity theory addresses 3 main concepts: psychological processes that differentiate social from personal identity; strategies to derive a positive social identity; and how characteristics of various social structures determine which strategies apply.[8]

Social categorization is the process through which individuals are placed into groups. Classifying individuals into a finite number of social categories helps organize socially relevant information, which may help in understanding and predicting behaviors. When individuals "belong" to a particular group, they are thought to share central group-defining characteristics that distinguish them from those outside of the group. For that reason, people typically notice similarities between individuals in the same category and differences between individuals in different categories. People are often judged in terms of characteristic features of the social group to which they are categorized, whereas unique traits of the individual are ignored.[8] An individual may be categorized by geographic group (eg, by rural vs urban community, state, region, or country) as well as by various other criteria (eg, sex, race, ethnic group, or occupation). People tend to categorize themselves to the extent that they think the differences between group members are smaller than the differences between group members and those of other groups.

Social comparison is the process by which group characteristics are interpreted and assigned value, usually by comparing defining characteristics of one group with those of other groups. Social comparisons define how each group is distinguished from others, not to be confused with social categorization, which determines how individuals are classified.

Social identification is the means by which an individual defines social reality by their group membership and how their group compares to others. Specific features associated with their group, and the social value of these features, determine how group membership reflects on the individual. Those belonging to a privileged group are often motivated to promote their group's social identity and distinguish it from others. Those belonging to a devalued group must use various strategies to define themselves in a positive light in despite the affiliation.

One strategy used to improve one's social status is *individual mobility*, in which a person of a devalued group pursues an activity that helps grant inclusion into a group of higher social standing. Examples of such activities include achievement in education, a profession, athletics, and accumulation of wealth. Individual mobility allows for specific group members to attain a more positive social identity, but does not benefit the entire group.

Social creativity is the process by which members of a devalued group transform group comparisons by redefining distinctive group characteristics as positive rather than negative. The meaning may be changed by focusing on more favorable dimensions of the comparison, broadening the comparison to include other groups, or by changing the meaning of a low-status group membership. Although this strategy may help people in a devalued group cope, it typically fails to change the status quo.

Social competition occurs when group members join together to wage conflict intended to change the status quo (eg, gain equal rights). Social competition consists of collective group action oriented toward the improving social status for the entire group, rather than for that of certain individual.[8]

The way in which individuals respond to their group's circumstances depends in part on how it is perceived by the prevailing social structure. *Permeability of group boundaries* refers to ease of social mobility and individual freedom to access groups to which one is not a member. If group boundaries are permeable, individual mobility is more likely to be successful and more commonly pursued. If boundaries are impermeable, individuals are more likely to feel bound to and by their group.[8]

THE ECHO CHAMBER

Erik Erickson wrote "the growing and developing youth, faced with this physiological revolution within them, and with tangible adult tasks ahead of them, are now primarily concerned with what they appear to be in the eyes of others as compared with what they feel they are, and with the question of how to connect the roles and skills cultivated earlier with the occupational prototypes of the day."[10] Modern youth have access to online social networking, a social outlet in which opinions of those outside one's defined group (eg, adults, those of other ethnic groups, or of another political persuasion) can be largely ignored in favor of a coconstructed reality called an echo chamber. Here, group opinions and identities can take on exaggerated importance, protected from exposure to differing views, which may compel compromise or understanding. In such an echo chamber, slights and negative comments also take on greater importance and can be difficult to ignore.

Social norms and identity are constructed through interactions between individual members of one's own group as well as with those of different groups. Online, youth are more able to censor or ignore alternative opinions, and therefore, find it easier to accept norms that are intolerable to general society, for better or worse. According to Landry and colleagues,[5] the anonymous nature of social media may "have negative health consequences due to a false belief of privacy leading to more provocative behavior and discussion around drinking, sex, violence, suicide ideation, and bullying, coupled with less parental monitoring." Youth with less adult supervision tend to engage more with screen media. Those who spend more time interacting with peers online, as evidenced by hyper-texting (ie, as sending or receiving more than 120 messages per day) or hyper-networking (ie, spending 3 or more hours per day on social networking sites), engage in more behaviors risky to their health and report poorer health.[11] Seventy-six percent of hyper-texters and 72% of hyper-networkers send messages or photographs they would not want their parents to see, and 56% use texting or social networking sites to plan a physical meeting free of parental supervision, often to drink alcohol (41.5%) or have sex (27.4%). The teens most likely to engage in hyper-texting and hyper-networking are those who identify as minorities, whose parents have less education, and who live in homes without a father.[11] Hyper-texters are at higher risk for sexual behavior, whereas parental monitoring, measured by knowledge of the teen's whereabouts, is protective.[5]

CO-CREATED REALITIES

Adolescent engagement with social media may be best understood as a coconstructed reality, as explained by Underwood and Ehrenreich.[4] Through social interactions and using search engines that tailor results via users' preferences, adolescents co-create their online environment. The online world of adolescents is intimately connected with their offline social world.[6] Online social interactions influence adolescents' self-concept, through posts and comments, browsing social media feeds, monitoring others' social activity, sharing thoughts, as well as receiving peer feedback via the amount and quality of "friends," followers, "likes," and comments.[4]

Adolescents actively, but unconsciously, refine self-identity through observing and interacting with peers both online and off. Youth experiment with different parts of their identity via expressing themselves, exploring others, as well as establishing and maintaining relationships.[5] Social media feeds an inherit appetite of youth: to connect with peers in order to explore themselves.[4] Social media can be an important vehicle for adolescents to understand how they fit into various peer groups. The ability to instantly interact with peer groups at any time engages many adolescents in continuous self-appraisal, gauged by how many friends they have, how many and what kind of comments they receive, and how they compare with peers in these measures.

NEWS MEDIA COVERAGE AND PERCEPTIONS OF RACE

In recent years, multiple incidents involving police have led to injury or death of African Americans. These tragedies have been the subject of extensive media coverage, bringing mainstream public attention to the issue of race relations in America. Similar to the trial of O.J. Simpson for the murder of his ex-wife Nicole Brown 20 years ago, there is a wide gap in attitudes toward these incidents between different racial and ethnic groups. In 2015, the Kaiser Family Foundation and CNN surveyed 2000 Americans to gauge attitudes about discrimination and racism. The results were representative of the US adult population, although responses of some groups such as Asian Americans were excluded from the analyses because they were not numerous enough to be statistically significant.

Most African Americans surveyed indicated the major reasons for recent protests were anger over the following:

1. The treatment of African Americans by the police (81%),
2. How government officials handled the incidents (73%), and
3. Poverty and lack of opportunity in some neighborhoods (61%).

Although most European Americans and Hispanic Americans agreed that these factors were a reason for protests, they were less likely to consider each a major reason. These incidents involving police and African Americans brought about the Black Lives Matter movement, which is supported by 58% of African Americans but only 35% of the general public.[12] Of note, 1 in 5 African Americans and Hispanic Americans report suffering unfair treatment by the police in the past 30 days, compared with just 3% of European Americans, which may engender greater support for the movement among African Americans. Thirteen percent of African Americans report having attended a Black Lives Matter event, compared with 4% of European Americans and Hispanic Americans.

The Kaiser Family Foundation/CNN Survey found that racism continues to be a reality for African Americans and Hispanic Americans. A third of adult African Americans report having been victims of racial discrimination at some point, and 45% endorse having been afraid their life was in danger because of their race. Fifty-three percent indicated having been treated unfairly in the last month alone. Among Hispanic Americans, 26% state that they have been discriminated against; 20% felt their life was in danger because of their ethnicity, and 36% report being treated unfairly in the last month because of ethnicity. In contrast, only 11% of European Americans indicated experiencing discrimination, 27% having been afraid their life was in danger because of their race or ethnicity, and 15% having been treated unfairly in the last 30 days because of these factors. Sixty-four percent of Americans feel that racial tensions have increased in the past 10 years, but only 23% feel that tensions have increased in their local community. African Americans (66%) and Hispanic Americans (64%) are more likely than Americans overall (49%) to classify racism as a big problem. Racism is now considered a problem by more Americans than in 2011, when only 28% considered race relations a problem. The change may indicate that more visible news media coverage of the issue increases public concern.[12]

Many communities in the United States continue to reflect racial imbalance and lack of diversity. Only 37% of European Americans indicate that there are people of a different race in their neighborhood or they socialize with people a different race, compared with 72% of Hispanic Americans and 70% of African Americans. Higher-income African Americans and lower-income European Americans are more likely to live or socialize in diverse communities.[12] This separation of races in America likely contributes to misunderstandings between ethnic and racial groups.

Considering the separation of many Americans into ethnically and racially homogenous communities, especially in rural areas and in the country's center, many European Americans have exposure to those of different races and ethnicities only through the media. Media portrayals therefore inform how such individuals understand those of other racial/ethnic groups and may contribute to a sense of "otherness," especially when these representations are caricatures or one dimensional. For members of a minority group, limited exposure to media characters that are "like them" may poorly reflect the complex social reality they experience from interactions with people in their defined social group, leading to a warped social identification. Geographic separation of various groups impairs communication and resolution regarding differences of opinion, so group differences as portrayed in the media can take on an exaggerated importance. As the 2 largest minority groups in the United States, African Americans and Hispanic Americans could expect the mainstream media to fairly portray members of these groups, and to be well represented as characters, writers, producers, and directors, which unfortunately is not a reality. About 7 in 10 African Americans and Hispanic Americans feel the news and entertainment media portray people of their racial and ethnic background accurately at least some of the time. However, 31% of African Americans and 24% of Hispanic Americans say they are never or rarely portrayed accurately, compared with 14% of European Americans.[12]

FROM RACIST STATEMENTS TO HATE CRIMES

Racism is an unfortunate reality that affects all Americans, particularly for racial and ethnic minorities. Racist remarks and micro-aggressions are insidious examples of a continuum that extends to extremist groups and hate crime. Hate groups in the United States have recently received greater media attention, because members of such groups have spoken out and protested publicly in response to events such as the presidential election, divisive rhetoric involved with the campaign, the removal of Confederate monuments in New Orleans and other Southern cities, and a commission by the mayor of Richmond to reassess that city's Confederate monuments. The Southern Poverty Law Center defines hate groups as those with "beliefs or practices that attack or malign an entire class of people, typically for their immutable characteristics." The Center indicates that as of July 1, 2017, 917 hate groups were active in the United States, and in 2013, approximately 260,000 reported and unreported hate crimes took place nationally.[13] There is little evidence regarding what drives hate crimes, although economic hardship may be related.[14] Surprisingly, there is also little evidence to indicate whether an increase in hate groups leads to an increase in hate crimes.[14] Even as the number of hate groups have increased between 2002 and 2020, the number of hate crimes decreased slightly, although the considerable media coverage these events garner risks misleading the public into thinking otherwise (eg, the events of San Bernardino and Orlando).[14]

Students at Humboldt State University tallied geotagged tweets that contained homophobic, racist, or anti-disability slurs in the United States between June 2012 and April 2013.[4] This project was inspired by an increase in hate speech following President Obama's reelection. The students read each individual tweet to determine if the slur it contained was used in a positive, negative, or neutral way. They then plotted the resulting data in a map called the "Geography of Hate." Researcher and geographer Monica Stephens writes: "debates around online bullying and the censorship of hate speech prompted us to examine how social media has become an important conduit for hate speech, and how particular terminology used to degrade a minority group is expressed geographically. As we've documented in a variety of cases, the virtual spaces of social media are intensely tied to particular virtual space in the offline world, and as this work shows, the geography of online hate speech is no different." They determined 150,000 tweets contained a slur with a hateful connotation. The report notes that probably only about 1.5% of all hateful tweets were geotagged, because most tweets are made by users who are not logged into location services.

The results showed a disproportionate number of hateful tweets came from the Midwest and the Southeastern United States, which may indicate that hateful ideology is more active in these regions.[15] Considering the populations and histories of these regions, it is interesting to ponder why residents of these areas in particular make more of these comments, as opposed to areas that may be more racially and ethnically homogenous or diverse. A complex discussion of this data is beyond the scope of this article; it seems likely that the interplay between local history, population, and culture affects the frequency of online hate speech in particular areas.

ONLINE VERSUS OFFLINE RACISM

Discriminatory experiences can have a lasting impact on youth development. Up to 94% of African American, Hispanic American, and Asian American youth have experienced discrimination associated with their racial or ethnic identity.[16] Like any other social institution, the Internet both reflects and shapes the prejudices of perpetrators. Online anonymity decreases the inhibiting effect of social norms and possibility of repercussions that traditionally constrain cruelty in social interactions. Online interactions are often accompanied by psychological and emotional detachment, creating an atmosphere in which users who make racist and other hurtful statements feel little or no accountability.[17] Due in part to this detachment from reality, explicit racist speech is more commonplace online. Individuals may feel freer to make discriminatory or racist statements because of ineffective Web site moderation, increased anonymity, and the distance offered by interacting online.[18] Earlier investigators hoped that discrimination would be rare online, mitigating the effects of discrimination minorities experience offline, but recent studies have found that discrimination occurs online as well, in new forms.[19]

Keum and Miller[18] highlight several factors that distinguish online from offline racism. Online racism is more pervasive, due to the abundance of racist content that is often inadvertently encountered. Racist messages, photographs, and videos are constantly posted and shared online, where they are easily found. Regular exposure to online racist messages, whether minor or major, local or distant, can cause racism to seem even more commonplace than it is. The Internet provides ready access to a vast number of vicarious experiences of racism, the extent of which one is unlikely to encounter offline. The sheer volume of these experiences documented online is a potent discrimination-related stressor.

The removal of online racist messages often requires an involved process and is typically left undone, so such content is often preserved indefinitely. Racist incidents are often shared, retweeted, and commented on, which compounds the resulting audience and may result in reexposure. Therefore, online racism is not bound to a specific point in time and may be reexperienced through repeated contact. For heavy Internet users, recurring exposure to discrimination may be especially harmful.[18] Vicarious exposure to discrimination is associated with feelings of helplessness and anger.[20] Encountering online discrimination is associated with depression, anxiety, lower academic motivation, and problematic behaviors.[19]

Tynes and colleagues[21] reviewed 38 half-hour transcripts of teen chat rooms and found that 37 contained at least one racial/ethnic utterance, most of which had a neutral or positive valence. Fifty-nine percent of transcripts from chat rooms lacking monitors included negative racial/ethnic discourse, compared with 19% of those with monitors. European American teens were as likely to be victims of racial attacks as other adolescents. Hispanic American participants endured 16 attacks of a racist nature in online discourse, European Americans 13, African Americans 8, biracial teens 2, and Native Americans 1. These chat rooms were not created for discussions on race, so the frequency of race-related comments confirms that race is a significant aspect of the adolescent identity and focus. In visual chat rooms, biracial teenagers were excluded from one or both racial groups unless they identified with one or the other.[6] In nonvisual chat rooms, biracial teens were more accepted. Most racial discussions in chat rooms were either positive or neutral in tone, although negative racial attitudes and behaviors were found as well.[6]

Adolescents often encounter stereotyping and racist comments online, but may lack the media literacy to assess the source.[22] Hate group Web sites sometimes have ambiguous names and are easily mistaken for factual sites, while conveying misinformation intending to disparage a race. These "cloaked sites" exist to spread racist ideology. Youth are often poorly able to differentiate fact and fiction and may accept hateful messages as truthful rather than propaganda.[16]

Tynes[19] reviewed surveys, interviews, and samples of online experiences of 340 sixth through 12th grade students. The study identified incidents of discrimination, defined as denigrating or excluding others on the basis of race or ethnicity "through the use of symbols, voice, video, images, text and graphic representations." Online discrimination was directly experienced by 42% of minority students within the first year of the study, 55% in the second, and 58% in the third. Discrimination was experienced vicariously by 64% of minority youth in the first year, 69% in the second, and 68% in the third. Examples of discrimination included: racial epithets; untrue statements, stereotyping, implicitly racist statements; racist jokes; symbols of hate (eg, the Confederate flag), threats of physical harm or death; and representations or photographs of dead black bodies. The most common direct incident was being sent a racist image, and the most common vicarious incident was witnessing rude or mean remarks about a person's ethnicity. The least common events were exclusion from a site (9%–13% over 3 years) and threats of violence (7%–13% over 3 years). Discrimination was most likely to occur on social networking sites or via text messaging.[19] Encountering racial discrimination online has become a typical experience of adolescence and bears significant implications.

Media depictions of minority characters also contribute to discrimination. Several studies of popular media have found that African American characters are often portrayed engaging in violent behaviors, particularly in video games.[23] European American violent video game players using an African American avatar demonstrate stronger negative attitudes toward African Americans, such as linking African Americans to weapon use.[24] Furthermore, evidence suggests that European American players playing as a racially stereotyped African American video game character subsequently have more negative perceptions of African Americans and feel less support for African Americans.[25]

EFFECTS OF RACISM ON IDENTITY FORMATION

Racism is not just a rare phenomenon for Americans of racial and ethnic minorities; it permeates society and colors everyday social interactions. Interpersonal discrimination is a common experience with negative effects on the physical and mental health of minorities, especially African Americans.[26] Dealing with racism on a regular or daily basis frequently causes emotional distress. A constant barrage of negativity directed at one's identity can cause depressive symptoms, including impatience, irritability, hopelessness, reduced self-regulation, and disinterest in long-term goals.[26] Many studies link racism with internalizing and externalizing disorders. Involvement in disrespectful or abusive relationships can engender the belief that others are untrustworthy, with hostile and selfish intentions. These views may persist in inappropriate situations and negatively shape one's behavioral responses.[27]

PROTECTIVE FACTORS

A primary task of families and communities is to prepare children to function in society. Effective socialization teaches children the values and rules of society and how to locate themselves in the social structure. As youth explore their identities and interact with peers, their family values are present, consciously or otherwise. Effective socialization gives youth the necessary skills to function in society and form a protective identity that can withstand negative social interactions.[26] In the case of racial and ethnic minorities, socialization includes promoting pride in one's minority status and learning how to deal with racism and prejudice.[28] This ethnic-racial socialization incorporates the aforementioned social creativity and social competition, because individuals develop pride despite a "devalued" status in the larger society and learn when and how to challenge the status quo. Parents and communities must help children maintain a positive identity and cope with hostility, which is based in part on racism.[26]

Cultural socialization consists of "parental practices that teach children about their racial or ethnic heritage; that promotes cultural customs and traditions; and that promote children's cultural, racial, and ethnic pride, either deliberately or implicitly." Examples include talking about important historical and cultural figures; exposing children to culturally relevant books, artifacts, music, and stories; and celebrating cultural holidays.[28] These practices can help buffer against the absence of minority tradition or overt denigration of the minority in the larger mainstream culture. Cultural socialization in African Americans, for example, has been linked to higher self-esteem, higher academic achievement, more positive views of African Americans, and fewer externalizing and internalizing problems.[29]

In addition to cultural socialization, minority parents can prepare their children for bias in mainstream society and how to deal with its manifestations. Parents and caregivers can anticipate exposure to various social situations and explain strategies likely to help, enhancing children's capacity to cope with them. The few studies examining the effects of this preparation for bias indicate mixed results: higher self-esteem and lower depressive symptoms, but also lower academic performance, increased experience of stigmatization, and more frequent conflicts.[30] Preparation for bias warns youth they may face discrimination, making it less likely that if it occurs they are unprepared, misinterpreted, or feel alone, and provides adaptive coping strategies, possibly bolstering resilience.[26] This preparation involves a delicate balance of expectations, however, for an overemphasis on bias without supportive parenting and cultural socialization may lead to self-fulfilling expectations of hostility in relationships, lack of trust, and an overall sense of cynicism. Therefore, preparation for bias should be done in the context of cultural socialization and supportive, authoritative parenting in order to maximize the possibility of success while maintaining positive relationships.[26]

Several studies have consistently found a positive association between ethnic identity and self-esteem. Both factors are protective against the anxiety-provoking effects of online racial discrimination for African American adolescents.[31] Racial/ethnic identity can be an important strength for minority youth: minimizing the negative effects of discrimination and preventing the internalization of negative stereotypes. Having a positive impression of one's racial/ethnic group is associated with better psychological functioning and minimizes the negative impact of racism.[16] Youth with a positive impression of their ethnic group may better evaluate critical or cruel comments. This idea is consistent with Erikson's theory that greater clarity and commitment regarding identity provide a sense of connectedness, which promotes adjustment.[32,33]

One manner in which individuals of devalued minority groups have found to promote a positive sense of self is to connect with other group members through Web sites, private social media groups, and gaming guilds. These online affiliations can help create a sense of belonging, understanding, and safety in what can be a harsh and critical world. For example, African American women playing online video games have reported experiencing prevalent linguistic profiling and subsequent racism and often mitigate this impact by gaming in ethnically-like female groups.[23] By gathering with an accepting group in a semi-private "safe space," individuals can recharge and be themselves without worrying about negative judgment related to their group membership. Such groups can provide a reprieve from negative experiences related to discrimination or misunderstanding between groups, but can risk becoming an echo chamber as well.

Ethnic-racial identity develops through exploration (learning about one's ethnic-racial group), resolution (understanding what membership to this group means in one's life), and affirmation (the affect connected with group membership). This process has been shown to promote positive adjustment and protect against the effects of discrimination, leading to positive outcomes despite the context of risk.[34] The exploration of what it means to belong to one's racial-ethnic group through understanding its history, resolving its differing representations, and affirming its positive characteristics can give one a sense of agency and purpose. The likelihood of experiencing discrimination online is high, so caregivers and professionals should help prepare minority youth for this eventuality while guiding their choices to minimize exposure. In addition, caregivers and professionals should help prepare youth of all ethnicities and races to be wary of stereotypes, simplistic characterizations of "the other" and to recognize that all people share much in common beyond simple group identification.

SUMMARY AND RECOMMENDATIONS FOR PROFESSIONALS

As screen media in its many forms continues to gain influence in the lives of youth, caretakers and professionals are often frustrated in the desire to steer them toward positive media choices. Guidance and monitoring by parents and caregivers significantly influence the online interactions and content that youth experience. It is imperative that caregivers understand what media their children or teens engage in, share an ongoing dialogue on the content, and limit content and access when necessary. Youth should be exposed to material that is appropriate to intellectual development in a graded manner over time, which will allow them a healthy understanding of media content, which can be productively incorporated into their lives.

Youth will likely witness racism and discrimination in their online as well as offline lives. Caregivers and professionals have a duty to model appropriate behavior and offer guidance on acceptable conduct toward others. Caregivers and professionals should maintain an active dialogue with children and teens concerning interactions with others and place limits on immoral, unhealthy, or risky behavior. This dialogue should include discussion of discrimination and direction regarding how to handle the situation, whether the youth finds him or herself a bystander, victim, or perpetrator. This discussion should be done with care to avoid instilling a general mistrust of others, allowing for healthy, positive relationships with others regardless of their group membership.

Child psychiatrists and mental health professionals must recognize that racism is a fact of life, online as well as offline. We should stay informed about current issues regarding discrimination, be prepared to discuss it with our patients as they experience or perpetuate the problem, and guide families through the fallout. Professionals can assist parents in preparing patients for such bias, and promoting positive identity formation, ethnic and cultural pride, and a sense of agency in their lives. Youth are often unable to distinguish racist propaganda and fake news from reliable information, so caregivers and professionals must teach youth to discern the difference, steering them toward factual sources. Caregivers and professionals can also advocate for schools to teach these skills that youth may better judge for themselves.

Finally, child psychiatrists and mental health professionals should recognize that only with a change of the status quo will life improve for all patients and promote social competition in any number of ways. One should encourage youth to maintain supports both inside and outside their racial/ethnic group, focusing on those with whom they can share their authentic selves. With such companions, youth will best mitigate effects of discrimination and navigate both positive and negative experiences of life.

REFERENCES

1. Rideout V. The common sense consensus: media use by tweens and teens. San Francisco (CA): Common Sense Media, Inc; 2015. Available at: CSM_TeenTween_MediaCensus_FinalWebVersion_1.pdf.
2. Rideout V, Foehr U, Roberts D. Generation M2: media in the lives of 8- to 18-year-olds. Kaiser Family Foundation; 2010. p. 1–101.
3. Lenhart A, Duggan M, Perrin A, et al. Teens, social media & technology overview. Pew Research Center; 2015.
4. Underwood M, Ehrenreich S. The power and the pain of adolescents' digital communication: cyber victimization and the perils of lurking. Am Psychol 2017; 72:144–58.
5. Landry M, Turner M, Vyas A, et al. Social media and sexual behavior among adolescents: is there a link? JMIR Public Health Surveill 2017;3:e28.
6. Subrahmanyam K, Smahel D, Greenfield P. Connecting developmental constructions to the internet: identity presentation and sexual exploration in online teen chat rooms. Dev Psychol 2006;42:395–406.
7. Jackson LA, Fitzgerald HE, Zhao Y, et al. Information technology (IT) use children's psychological well-being. Cyberpsychol Behav 2008;11:755–7.
8. Ellemers N, Haslam A. Social identity theory. In: Van Lange PAM, Kruglanski AW, Tory Higgins E, editors. Handbook of theories of social psychology, vol. 2. SAGE Publications; 2011. p. 379–98.
9. Tajfel H, Turner J. The social identity theory of intergroup behavior. In: Austin W, Worchel S, editors. Psychology of intergroup relations. 2nd edition. Chicago: Nelson-Hall; 1986. p. 2–74.
10. Erikson E. Childhood and society. Eight stages of man. New York: W. W. Norton; 1950. p. 247–74.
11. Frank S. Hyper-texting and hyper-networking: examining why too much texting and social networking is associated with teen risk behavior. 141st APHA Annual Meeting and Exposition. Boston, November 2-6 2013 (November 5). 2013.
12. DiJulio B, Norton M, Jackson S, et al. Kaiser Family Foundation/CNN Survey of Americans on Race. 2015. p. 1–29. #8805 Available at: www.kff.org. Accessed July 10, 2016.
13. Southern Poverty Law Center. Southern Poverty Law Center hate map. Southern Poverty Law Center; 2017. Available at: https://www.splcenter.org/hate-map. Accessed July 1, 2017.

14. Ryan M, Leeson P. Hate groups and hate crime. Int Rev Law Econ 2011;31: 256–62.
15. Stephens M. FAQ geography of hate. Floating Sheep; 2013. Available at: http://www.floatingsheep.org/2013/05/faq-geography-of-hate.html. Accessed July 15, 2017.
16. Tynes BM, Rose CA, Hiss S, et al. Virtual environments, online racial discrimination and adjustment among a diverse, school-based sample of adolescents. Int J Gaming Comput Mediat Simul 2016;6:1–16.
17. Suler J. The online disinhibition effect. Cyberpsychol Behav 2004;7(3):321–6.
18. Keum BT, Miller MJ. Racism in the digital era: development and initial validation of the Perceived Online Racism Scale. J Couns Psychol 2017;64:310–24.
19. Tynes BM. Online racial discrimination: a growing problem for adolescents. American Psychological Association: Psychological Science Agenda: Science Brief; 2015. Available at: http://www.apa.org/science/about/psa/2015/12/online-racial-discrimination.aspx. Accessed July 1, 2017.
20. Harrell SP. A multidimensional conceptualization of racism-related stress: implications for the well-being of people of color. Am J Orthopsychiatry 2000;70(1): 42–57.
21. Tynes B, Reynolds L, Greenfield PM. Adolescence, race, and ethnicity on the internet: a comparison of discourse in monitored vs. unmonitored chat rooms. J Appl Dev Psychol 2004;25:667–84.
22. Daniels J, Hughey MW. Good ideas and new dilemmas: hurdles for studying racism at online news sites. Paper presented at Annual Meetings of the American Sociological Association. Denver, CO, August 16, 2012.
23. Burgess MCR, Dill KE, Stermer SP, et al. Playing with prejudice: the prevalence and consequences of racial stereotyping in video games. Media Psychol 2011; 14:289–311.
24. Yang GS, Gibson B, Lueke AK, et al. Effects of avatar race in violent video games on racial attitudes and aggression. Soc Psychol Personal Sci 2014;5:698–704.
25. Behm-Morawitz E, Hoffswell J, Chen SW. The virtual threat effect: a test of competing explanations of the effects of racial stereotyping in video games on players' cognitions. Cyberpsychol Behav Soc Netw 2016;19:308–13.
26. Burt C, Simons R, Gibbons FX. Racial discrimination, ethnic-racial socialization, and crime: a micro-sociological model of risk and resilience. Am Sociol Rev 2012;77:648–77.
27. Dodge KA. Translational science in action: hostile attributional style and the development of aggressive behavior problems. Dev Psychopathol 2006;18: 791–814.
28. Hughes D. Correlates of African-American and Latino parents' messages to children about ethnicity and race: a comparative study of racial socialization. Am J Community Psychol 2003;31:15–33.
29. Bynim MS, Burton E, Thomaseo BC. Racism experiences and psychological functioning in African-American college freshman: is racial socialization a buffer? Cultur Divers Ethnic Minor Psychol 2007;13:64–71.
30. Stevenson HC, Reed J, Bodison P, et al. Racism stress management: racial socialization beliefs and the experience of depression and anger in African-American youth. Youth Soc 1997;29:197–222.
31. Tynes BM, Umaña-Taylor AJ, Rose CA, et al. Online racial discrimination and the protective function of ethnic identity and self-esteem for African-American adolescents. Dev Psychol 2012;48:343–55.

32. Umaña-Taylor AJ, Tynes BM, Toomey RB, et al. Latino adolescents' perceived discrimination in online and offline settings: an examination of cultural risk and protective factors. Dev Psychol 2015;51:87–100.
33. Gray KL. Intersecting oppressions and online communities: examining the experiences of women of color in Xbox Live. Information, Communities and Society 2012;15:411–28.
34. Masten AS, Desjardins CD, McCormick CM, et al. The significance of childhood competence and problems for adult success in work: a developmental cascade analysis. Dev Psychopathol 2010;22:679–94.

Risky Business
Talking with Your Patients About Cyberbullying and Sexting

Elizabeth K. Englander, PhD

KEYWORDS

• Bullying • Cyberbullying • Sexting • Social media

KEY POINTS

- Physicians who treat children and adolescents today are more aware than ever that digital technology use can be associated with several new social problems, notably, cyberbullying (repetitive, deliberate digital cruelty) and sexting (the sending of nude photos to a peer using digital technology).
- This article reviews existing research on both behaviors and presents new research that explores relatively neglected areas of concern: cyberbullying and cell phone ownership among children aged 8 to 11 year old, and outcomes following sexting, including positive and mixed outcomes.
- Two samples are studied, the first consisting of 4584 elementary school-aged children, and the second of 1332 college freshman, both studied between 2014 and 2017.
- Findings were as follows: owning a cell phone significantly increased the risk of becoming involved in cyberbullying, both as a victim and as a perpetrator, among children in grades 3, 4, and 5, but especially among children in grades 3 and 4.
- Among college freshman who engaged in sexting, 61% reported no outcomes of any kind. Of the 39% who did report consequences following sexting, 19% reported negative outcomes only (ie, feeling worse or embarrassed, or being bullied or harassed), 13% reported only positive outcomes (ie, an improved relationship with the picture's recipient or increased self-confidence), and 7% reported both negative and positive outcomes (mixed).

INTRODUCTION

Pediatric practitioners today are more aware than ever of the importance of addressing public health threats with patients and parents. Issues such as weight, automobile safety, and drug and alcohol use are now a standard part of many well-child visits. But newer threats to public health are treated with more trepidation. Most physicians who treat children and adolescents today are aware of certain

Disclosure Statement: The author has no disclosure.
Massachusetts Aggression Reduction Center, Bridgewater State University, Maxwell Library, 201, Bridgewater, MA 02325, USA
E-mail address: englander@marccenter.net

Child Adolesc Psychiatric Clin N Am 27 (2018) 287–305
https://doi.org/10.1016/j.chc.2017.11.010
1056-4993/18/© 2017 Elsevier Inc. All rights reserved.

childpsych.theclinics.com

risks posed by digital technology use, notably, cyberbullying (repetitive, deliberate digital cruelty) and sexting (the sending of nude photos to a peer using digital technology). Although awareness of these issues has grown, 2 significant gaps in the research literature still limit a practitioner's ability to successfully treat patients and help them avoid unnecessary risk. First, both cyberbullying and sexting are still viewed as problems of adolescence; therefore, related screening and preventative education are often neglected among younger children. Second, sexting may be viewed as a monolithic activity resulting from emotional difficulties, whereas newer data suggest that different youth sext for different reasons and experience different outcomes. To be effective in discussions with youth, new findings concerning these issues must be taken into account.

This article reviews cyberbullying and sexting separately. Within each section, background research ("Previous research") is briefly reviewed and, when available, new findings ("New research") are presented that can help to fill gaps in the literature and thus guide conversations with patients. The "New research" sections report data from 2 recent studies conducted at the Massachusetts Aggression Reduction Center (MARC). The first study, examining cyberbullying in young children, surveyed 4584 students in grades 3, 4, and 5 between 2014 and 2016.[a] This sample was drawn from children in Massachusetts, Virginia, Oregon, New York, and New Jersey. In the second study, examining the phenomenon of sexting, 1332 college freshmen at a medium-sized public university were studied between 2014 and 2017. These subjects were surveyed anonymously about their high school social experiences, including digital interactions, sexting, and coerced or pressured sexting. These 2 new studies provide valuable information that can help practitioners feel confident in their ability to discuss these digital technology risks with patients.

CYBERBULLYING

Cyberbullying is strongly associated with mental health disorders and contributes to negative outcomes such as suicide.

Cyberbullying has no universally accepted definition, but most researchers define it as a form of intentional, repeated aggression, using electronic forms of contact, such as text messaging and social media.[1] Cyberbullying and digital forms of harassment are serious public health issues that have been linked to a variety of mental and physical health problems.[2,3] Problems caused by cyberbullying include anger, frustration, humiliation, social isolation, and depression. Cyberbullying has also been associated with other affective disorders and with substance abuse.[4–8] The data detailing the relationship between cyberbullying and health problems are not only cross-sectional; a few longitudinal studies

---

[a] The electronic survey asked children to self-report regarding their ownership of cell phones and their experiences with bullying and cyberbullying victimization and perpetration. Bullying was defined as cruel acts, words, postings, pictures, or messages between children. Children were asked about the repetitive nature of any related behaviors they reported. Wording was simple, age-appropriate, and piloted to maximize comprehension. After the pilot, minor alterations were made to some questions. Cronbach's alpha for the 7 items measuring involvement in bullying and cyberbullying was $\alpha = .76$ (indicating adequate reliability). Analyses were completed using SPSS (Statistical Package for the Social Sciences), version 23. Chi square tests with Bonferroni corrections were used to compare cell phone owners with nonowners (chi square values using the continuity correction are listed in this report). In addition, binary logistic regression tested a model in which cell phone ownership and traditional bullying involvement predicted cyberbullying behaviors and victimization.

with prospective data have found that cyberbullying predicted depression months or years later.[9–11] Cyberbullying can exacerbate physical health problems and lead to suicidal ideation.[1,12] Both perpetrators and victims are at much higher risk for health problems and behavioral disorders.[13]

Cyberbullying Prevalence

Previous research

Cyberbullying seems to be less common than traditional bullying, but not rare, although prevalence rates vary across studies. Studies published in the last 5 years include a metaanalysis of 80 studies from several countries, which found that the average prevalence rate was approximately 15%.[14] A study that examined more than 20,000 high school students found similar cyberbullying victimization rates (almost 16%); further, many victims of cyberbullying were also victims of traditional bullying.[15] Other recent research has found higher rates; a study of 1141 students aged 6 to 11 years old found that 25% reported being cyberbullied at least monthly.[16] Finally, a 2011 retrospective study of several hundred college students found that 41% reported being victims of cyberbullying at some point during the 4 years of high school.[17] The different prevalence rates seem to be attributable, at least in part, to 3 factors: the different definitions used in the research, the variable age of the subjects (eg, 10-year-olds vs 16-year-olds), and the type and range of digital behaviors queried in the study.[18]

A few studies published since 2011 have reported data on children aged 11 years or younger separately from other age groups. Prevalence rates for this younger age group in these few studies ranged between 18% and 27%. One study of 660 Mid-western American children in grades 3, 4, and 5 found that almost 18% reported cyberbullying victimization and, further, that this was related to victimization in school through traditional bullying.[19] A study of Canadian 10- to 12-year-olds (grades 4, 5, and 6) found that 27% reported in June that they had experienced cyberbullying victimization during the preceding school year.[20] A study of British children (116 boys and 104 girls) aged 7 to 11 years found that 21% self-identified as cybervictims and 5% reported being a cyberbully.[21] Finally, a study of 372 Turkish children aged 8 to 11 years old found that 27% of the children studied were victims of cyberbullying, 18% reported being cyberbullies, and an additional 15% reported being both cyber-bullies and cyber-victims.[22]

New research

New findings are consistent with previous research. Almost one-quarter (24%) of all grade 3, 4, and 5 students (25.7% of boys and 22.4% of girls) reported experiencing some type of digital cruelty, either cyberbullying or transient, less serious, and 1-time incidents of digital cruelty. Overall, 5.8% of elementary school students in this sample also admitted to cyberbullying their peers. Cyberbullying may once have been a problem reserved for adolescence but that is clearly no longer the case.

Fig. 1 presents the short form of the Bullying and Cyberbullying Checklist, developed by the MARC and the Bullying and Cyberbullying Prevention and Advocacy Collaborative (BACPAC) at Boston Children's Hospital. It is designed as a screening device to guide practitioner queries during a behavioral assessment, for use with children younger than 12 years old. The full version, which can be downloaded at http://www.MARCcenter.org, includes a guide for reviewing these issues with parents, and ways that a practitioner can help a child who is a victim of bullying or cyberbullying.

MARC/BACPAC Pediatric Questionnaire:
BULLYING & CYBERBULLYING

Date of Office Visit: _____

Gender: Male ☐   Female ☐

Child's age: [_____] years : [_____] months

Child's grade: _____ IEP? Yes ☐ No ☐

Neurodev / Psych Dx (if established): _____

Parent Present during interview?

Yes ☐ No ☐

Subjective complaints
(eg, H/A, tics, sleep):

_____

_____

SECTION 1: SOCIAL SKILLS ASSESSMENT.
1. Are the kids in your school friendly?
2. Tell me about one child at your school who you like.
3. Who is your best friend in school? Do you ever play or see each other when you're NOT in school?

Note if the child states or suggests that he or she has no friends.

_____

SECTION 2: Cell Phone Use
4. Some kids your age have cell phones but some use their parents' or friends'. That's normal. Do you have your own cell phone?
   - IF YES: Do you carry it with you every day, to school?
   - Do you keep it in your room at night?
   - IF NO: How often do you take your parents' cell phone to school?

Make a note if the child has frequent or daily access to a cell phone.

_____

Assess for sleep deprivation:

_____

SECTION 3: Social Media Use (Note: minimum age by FTC Regulation is 13 y old)
5. Do you use Instagram, SnapChat, Musica.ly, AskFM, or other social media with your friends?
   - IF YES: Do you use it every day? Do you post messages / pictures?

Make a note if the child uses social media, and which app they use.

_____

Fig. 1. MARC and Bullying and Cyberbullying Prevention and Advocacy Collaborative (BAC-PAC) checklist. FTC, Federal Trade Commission; IEP, individualized education program; Neurodev/Psych Dx, Neurodevelopment or psychiatric diagnosis. (*Courtesy of* Elizabeth Englander, PhD, Peter C. Raffalli, MD, Bridgewater State University, Bridgewater, Massachusetts & Boston Children's Hospital, Boston, MA.)

Key question

Are experiences with cyberbullying common among elementary school children?

Key research finding

Between 20% and 25% of children younger than 12 years old have experienced cyberbullying victimization.

How this finding affects clinical practice

Because of its association with depression, anxiety, and other serious problems, cyberbullying should be explored as part of a behavioral health assessment.

SECTION 4: ASSESSMENT OF BULLYING OR CYBERBULLYING INVOLVEMENT

**BEGIN BY STATING: "You probably know that grownups today are very worried about bullying. I'd like to ask you a little bit about that, but I want to make sure you understand what I mean. When I ask about bullying, I mean another kid (or group of kids) who picks on someone or is mean to them *on purpose, over and over again* – not just one time."

1. Do you ever see bullying happen between kids? It could be at your school, on an app, OR online (like in a game)?

☐ YES   ☐ NO   NOTE: **It is unusual for a child to respond "no" to this question.**

2. Is there any one kid or a bunch of kids that pick on <u>you</u> or make <u>you</u> feel bad over and over again?

☐ Yes **(inquire as to the frequency) :** (___x daily; ___ times a week; ___times a month; ___times a year).

IF NO, SKIP TO END

IF YES....

Where does this happen? (check all that apply):

☐ classroom	☐ lunchroom	☐ hallways
☐ stairwell	☐ bathroom	☐ locker-room
☐ playground	☐ bus	☐ Website:
☐ App: _____	☐ Game: _____	
		☐ other:
		☐

What did he or she do to you? (check all that apply):

☐ MADE FUN OF ME	☐ KIDS LAUGHED	☐ NAME-CALLING
☐ RUMORS	☐ MADE UP LIES	☐ GOT ME IN TROUBLE
☐ PUSHED,SHOVED,HIT,THREW STUFF	☐ POSTED A PICTURE OF ME	
	☐ OTHER:	

RECORD ALL DETAILS OF BULLYING HERE:

Fig. 1. (*continued*).

Cell Phone Ownership

Previous research

In the United States, 8- to 10-year-olds experience almost 8 hours of media per day.[23] A nationally representative sample of American families with children 8 years old or younger revealed that the number of children who used mobile devices nearly doubled between 2011 and 2013 (from 38% to 72%). Young children are also increasingly the owners of mobile devices. A study of several thousand 8-year-olds in Massachusetts in 2011 found that 20% owned cell phones.[24] More recent studies in Europe have found that between 10% and 45% of 9- to 11-year-olds owned smartphones (with 1 notable outlier: Denmark, where an astonishing 70% of 9-year-olds own smartphones).[25]

3

3. It's very important that you understand that if you are being bullied that it is _never_ your fault. Bullying is wrong and people should _never_ bully others. Have you told anybody about the kids that are bothering you?

☐ Yes **(Who have you told? Circle: Peer / Friend / Parent / Teacher / Other)** :

_____

IF Yes.....Were the adults able to stop the bullying?

No. (How did they try to help?)	Yes. (What actions did they take that were helpful?)

Did talking about it make you feel better?
☐ **No ("That's ok. Sometimes talking does help though.")**
☐ **Yes**

4. "Sometimes it feels good just to talk about things. I wish you and I had more time to talk about it today. Would you like to have a chance to talk about it sometime soon?"

☐ Yes **(If "Yes," refer to:)**

_____
_____

IF NO.....
..."Would you like me to try to help? As your doctor, I can talk with the school officials and try to make sure that the bullying stops. While I cannot promise that everything will be better, I know that _if we do nothing_ the bullying will likely continue and probably get worse. I want you to be happy and safe at school – is it okay with you if I talk to your school about this?"

☐ Yes **(Who would you like me to talk to? Principal / Nurse / Counselor / Teacher / Other:**

Fig. 1. (_continued_).

New research

In the study being reported here, 49.6% of elementary students reported owning their own cell phone. Genders were very similar: 49.7% of boys and 49.5% of girls reported owning their own cell phone. Older students were significantly more likely to report ownership: 59.8% of fifth graders, 50.6% of fourth graders, and 39.5% of third graders reported owning their own cell phone.[b]

Key question

Do elementary school children own their own cell phones?

Key research finding

Approximately 40% of third graders, 50% of fourth graders, and 60% of fifth graders reported owning their own cell phone.

How this finding affects clinical practice

Because cell phone ownership in young children is now so common, its risks should be addressed with young patients and their caregivers.

---

[b] ($\chi^2 = 124.727$ [2], $P<.000$).

4

REVIEW WITH PARENTS/CAREGIVERS

Factors that may increase this child's risk of being involved in cyberbullying or bullying:
- Delayed or challenged social skills (see answers to SECTION 1)
- Cell phone ownership (see answers to SECTION 2)
- Is a device interrupting the child's sleep? (see answers to SECTION 3)
- Use of social media prior to age 13 (see answers to SECTION 3)

Has the child disclosed being a victim of bullying or cyberbullying? (see answers to SECTION 4)
- If YES, has the child spoken to a peer or friend?
- If YES, has the child spoken to an adult?
- What actions have peers or adults taken that were helpful?

Actions going forward:
- Encourage attention to social skills development if warranted (school programs; independent practitioners; extracurricular activities)
- Encourage parental discussions about social media, cell phone use, bullying and cyberbullying
    - Encourage consideration of parental control software (parents can check their child's cell phone provider for this)
    - Distribute materials to help with these discussions (parent downloads from WWW.MARCCENTER.ORG)
- Discussion actions to be taken if bullying or cyberbullying were disclosed
    - Contact school?
    - Encourage / facilitate social skills, friendships?
    - Refer for psychological counseling or support?
- Plan follow-up if bullying or cyberbullying were disclosed

5

GUIDE TO THE BULLYING/CYBERBULLYING CHECKLIST/INTERVIEW

WHEN A CHILD IS BEING BULLIED

THERE ARE THREE VENUES THROUGH WHICH YOU CAN HELP THIS CHILD:

- **BY GIVING THEM A "SAFE ADULT" AT SCHOOL THEY CAN ALWAYS SPEAK WITH (EG, THE SCHOOL NURSE, THE SCHOOL ADJUSTMENT COUNSELOR);**

- **BY GIVING THEIR PARENTS GUIDANCE ABOUT HOW TO COPE (THROUGH HANDOUTS, WEBSITES); AND**

- **BY OFFERING THEM SUPPORT FROM YOURSELF.**

**If child consents to your involvement, seek written parental consent to share information with the school in writing. The more details the child can provide as to who, what, where, how, the more power the school will have to act. Explain this to the child/parent and do your best to gently get details for your letter to the school. If child or parent will not consent to communication with school, provide advice / handouts (www.MARCcenter.org) to help the parent advocate themselves for their child with the school. Always document in your note the conversation in the office.

WEBSITES FOR PARENTS/TEACHERS/STUDENTS:

1. The **Massachusetts Aggression Reduction Center (MARC)**: www.MARCcenter.org

2. Bullying And Cyberbullying Prevention and Advocacy Collaborative (**BACPAC**) at Children's Hospital Boston: www.childrenshospital.org/BACPAC

3. Stop Bullying Now from the U.S. government: http://stopbullying.gov

Fig. 1. (continued).

Is There Any Increased Risk for Young Children in Owning Cell Phones?

Previous research

There are suggestions (based on both common sense and research evidence) that simply owning a cell phone seems to translate into increased time spent online and more use of social media.[26,27] Among adolescents, increased access and usage of digital technology may increase the odds of becoming a victim or perpetrator of cyberbullying.[28–31] Theoretically, increased access and use increases digital exposure to a potential cyberbully, in much the same way that greater exposure to a traditional aggressor can increase the odds of in-person victimization.[32,33]

New research

In this study of third, fourth, and fifth graders, cell phone owners were more likely to report experiencing digital cruelty from peers (28.2%) compared with nonowners (19.9%).[c] This relationship was true for both boys and girls,[d] and for all 3 grades.[e] Cell phone owners as a group were significantly more likely to report being a victim of cyberbullying specifically,[f] although that was only true for children in grades 3 and 4.[g]

Cell phone owners were also more likely to admit to cyberbullying others.[h] Cyberbullying behaviors were associated with cell phone ownership in all 3 grades (3, 4, and 5). More cell phone owners reported being a cyberbully compared with nonowners; this was true for all 3 grades.[i]

Of course, in the real world, children can be both cyberbullies and victims of cyberbullying. Children who were only cyberbullies, cyberbullies and cybervictims, and only cybervictims were all more likely to be cell phone owners in comparison with children who were uninvolved in cyberbullying.[j] However, this relationship was not true for fifth graders.

Key question

Is cell phone ownership in elementary school children associated with increased risk for cyberbullying involvement?

Key research finding

Among elementary school children, owning a cell phone was associated with an increased likelihood of both being a victim of cyberbullying, and of cyberbullying others. This was true for all elementary-aged children but most true for third and fourth graders.

How this finding affects clinical practice

Most parents are unaware of the link between cell phone ownership and cyberbullying. They should be made aware of this risk when they consider whether or not to permit their child to carry a cell phone daily (Table 1).

---

[c] ($\chi^2 = 43.669$ [1], $P<.000$).

[d] Boys ($\chi^2 = 11.49$ [1], $P<.001$); girls ($\chi^2 = 43.669$ [1], $P<.000$).

[e] Third graders ($\chi^2 = 23.626$ [1], $P<.000$); fourth graders ($\chi^2 = 13.674$ [1], $P<.000$); and fifth graders ($\chi^2 = 4.913$ [1], $P<.027$).

[f] ($\chi^2 = 12.626$ [1], $P<.000$).

[g] Grades 3 & 4: ($\chi^2 = 8.785$ [1], $P<.003$; $\chi^2 = 4.284$ [1], $P<.038$).

[h] ($\chi^2 = 28.206$ [1], $P<.000$).

[i] Third graders ($\chi^2 = 22.736$ [1], $P<.000$), fourth graders ($\chi^2 = 5.218$ [1], $P<.022$), and fifth graders ($\chi^2 = 3.903$ [1], $P<.048$).

[j] ($\chi^2 = 35.611$ [3], $P<.000$ and $\chi^2 = 35.611$ [3], $P<.000$).

Table 1
Prevalence of cell phone ownership among cyberbullies, cybervictims, and cyberbully victims

	Cyberbullies % (N)	Cyberbully Victims % (N)	Cybervictims % (N)	Uninvolved % (N)	Significance
Cell phone owners	64.6 (115)	67.4 (60)	55.2 (192)	48 (1906)	$P<.000$
3rd grade owners	59.7 (40)	73.1 (19)	46.6 (54)	37.2 (512)	$P<.000$
4th grade owners	62.5 (35)	63.6 (21)	57.6 (68)	49.2 (680)	$P<.032$
5th grade owners	72.7 (40)	66.7 (20)	61.4 (70)	58.9 (714)	$P = 0$

SEXTING

A second digital behavior that has emerged as potentially risky is sexting, the sending of nude or sexual texts, photos, or videos to a peer via digital technology. Sexting is not, of course, the only sexual use of the Internet. Other sexual uses include pornography, seeking factual sexual information, visiting virtual sex shops (purchasing goods), entertainment, seeking out sex therapists, and connecting with partners or potential partners.[34] Some uses even extend to criminal behavior.[35] However, legal challenges are not the only area of interest, particularly when children and adolescents are involved. Sexting may also entail social, psychosexual, and mental health risks. James and Khadr[36] (2016) emphasized the necessity of physicians assessing for sexting because the presence of sexting behaviors may at times indicate exploitation and can be linked to serious outcomes. That even children in seventh grade report sexting and associated health risks underscores the need for clinicians to ask patients about sexting.[37]

Sexting has been studied in a variety of forms (eg, sexualized text, photos, and videos) but, as with cyberbullying, there is no consensus definition. This has hampered the field but some conclusions are nevertheless beginning to emerge.

First: Sexting Is Neither Rare nor Ubiquitous

Previous research

Estimates of the frequency of sexting among youth range from 5% among middle schoolers to 44% of young adults.[38–40] The older subjects are, the higher their proportional involvement, at least through young adulthood. An MTV (Music Television) study found that 24% of 14- to 17-year-olds and 33% of 18- to 24-year-olds admitted having sexted; that pattern is typical.[41] Most estimates of the frequency of adolescent sexting neither fall below 10% nor exceed 40%, with clustering around the teens and low 20s percent. Klettke and colleagues[42] found only 6 studies that had examined adolescents using random or nationally representative samples. The prevalence estimates from these studies were between 10% and 16% (depending on which specific behaviors were examined). In every study examined, receiving was more common than sending. The potential significance of sending, versus receiving, a sext has not been specifically examined.

New research

Each year between 2014 and 2017, a higher percentage of subjects reported having sexted at some time in their lives. In 2014, 38.6% reported having sexted; by 2017, that percentage was 51.1%.

> *Key question*
>
> Is sexting frequent enough to consider discussing it with patients?
>
> *Key research finding*
>
> One-quarter to one-half of teens report having sexted. Sexting is being reported more frequently over the past few years.
>
> *How this finding affects clinical practice*
>
> Sexting may be the new first base. As with all emerging forms of sexuality, youth need to discuss risks and questions with their physicians.

Second: Sexting Is Not Confined to Adolescence

Previous research

Sexting occurs in middle school and among adults over 18 years of age.[39,40] One study found that poor outcomes were significantly more common among middle-school sexters, relative to their high-school counterparts.[43] In that study, youth who engaged in sexting while in middle school reported significantly higher rates of having sexted because of negative peer pressure, and regretting it after the picture was sent. Another study found that the middle school sexters were far more worried and depressed compared with their high school counterparts, and were more likely to report that they had no adults to talk to about sexting.[44]

> *Key Question*
>
> Does sexting occur before high school?
>
> *Key Research Finding*
>
> Sexting is less common among middle schoolers, but 10% to 15% seem to send nude photos. The emotional impact seems to be more negative among these preteens and young teenagers.
>
> *How this finding affects clinical practice*
>
> Sexting can be explored with preteens by asking questions about the inappropriate use and sharing of photos, including private photos.

Third: Media Reports of the Risks Associated with Sexting May Not Be Reliable

Previous research

One study showed that sexters had a higher number of sexual partners compared with nonsexters, but this was only true for females.[45,46] Another study found no association between sexting and high-risk sexual behaviors, such as age of first sexual intercourse and number of partners in the past 3 months.[47]

Contrary to many media reports, wide redistribution of sexts (nude or sexual photos or videos) and other dire sexting consequences may be exceptions rather than rules. Studies of youth and young adults who sext suggest that approximately 25% (or fewer) report that the pictures they sent were ultimately redistributed to others.[48-50] Research examining outcomes such as harassment or bullying by peers, lost opportunities, trouble with parents or school authorities, or having the picture posted online found such outcomes to be unusual, often endorsed by fewer than 5% of sexters.[46,51] Most sexters report that nothing happened after they sexted, either positive or negative.[46,51,52]

Key question

Is sexting a high-risk behavior?

Key research findings

Sexting is associated with sexual activity, but not necessarily with high-risk activity. Some of the highly publicized negative outcomes, such as redistribution or criminal prosecution, are actually rare and are not perceived by teens as likely.

How these findings affect clinical practice

The long-term impacts or consequences of sexting are unknown and negative consequences can occur even in the short term.

Motivations for Sexting

Previous research

Sexters are not a uniform group, and motivations, risk, and context vary significantly. Contrary to assumptions often expressed in the media, sexting is not uniformly associated with poor self-esteem or depression. Some studies have found a relationship between sexting and depression, even when gender, family status, and socioeconomic status were controlled.[47,53] Other studies have failed to find that association.[54]

Motivations to sext include enhancing intimacy or sexuality in a relationship, testing levels of trust, a partner's happiness or satisfaction, gaining attention or interest, and pressure from peers or from the recipient.[55] These motivations may differ between the genders. For example, female responders seem to be more likely to report feeling pressure to sext.[55,56]

The relationship between a sexter and the picture's recipient seems to be key, and sexting between established partners seems to be different than other types of sexting.[57,58] In a few studies, researchers noted that most sexters felt positively about the experience and that positive outcomes seem to be associated with sexting within established relationships.[51,59,60] The likelihood of a negative outcome seems to increase when sexters also report negative pressure to sext.[61]

Outcomes After Sexting

Previous research

Several studies have noted that most sexters report no outcomes or consequences following sexting.[46,61–63] However, most research focuses solely on negative outcomes.

New research

This study goes further in examining positive, negative, and mixed outcomes following sexting. More than half of the 1332 college freshman who had sexted (61%) reported that there were no outcomes or consequences after sending the picture. Of the sexters who did report consequences, 48% reported negative outcomes only, 18% reported both negative and positive outcomes, and 33% reported only positive outcomes. This study is among the few that reports positive outcomes following the sending of a nude picture.

One negative outcome dominated the findings: 74% of mixed outcome sexters and 83% of negative-only outcome sexters reported "feeling worse" or "embarrassed." **Table 2** reports the different outcomes studied and their frequencies among negative-only, positive-only, and mixed outcome sexters.

Key question

Does sexting inevitably result in negative consequences?

Key research finding

Approximately 6 in 10 sexters reported no consequences of any type. Of the 4 in 10 who did experience consequences, approximately half reported they were negative; however, another third reported only positive outcomes following sexting and 18% reported mixed outcomes (both positive and negative).

How this finding affects clinical practice

Physicians should discuss sexting with patients; however, do not assume that the aftermath is always negative. Be open-minded about the possible positive outcomes that might have occurred.

Pressure and Negative Outcomes

Previous research

Pressure to sext has been associated with negative outcomes following sexting.[61,64,65] More than a quarter of sexters in 2014 (27%) and 22% of sexters in 2015 reported that their nude picture had been forwarded via texting or posting online without their consent. Interestingly, this did not seem to occur primarily following the demise of established relationships; instead, it most often seemed to target sexters who declined to

Table 2
Different outcomes after sexting and their frequencies among negative-only, positive-only, and mixed-outcome sexters

	Positive-Only Outcomes (%)	Negative-Only Outcomes (%)	Mixed Outcomes (%)
Negative Outcomes			
Harassed or bullied	—	24	15
Someone broke up with me	—	4	—
Friends dumped me	—	2	8
Got in trouble with parents	—	14	28
Got in trouble at school	—	3	—
Avoided work or school	—	4	5
Lost an opportunity	—	0	3
Felt worse after	—	78	67
I was embarrassed	—	28	44
Picture posted online	—	10	3
Positive Outcomes			
Became closer in my relationship	40	—	18
Someone decided they liked me after they saw the picture	34	—	69
I became more popular	15	—	13
I felt more self-confident or better after sending the picture	44	—	26
Got a new boyfriend or girlfriend	9	—	18

date someone. Sexting before age 18 years, sexting to multiple persons, and sexting under pressure all increased the risk of unauthorized distribution. Pressured sexting is actually more common than voluntary just-for-fun sexting. As might be expected, subjects reported experiencing different degrees of pressure or coercion. Only a small proportion of sexting occurs in response to serious threats or because of intense fear. On the other hand, sexting at least partially because of peer pressure does seem to be very common. Male responders were more likely to sext multiple times and more likely to report that they sexted entirely because they wanted to. Female responders were more likely to report having sexted once and were more likely to report feeling some degree of pressure or coercion. The subjects who reported sexting only because of pressure or coercion were all female responders.

Female responders who felt pressured or coerced to sext were most likely to report that the source of that pressure was someone they were attracted to, who they wanted as a boyfriend. In the field, as these issues are discussed with teenagers, practitioners frequently understand from both genders that it is not unusual for some boys to request a nude picture from a girl before they will consider dating or entering a relationship with her. It seems possible that teenage girls are feeling pressured to sext by boys who see a girl's interest in them as leverage for getting a naked picture.

New research

As mentioned previously, any relationship between pressure to sext and positive outcomes has not been previously explored. This study of 1332 college freshman found that pressure to sext was related to negative and mixed outcomes but was also observed among subjects who reported positive-only outcomes. That is, negative-only and mixed-outcome sexters were almost all pressured to sext, whereas only approximately 60% of positive-outcome sexters were pressured to sext. Subjects who reported no outcomes of any kind were the least likely to report being pressured to sext but, even among those sexters, slightly fewer than half reported such pressure.

Key question

If someone is pressured to sext, is that always a cause for serious concern?

Key research finding

Some sexters who reported only positive outcomes following sexting also acknowledged that they were pressured, at least in part, to sext.

How this finding affects clinical practice

If a patient reports that they were pressured to sext, further discussion is warranted, and the patient's risk of negative emotional outcomes is increased (but not inevitable).

Subjects' Perceptions Regarding Risk and Education

As several subjects noted in focus groups, sexting is often perceived by teens as a relatively safe activity. "You can't get pregnant and you can't get a disease" was a relatively common refrain. Other dangers, such as the possibility that a photo would reduce future opportunities, were seen as increasingly unlikely between 2014 and 2017. This is not to say that no subjects perceived any dangers. More than three-quarters of subjects agreed that a nude picture may be shown around to peers but, interestingly, subjects were less likely to report feeling upset if a peer saw the picture and more likely to feel upset if an adult saw it.

Subjects were also very likely to report taking steps to mitigate any risk. Almost 80% reported that they either took the photo without their face showing or with their face and/or head obscured, suggesting that making the photo unidentifiable is perceived as a precautionary measure. Finally, although subjects did not report an increase in school education about sexting between 2014 and 2017, they did report a fairly dramatic increase in discussions with parents. The percentage of subjects who reported discussing sexting with their caregivers increased from 17% in 2014 to 37% in 2017. Such discussions may have made subjects more aware of some risks associated with sexting and more likely to take steps to reduce those risks.

ROLE OF PEDIATRIC PRACTITIONERS IN DISCUSSING CYBERBULLYING AND SEXTING

Topics concerning digital technology should be approached with care. Although both patients and parents are generally concerned about cyberbullying, parents may believe that cell phones only increase safety. They may also believe that carrying a cell phone will increase their child's social success. It is important to acknowledge parental concerns while increasing their awareness about the possibility of negative effects following cell phone acquisition and providing some guidance on how to mitigate these risks through discussion. (Parental guidance downloads are available on-line at www.MARCcenter.org.) Sexting is a topic that tends to also engender parental anxiety. First and foremost, physicians should not dismiss all risks potentially associated with sexting, even though current research does suggest that this risk has been overestimated. Instead, physicians can explore sexting and any association with mental health problems or high-risk sexual activity, and can emphasize the importance of discussing parental values about nudity and sexuality with teens. Importantly, there is a lack of knowledge about long-term risks associated with sexting (regarding which there is no current research).

Physicians can benefit from awareness of the factors that may increase their uncertainty and thus decrease the odds that they will approach these topics with patients. First, a practitioner may feel uncertain about whether or not digital behaviors constitute a new threat to health or are simply extensions of already-existing threats.[66] It is now apparent that contemporary media and screen habits are not functionally equivalent to the television watching that previous generations experienced. For this reason, applying television rules is likely to be ineffective. For example, simply recommending that parents limit screen time for a 12-year-old to 1 hour a day may be very difficult to implement. Does online homework count? What about reading books on a digital device? How are text messages counted? What about the screens children encounter in every friend's house? Of course, with younger patients, parents can exert much more control over screen time and evidence consistently suggests that doing so is a positive intervention.

Second, a physician may feel less tech-savvy than his or her patients, which can result in a reluctance to speak to patients about digital behaviors that could affect health, even cyberbullying and sexting.[67] It is hoped that this article will help increase the self-confidence of practitioners. It is important that a practitioner's lack of technical knowledge should not simply lead to the idea that all technology is just bad and should be stopped. Like it or not, children today will live with technology their entire lives. The practitioner's job is to prepare them to cope with it, not to retreat by denying its importance. Having said that, encouraging a reasonable balance between screen and non-screen time is a very worthwhile conversation to have with youth.

Third, a physician may find that some patients are at higher risk than others. For example, patients with sexual minority status may be at increased risk of mental and sexual health problems following digital victimization, including substance abuse and depression.[68,69] Yet, digital technology and social networks can play an important supportive role in the lives of sexual minority youth, which makes it even more important to discuss safer and more sensible ways of using digital technology while minimizing risk.

SUMMARY

It is very unlikely that either cyberbullying or sexting will go away. The fascination that youth have with technology, social status and dynamics, and sexuality, suggest that these issues are more likely to be managed and minimized, rather than eliminated. Encouragingly, youth often want very much to discuss how to avoid these problems; however, ways to minimize risk that seem obvious to adults are not only always so obvious to children and adolescents. For example, adults know that despite the intensity of teenage relationships these pairings are unlikely to be permanent; however, teens may need to be reminded of this. Adolescents may not consider that long-term consequences of sexting are unknown, even though short-term risk may not seem significant. Both younger and older children can forget that a face-to-face conversation can help defuse a tense social situation occurring online (or off) and, in the midst of emotional angst, it can be difficult to remember how much the support of friends, families, and physicians can help someone cope. It can be helpful for practitioners and parents to remember that all of these truisms are based on life and social experience, rather than on technical knowledge per se.

REFERENCES

1. Hinduja S, Patchin JW. Bullying, cyberbullying, and suicide. Arch Suicide Res 2010;14(3):206–21.
2. Beckman Linda. Traditional bullying and cyberbullying among Swedish adolescents: gender differences and associations with mental health. Karlstad University, Faculty of Health, Science and Technology; 2013. p. 639930. Available at: http://www.diva-portal.org/smash/record.jsf?pid=diva2.
3. Moreno MA, Whitehill JM. New media, old risks: toward an understanding of the relationships between online and offline health behavior. Arch Pediatr Adolesc Med 2012;166(9). https://doi.org/10.1001/archpediatrics.2012.1320.
4. Ahuja A. LGBT adolescents in America: depression, discrimination and suicide. Eur Psychiatry 2016;33:S70.
5. Goebert D, Else I, Matsu C, et al. The impact of cyberbullying on substance use and mental health in a multiethnic sample. Matern Child Health J 2011; 15(8):1282–6.
6. Hinduja S, Patchin JW. Cyberbullying: an exploratory analysis of factors related to offending and victimization. Deviant Behav 2008;29(2):129–56.
7. Mitchell KJ, Ybarra M, Finkelhor D. The relative importance of online victimization in understanding depression, delinquency, and substance use. Child Maltreat 2007;12(4):314–24.
8. Ortega R, Elipe P, Mora-Merchán J, et al. The emotional impact on victims of traditional bullying and cyberbullying: a study of Spanish adolescents. J Psychol 2009;217(4):197–204.
9. Cross D, Lester L, Barnes A. A longitudinal study of the social and emotional predictors and consequences of cyber and traditional bullying victimisation. Int J Public Health 2015;60(2):207–17.

10. Gámez-Guadix M, Orue I, Smith PK, et al. Longitudinal and reciprocal relations of cyberbullying with depression, substance use, and problematic internet use among adolescents. J Adolesc Health 2013;53(4):446–52.
11. Anja Schultze-Krumbholz, Jäkel A, Schultze M, et al. Emotional and behavioural problems in the context of cyberbullying: a longitudinal study among German adolescents. Emotional and Behavioural Difficulties 2012;17(3–4):329–45.
12. Kowalski RM, Limber SP. Psychological, physical, and academic correlates of cyberbullying and traditional bullying. J Adolesc Health 2013;53(1):S13–20.
13. Nixon CL. Current perspectives: the impact of cyberbullying on adolescent health. Adolesc Health Med Ther 2014;143. https://doi.org/10.2147/AHMT.S36456.
14. Modecki KL, Minchin J, Harbaugh AG, et al. Bullying prevalence across contexts: a meta-analysis measuring cyber and traditional bullying. J Adolesc Health 2014;55(5):602–11.
15. Schneider SK, O'Donnell L, Stueve A, et al. Cyberbullying, school bullying, and psychological distress: a regional census of high school students. Am J Public Health 2012;102(1):171–7. Available at: http://ajph.aphapublications.org/cgi/content/abstract/AJPH.2011.300308v1.
16. Ybarra ML, Boyd D, Korchmaros JD, et al. Defining and measuring cyberbullying within the larger context of bullying victimization. J Adolesc Health 2012;51(1):53–8.
17. Englander Elizabeth. Research findings: MARC 2011 survey grades 3–12amprdquosemicolon. Bridgewater (MA): Massachusetts Aggression Reduction Center, Bridgewater State University; 2012. Available at: http://webhost.bridgew.edu/marc/MARC%20REPORT-Bullying%20In%20Grades%203-12%20in%20MA.pdf.
18. Englander Elizabeth. Bullying and cyberbullying: what every educator needs to know. Cambridge, (MA): Harvard Education Press; 2013.
19. DePaolis K, Williford A. The nature and prevalence of cyber victimization among elementary school children. Child Youth Care Forum 2014;44(3):377–93.
20. Holfeld B, Leadbeater BJ. The nature and frequency of cyber bullying behaviors and victimization experiences in young Canadian children. Can J Sch Psychol 2015;30(2):116–35.
21. Monks C, Robinson S, Worlidge P. The emergence of cyberbullying: a survey of primary school pupils' perceptions and experiences. Sch Psychol Int 2012;33(5):477–91.
22. Arslan S, Savaser S, Hallett V, et al. Cyberbullying among primary school students in Turkey: self-reported prevalence and associations with home and school life. Cyberpsychol Behav Soc Netw 2012;15(10):527–33.
23. Rideout VJ, Foehr UG, Roberts DF. Generation M [Superscript 2]: media in the lives of 8-to 18-year-olds. Menlo Park (CA): Henry J. Kaiser Family Foundation; 2010.
24. Englander E. Research findings: MARC 201, survey grades 3-12. Bridgewater (MA): Massachusetts Aggression Reduction Center, Bridgewater State University; 2012. Available at: http://webhost.bridgew.edu/marc/MARC%20REPORT-Bullying%20In%20Grades%203-12%20in%20MA.pdf. Accessed December 20, 2017.
25. Mascheroni G, Olafsson K. The mobile internet: access, use, opportunities and divides among European Children. New Media Soc 2016;18(8):1657–79.
26. Zero to eight: children's media use in American 2013. Common Sense Media; 2013. Available at: https://www.commonsensemedia.org/file/zero-to-eight-2013pdf-0/download.

27. Mascheroni G, Olafsson K. The mobile Internet: access, use, opportunities and divides among European children. New Media & Society 2016;18(8):1657–79.
28. Hinduja and Patchin, Cyberbullying.
29. Holfeld B, Leadbeater BJ. The nature and frequency of cyber bullying behaviors and victimization experiences in young Canadian children. Canadian Journal of School Psychology 2015;30(2):116–35.
30. Mishna F, Cook C, Gadalla T, et al. Cyber bullying behaviors among middle and high school students. Am J Orthopsychiatry 2010;80(3):362–74.
31. Smith PK, Mahdavi J, Carvalho M, et al. Cyberbullying: its nature and impact in secondary school pupils. J Child Psychol Psychiatry 2008;49(4):376–85.
32. Fisher BS, Cullen FT, Turner MG. Being pursued: stalking victimization in a national study of college women. Criminology 2002;1(2):257–308.
33. Wilcox P, Jordan CE, Pritchard AJ. A multidimensional examination of campus safety: victimization, perceptions of danger, worry about crime, and precautionary behavior among college women in the post-clery era. Crime Delinquen 2007;53(2):219–54.
34. Griffiths Mark. Sex on the internet: observations and implications for internet sex addiction. J Sex Res 2001;38(4):333–42.
35. Internet-Facilitated Sexual Offending | ATSA. 2010. Available at: http://www.atsa.com/internet-facilitated-sexual-offending. Accessed April 28, 2017.
36. James D, Khadr S. New challenges in child protection. The child protection practice manual: training practitioners how to safeguard children. Oxford: Oxford University Press; 2016. p. 11.
37. Houck CD, Barker D, Rizzo C, et al. Sexting and sexual behavior in at-risk adolescents. Pediatrics 2014;133(2):e276–282.
38. "Rare Disease," Wikipedia, the Free Encyclopedia. 2016. Available at: https://en.wikipedia.org/w/index.php?title=Rare_disease&oldid=737022093. Accessed April 28, 2017.
39. Rice E, Gibbs J, Winetrobe H, et al. Sexting and sexual behavior among middle school students. Pediatrics 2014;134(1):e21–28.
40. Benotsch EG, Snipes DJ, Martin AM, et al. Sexting, substance use, and sexual risk behavior in young adults. J Adolesc Health 2013;52(3):307–13.
41. AP - MTV digital abuse study, executive summary. Associated Press and MTV; 2009. Available at: http://www.athinline.org/MTVAP_Digital _Abuse_ Study_Executive_Summary.pdf.
42. Klettke B, Hallford DJ, Mellor DJ. Sexting prevalence and correlates: a systematic literature review. Clin Psychol Rev 2014;34(1):44–53.
43. Englander E, McCoy M, Dubois-Iredale V, et al. Sexting: research across four years. Munster (Germany): European Society of Criminology; 2016.
44. Ringrose J, Gill R, Livingstone S, et al. A qualitative study of children, young people and 'sexting'. London: NSPCC; 2012. Available at: http://www2.lse.ac.uk/media@lse/documents/MPP/Sexting-Report-NSPCC.pdf. Accessed December 12, 2017.
45. Fleschler Peskin M, Markham CM, Addy RC, et al. Prevalence and patterns of sexting among ethnic minority urban high school students. Cyberpsychol Behav Soc Netw 2013;16(6):454–9.
46. Temple JR, Choi H. Longitudinal association between teen sexting and sexual behavior. Pediatrics 2014;134(5):e1287–92.
47. Mark K, Longinaker N, Collinetti E, et al. Gender differences in sexting behaviors among chlamydia positive adolescents and young adults. J Adolesc Health 2014;54(2):S52.

48. Associated Press, MTV. AP - MTV Digital abuse study, Executive Summary 2009. Available at: http://www.athinline.org/MTVAP_Digital _Abuse_Study_Executive_ Summary.pdf. Accessed December 20, 2017.

49. Drouin M, Landgraff C. Texting, sexting, and attachment in college students' romantic relationships. Comput Human Behav 2012;28(2):444–9.

50. Englander E, McCoy M. Gender differences in peer-pressured sexting," in a socio-ecological approach to cyberbullying. Nova Science Publishers; 2016. p. 97–104.

51. Englander E, McCoy M, Dubois-Iredale V, et al. Sexting: research across four years. Presented at the European Society of Criminology, Munster (Germany) 2016.

52. Temple JR, Le VD, van den Berg P, et al. Brief report: teen sexting and psycho-social health. J Adolesc 2014;37(1):33–6.

53. Van Ouytsel J, Van Gool E, Ponnet K, et al. "Brief report: the association between adolescents' characteristics and engagement in sexting. J Adolesc 2014;37(8): 1387–91.

54. Temple JR, Le VD, van den Berg P, et al. Brief report: teen sexting and psycho-social health. Journal of Adolescence 2014;37(1):33–6.

55. Englander E. Sexting: first base in the 21st Century?. Teen pregnancy and pre-vention partnership annual conference held at St Louis (MO), April 12, 2017.

56. Henderson L, Morgan C. Sexting and sexual relationships among teens and young adults. McNair Scholars Research Journal 2011;7(1):9.

57. Drouin M, Tobin E. Unwanted but consensual sexting among young adults: rela-tions with attachment and sexual motivations. Comput Human Behav 2014;31: 412–8.

58. Gámez-Guadix M, Almendros C, Borrajo E, et al. Prevalence and association of sexting and online sexual victimization among Spanish adults. Sex Res Social Policy 2015;12(2):145–54.

59. Ferguson CJ. Sexting behaviors among young Hispanic women: incidence and association with other high-risk sexual behaviors. Psychiatr Q 2011;82(3):239–43.

60. Stasko E, Geller P. Reframing sexting as a positive relationship behavior. Presented at the American Psychological Association, Toronto, Canada 2015. Available at: https://www.apa.org/news/press/releases/2015/08/reframing-sexting. pdf. Accessed December 22, 2017.

61. Englander E, McCoy M. Gender differences in peer-pressured sexting. In: Wright MF, editor. A social-ecological approach to cyberbullying. Hauppauge (NY): Nova Publishing; 2016. p. 97–104.

62. Stasko, Geller. Reframing sexting as a positive relationship behavior.

63. Drouin, Tobin. Unwanted but consensual sexting among young adults.

64. Mark K, Longinaker N, Collinetti E, et al. Gender differences in sexting behaviors among Chlamydia positive adolescents and young adults. Journal of Adolescent Health 2014;54(2):S52.

65. Hinduja S, Patchin J. Sexting: a brief guide for educators and parents. Cyberbul-lying Research Center; 2014.

66. Moreno MA, Whitehill JM. New media, old risks: toward an understanding of the relationships between online and offline health behavior. Archives of Pediatrics & Adolescent Medicine 2012;166(9):868–9.

67. Peters TE, Herman T, Patel NR, et al. Technology and adolescent behavioral health care. In: Dewan NA, Luo JS, Lorenzi NM, editors. Mental Health Practice in a Digital World. Cham (Switzerland): Springer International Publishing; 2015. p. 141–58.

68. Hatzenbuehler ML, McLaughlin KA, Keyes KM, et al. The impact of institutional discrimination on psychiatric disorders in lesbian, gay, and bisexual populations: a prospective study. Am J Public Health 2010;100(3):452–9.
69. Graham R, Berkowitz B, Blum R, et al. The health of lesbian, gay, bisexual, and transgender people: building a foundation for better understanding. Washington, DC: Institute of Medicine; 2011.

Internet and Video Game Addictions

Diagnosis, Epidemiology, and Neurobiology

Clifford J. Sussman, MD[a,b,*], James M. Harper, MD[c,d],
Jessica L. Stahl, MD[e], Paul Weigle, MD[f]

KEYWORDS

- Internet gaming disorder • IGD • Video game • Internet • Addiction • Digital
- Computer

KEY POINTS

- Proposed criteria for diagnosis of Internet gaming disorder and other digital technology addictions are analogous to those for substance use or gambling disorders.
- Diagnosis of Internet and video game addictions should include both screening tools and clinical interview for "red flags," such as academic decline, sleep disruption, and changes in real-life activities and relationships.
- Epidemiologic studies, limited by variation in diagnostic methods, yield prevalence estimates ranging from less than 1.0% to 26.8%.
- Internet and video game addictions are associated with psychological and social comorbidities, such as depression, attention-deficit/hyperactivity disorder, alcohol use, anxiety, and poor psychosocial support.
- Neurobiological evidence suggests a dual processing model of digital technology addictions characterized by an imbalance between the reactive reward system and the reflective reward system.

INTRODUCTION

With the increasing power and accessibility to digital technology and exploding range of online activities over the past 2 decades has come a great expansion of the amount of

Disclosure Statement: The authors have no disclosures.
[a] Private Practice, 5410 Connecticut Avenue, Northwest, Suite 112, Washington, DC 20015, USA; [b] Department of Psychiatry, George Washington University Medical School, 2300 I Street NW, Washington, DC 20052, USA; [c] Adolescent Inpatient Psychiatric Unit, Dominion Hospital, 2960 Sleepy Hollow Road, Falls Church, VA 22044, USA; [d] Private Practice, Columbia Associates in Psychiatry, 2501 North Glebe Road, Suite 303, Arlington, VA 22207, USA; [e] Pediatric Nephrology, University of Washington, MS OC.9.820, PO Box 5371, Seattle, WA 98145-5005, USA; [f] Department of Psychiatry, Natchaug Hospital, Hartford Healthcare, 189 Storrs Road, Mansfield Center, Mansfield, CT 06250, USA
* Corresponding author. 5410 Connecticut Avenue Northwest, Suite 112, Washington, DC 20015.
E-mail address: cliffordsussmanmd@gmail.com

time youth regularly spend engaging with it. The 2015 Common Sense Media Use Census found that teens ages 13 to 18 spent a daily average of more than 6.5 hours on screen entertainment (including TV, smart phones, computers, video games, streaming videos, and so forth) and the daily average of tweens ages 8 to 12 was more than 4.5 hours.[1] This represents a significant increase in youth screen habits, with a substantial minority developing excessive, problematic habits that interfere with functioning in work, academics, relationships, and other domains. The concept that it is possible to develop a behavioral addiction to the Internet was first proposed in the 1990s,[2] and interest in this topic has grown along with the influence of the Internet in our lives.

Numerous researchers have investigated Internet and video game addictions ("IVGA" for the remainder of this article) in the past decade.[3–6] A wide variety of online activities are engaging enough to be potentially addictive, including video games, social media, smartphone use, texting, streaming videos, and online pornography. Notably, we omitted online gambling, as its related addiction is typically classified as a subtype of gambling disorder. The subtype of IVGA that research has validated most is video game addiction, particularly to games played online, such as massively multiplayer online games (MMORPGs). Increased acceptance of video game addiction led the 2013 inclusion of "Internet gaming disorder" (IGD) in the *Diagnostic and Statistical Manual of Mental Disorders, Fifth Edition* (DSM-V) as a "condition for further study."[7] A growing body of evidence indicates commonalities between IVGA, including IGD, and more well-established addictions, including substance use disorders and gambling disorder. This paper provides an updated review of IVGA, focusing on the significant body of research published in the 4 years since the proposal of IGD. We explore diagnosis, epidemiology, and neurobiology, much of which overlaps substantially with that of substance use disorders. This article will help clinicians improve their awareness, understanding, and ability to diagnose IVGA.

DIAGNOSIS OF INTERNET GAMING DISORDER AND OTHER TYPES OF INTERNET AND VIDEO GAME ADDICTIONS

Behavioral addictions may be conceptualized as an excessive, uncontrollable, "repeated behavior leading to significant harm or distress."[8] Young[2] initially conceptualized Internet addiction in 1996 using criteria adapted from those of pathologic gambling, the only behavioral addiction recognized in the *Diagnostic and Statistical Manual of Mental Disorders, Fourth Edition, Text Revision*. Those meeting criteria had extreme online habits causing academic, occupational, relationship, and/or financial dysfunction.[2] Young's[2] original diagnostic questions served as a basis for many subsequent rating scales and proposed criteria for IVGA.

Most studies of IVGA use similar criteria, based on a conversion of DSM criteria or a well-validated scale for diagnosing substance use disorder or pathologic gambling. Resultant IVGA assessment scales and diagnostic criteria have been adapted for specific subtypes, including addiction to online gaming, the Internet in general, smartphones, online pornography, and others.[9–16] Griffiths'[17] similar conceptualization of addiction, based on the key components of salience, mood modification, tolerance, withdrawal, conflict, and relapse, forms the basis for a number of IVGA assessment scales as well.[18–22]

Romano and colleagues[23] demonstrated that Internet addicts are more likely than nonaddicts to experience withdrawal symptoms following a brief 15-minute Internet exposure. A pronounced decline in mood prompted addicts to rapidly reengage with the Internet. Addicts were also more likely to have depressive, impulsive, and autistic traits.

In 2013, the American Psychological Association proposed IGD, a type of IVGA related exclusively to online video game play, in the DSM-V as a "condition requiring further study" using comparable criteria (**Box 1**).[7]

These IGD criteria are nearly identical to those of the DSM-V's substance use disorder and gambling disorder, although the threshold for IGD is significantly higher. In addition to persistent use leading to distress or impairment, substance use disorder requires only 2 of 11 additional symptoms for diagnosis. Pathologic gambling requires 4 of 9, whereas IGD requires 5 of 9. IGD concerns only addiction to online video gaming, and excludes that of other potentially addictive screen habits included in IVGA. The DSM-V IGD criteria as written are stricter than most definitions of IVGA, and therefore yield lower prevalence rates, more reflective of moderate to severe addiction than a mild addiction or "at-risk" habit, as outlined later in this article.

Other studies of IVGA that were not limited to Internet gaming also validated the resultant loss of function and detrimental outcomes for the affected individual (eg, distress, withdrawal, tolerance, lying, and conflict resulting from use), as well as other symptoms, such as preoccupation and using the Internet to escape negative feelings.[24,25] When evaluating a case of possible IVGA in a patient who does not engage

---

Box 1

Diagnostic and Statistical Manual of Mental Disorders, Fifth Edition proposed criteria for Internet gaming disorder as a condition for further study

Persistent and recurrent use of the Internet to engage in games, often with other players, leading to clinically significant impairment or distress, as indicated by 5 (or more) of the following in a 12-month period:

1. Preoccupation with Internet games. (The individual thinks about previous gaming activity or anticipates playing the next game; Internet gaming becomes the dominant activity in daily life.) Note: This disorder is distinct from Internet gambling, which is included under gambling disorder.
2. Withdrawal symptoms when Internet gaming is taken away. (These symptoms are typically described as irritability, anxiety, or sadness, but there are no physical signs of pharmacologic withdrawal.)
3. Tolerance—the need to spend increasing amounts of time engaged in Internet games.
4. Unsuccessful attempts to control the participation in Internet games.
5. Loss of interest in previous hobbies and entertainment as a result of, and with the exception of, Internet games.
6. Continued excessive use of Internet games despite knowledge of psychosocial problems.
7. Has deceived family members, therapists, or others regarding the amount of Internet gaming.
8. Use of Internet games to escape or relieve a negative mood (eg, feelings of helplessness, guilt, anxiety).
9. Has jeopardized or lost a significant relationship, job, or educational or career opportunity because of participation in Internet games.
Note: Only nongambling Internet games are included in this disorder. Use of the Internet for required activities in a business or profession is not included; nor is the disorder intended to include other recreational or social Internet use. Similarly, sexual Internet sites are excluded.

Specify current severity:
Internet gaming disorder can be mild, moderate, or severe depending on the degree of disruption of normal activities. Individuals with less severe Internet gaming disorder may exhibit fewer symptoms and less disruption of their lives. Those with severe Internet gaming disorder will have more hours spent on the computer and more severe loss of relationships or career or school opportunities.

in Internet gaming, it is feasible, if not yet fully validated, to use the criteria in **Box 1** by substituting the name of the online habit, such as "social media," in place of the words "internet games" and "internet gaming."

CLINICAL CONSIDERATIONS IN ASSESSING FOR INTERNET AND VIDEO GAME ADDICTION

Moreno and colleagues[26] recently developed a brief screening tool for clinical diagnosis of IVGA in teens and young adults, which showed 100% sensitivity, although only 59% specificity. A positive screen indicates the need for a more thorough investigation to make or rule out an IVGA diagnosis. Use of this tool enables increased recognition of IVGAs in clinical practice. Their 3-item screen assesses the degree (scored on a 0–4-point scale for each item) that an individual

1. Experiences social anxiety related to a preference for Internet use to the exclusion of real-life relationships
2. Feels withdrawal when not using the Internet
3. Loses motivation to do other things that need to get done because of the Internet[26]

A more detailed screening would then be indicated if a subject's total score was 3 or more.

When performing a psychiatric assessment, it is essential to take a thorough media history (See Nicholas Carson and colleagues' article, "Assessment of Digital Media Use in the Adolescent Psychiatric Evaluation," in this issue).[27] The clinician must obtain a thorough collateral history from a parent or caregiver, as well as the young patient, to properly do so. This includes assessing time spent online, which teens may minimize in their reporting, neglecting to share that while ostensibly sleeping or doing homework on a computer they are actually engaging in online entertainment or social interaction. When assessing children and adolescents for IVGA, it is important to include the extent to which online activities are supervised by parents, where in the home they take place (ie, in a public area vs in the bedroom), what rules address technology use, to what extent conflicts arise regarding screen use, and whether academic performance has been impacted by screen habits.[28] Getting accurate information about screen habits directly from young adult patients living away from home may be more challenging, but focusing on academic or work performance, sleep quantity and quality, as well as "real-life" activities and relationships often provides insight into the influence of online habits on overall functioning. The clinician may elicit various other "red flags" that warrant further evaluation for IVGA. Reduced total sleep time, delay in sleep onset, decreased quality of sleep, and excessive daytime sleepiness lacking a clear cause could each point toward IVGA, as excessive time online often displaces and disrupts needed sleep.[9,10,29] A patient with few "real-life" interactions with friends, as most of his or her social connections are online, may also suffer from IVGA. However, many children and teens do not distinguish between real and virtual friends unless asked specifically to do so, as it has become more normative for most social interactions to occur online or via text.

EPIDEMIOLOGY OF INTERNET AND VIDEO GAME ADDICTION

The exact prevalence of IVGAs is difficult to assess. A lack of standard criteria for diagnosis of IVGA contributes to a substantial variability in population statistics. Prevalence may vary significantly by age, but many studies neglect to distinguish child, adolescent, and adult populations. The matter is further complicated by regional and cultural variability in online habits.

A recent review of cross-sectional and longitudinal studies of IVGA noted use of a variety of diagnostic instruments, as well as use of different cutoff values among studies using the same tool.[30] Mean prevalence estimates from that review and others like it reflect a wide range as well as regional diversity, as shown in **Fig. 1**.[30–39] Prevalence estimates of IGD, also displayed later in this article, indicate a narrower range, although regional divergence remains evident. In both IGD and IVGA, prevalence in Asia is generally higher than in North American or European studies.

It is notable that in studies that distinguish "high" or "definite" IVGA from "low" or "probable" IVGA, the lower prevalence of the former more closely matches that found in IGD, as seen in **Fig. 2**.[40–43]

In diagnosing IGD and other IVGAs, the requirement of clinically significant distress or impairment (or lack thereof) also creates estimate variations. One 2017 study including data from the United States, Canada, the United Kingdom, and Germany indicated a prevalence of 0.5% to 1.0% for those meeting full criteria for IGD, and an overall prevalence of 2.4% for those with "potentially dysfunctional gaming," defined as reporting at least 5 of 9 IGD criteria without related distress or impairment.[44] Similarly, a meta-analysis in 2011 found a significantly smaller mean video game addiction prevalence among studies that required functional impairment for diagnosis, compared with those studies that did not.[43] These differences reaffirm that further study is needed to establish standardized criteria before a more accurate prevalence is established.

The longitudinal stability of IVGA is unclear. Multiple studies demonstrate high rates of independent remission over 1 to 2 years.[30,45,46] One study from Hong Kong reported 46% of those with IVGA remitted after 1 year without intervention. Significant variability exists, however. A study of video game addiction in elementary age youth found a 2-year remission rate of only 15%.[47] The stability of IGD has not yet been investigated, to our knowledge.

RISK FACTORS AND COMORBIDITIES OF INTERNET AND VIDEO GAME ADDICTION

Conceptual models explain how an individual's biological and psychological characteristics interact with addictive features of digital technologies to result in IVGA. For

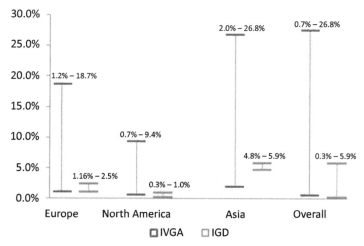

Fig. 1. Range of reported mean prevalence of IVGA and IGD by region.

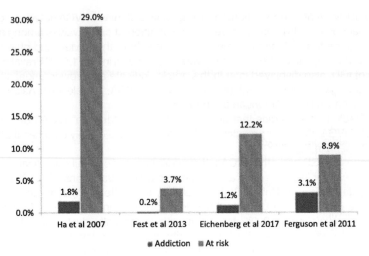

Fig. 2. Prevalence of IVGA categorized as "addicted" versus "at-risk."

example, one addictive aspect of the Internet may be the ability to represent oneself online in an idealized manner, whether by filtering aspects of one's self-representation on social media, or projecting a completely different self-image in the form of an individualized character or "avatar" in an online role playing game (RPG).[48–51] Another addictive factor of many online activities appears to be the incorporation of variable ratio reinforcement, a powerful method of operant conditioning.[50] These concepts, and others like them, need further empirical research for refinement or validation.[51] For clinical purposes, it will be useful for mental health professionals to recognize which features of digital technology draw individuals into addictive patterns of behavior, and to identify characteristics that may make an individual more susceptible to IVGA.

ADDICTIVE FEATURES OF VIDEO GAMES

RPGs, including massive multiplayer online RPGs (MMORPGs, or MMOs) are the game type most consistently related to IVGA, followed by "shooters," multiplayer online battle arena games, and real-time strategy games.[52–55] MMORPGs combine an especially potent mix of factors that makes players particularly vulnerable to developing IGD. These factors include escapism, socialization, competition, and "grinding," the process of perpetually "leveling up" or improving one's gaming character by accumulating in-game achievements and rewards. Together these elements may be synergistically habit forming.[56]

Another factor predisposing one to addictive play is an individual's sensitivity to environmental cues as well as perception of time relative to reward processing. Time cues within games are typically distinct from real-world cues. For example, players from vastly different time zones participate simultaneously in online games with day and night cycles that occur on a schedule unrelated to the physical world. Players become so focused on the constant, immediate feedback to their in-game actions that they become immersed in the game world and are less likely to respond to real-world cues.[57,58] Such players typically ignore real-world cues to stop playing (such as fatigue, social cues, or time of day), leading to excessive gaming times that encroach onto real-world responsibilities.

PSYCHOSOCIAL RISK FACTORS

Personal factors can also affect the likelihood of developing IVGA. Evidence suggests that individuals with social inhibitions or deficits tend to find online communication preferable to in-person interaction, possibly due to reduced risk of direct social confrontation or ability to follow "scripted" conversations focused on common themes.[59-61] Another individual factor that can lead to IVGA is the "fear of missing out" (FOMO). This occurs when the normative drive to be included and engaged in the social group is distorted by the perpetual 24/7 possibility of connections with peers (on social media sites, via text messages between friends, or in an online game). The individual with FOMO is anxiously compelled to excessively check these sources (to the detriment of offline endeavors) for fear of marginalization.[62,63] Other prosocial drives, including maintaining one's status in an online game or reputation within social groups that communicate online, may also contribute to IVGA.[64]

IVGA is particularly prevalent in individuals with a novelty-seeking personality trait, as online entertainment offers a combination of escapism and immediate and repeated reward gratification.[65] IVGA is also prevalent in those with the harm-avoidant personality trait, as online environments create a physically safe, anonymous space, detached from the risks of "real life."[21,40,65] Individuals with insecure, ambivalent, or anxious attachments are also especially vulnerable to developing IVGAs, possibly because they use online entertainment as a vehicle for escapism or immediate social gratification.[42,66,67] One study demonstrated lower rates of IVGA remission among individuals possessing comorbid Cluster B personality traits.[61] This may be because digital technology helps these individuals escape negative emotions, engage in dramatic self-presentation, or act out antisocial impulses in a relatively safe environment.[61]

Poor family support, poor family relationships, high family conflict, and poor psychosocial support are also disproportionally common in youth with IVGA.[37,46,68-70] Poor parent mental health is related to more severe IVGA.[71] Conversely, increasing parental involvement and social support is related to less severe IVGA.[32,72] Poor academic performance and less protective parenting style (as identified using subscales of the Parental Bonding Instrument) have been shown to be independent predictors for Internet addiction, even after controlling for family function (as measured by the "APGAR" instrument), autism, and attention-deficit/hyperactivity disorder (ADHD).[28]

Although many studies note a male predominance for IVGA[28,31,73-75] and IGD,[73,76] other studies find no significant gender differences[34,44,77]:

- Male individuals are more likely than female individuals to develop IVGA related to computer gaming.[33]
- Female individuals are more likely than male individuals to develop IVGA related to smart phone use or social networking,[75,78] and tend to have more psychiatric comorbidities.[79]

The following are other psychosocial risk factors found on reviewing the literature:

- Frequent, short-duration smartphone usage, including games and multiple applications, is highly correlated with IVGA.[34,80]
- Multiple studies agree that individuals with sleep disturbances are more likely to have IVGA.[81-83]
- Aggression,[84] poor social adjustment,[28] avoidant behaviors,[39] low empathy,[85] poor school performance,[32,47] student status,[52] and cyberbullying[86,87] all correlate with IVGA.
- Active religious practice is inversely correlated with IVGA.[88]

PSYCHIATRIC COMORBIDITIES

A number of psychiatric disorders are often comorbid with IVGA and IGD, although limited data exist to inform the causal relationship of these associations. A recent study of 330 Korean middle school students identified psychiatric comorbidity in 20% of those with IGD.[89]

- Depressive disorders: The most frequent comorbid disorders with IGD and IVGA in clinical studies are depressive disorders, such as dysthymia and major depressive disorder.[70,77–79,90–96] One study indicated that IVGA at baseline predicted new-onset depression 2 years later.[47] The relationship of IVGA to suicidal behavior is unclear. One study in adults found an association between IVGA and "suicide planning."[93] Conversely, a study of Turkish adolescents found no relationship between IVGA and suicide risk.[97]
- ADHD, impulsivity, and autism spectrum disorders (ASD): Higher general rates of IVGA have been found in those with ADHD.[28,81,98,99] One study found that 22% of patients with ADHD also suffer from IVGA.[98] Trait impulsivity is positively correlated with IVGA and 11% of those with IGD are impulsive.[76,100] Another study found that trait impulsivity at baseline predicted new-onset video game addiction 2 years later.[47] A final study found that the prevalence of IVGA in adolescents with comorbid ASD and ADHD was 20%, nearly twice that found in teens with either ASD (11%) or ADHD (13%) alone.[101]
- Bipolar disorder: Comorbidity of bipolar disorder with IVGA has been reported in multiple studies.[79,102] Rates of bipolar disorder have been found to be as high as 31% in those with IVGA, as compared with 6% in those with "excessive Internet use." Those with co-occurring IVGA and bipolar disorders are more likely to suffer comorbid substance use, conduct, and personality disorders, although these associations may be more related to bipolar diagnosis than IVGA.[102]
- Alcohol use: IVGA has been positively associated with alcohol use in multiple studies.[75,77,82,103] One study found a rate of alcohol abuse in those suffering IVGA of 13%.[98] Another discovered that adolescents with IVGA are significantly more likely to have problematic alcohol use (16%) than their peers without IVGA (5%).[77]
- Anxiety: Several studies have shown a positive correlation between IVGA and anxiety disorders.[24,76,78,79,91,93] Prevalence rates of IVGA in anxious youth has been reported as low as 9%[75] and as high as 23%.[98] A longitudinal study indicated that IVGA at baseline predicted new-onset social anxiety 2 years later.[47]
- Obsessive-compulsive disorder (OCD): In adults, OCD has been associated with IVGA.[78]
- Alexithymia: This inability to identify emotions in the self has been identified in up to 27% of adults with IVGA.[104] Rates are particularly increased in female individuals with a history of trauma and IVGA.[105]
- Trauma: Adolescents with a history of sexual abuse appear to be at greater risk of IVGA. One study found an IVGA prevalence of 44% in teens with such a trauma history compared with 33% in those without.[106]

NEUROBIOLOGY OF INTERNET AND VIDEO GAME ADDICTION
Importance of a Neurobiological Addiction Model

Advances in understanding reward circuitry of the brain have paved the way for a theory that has changed how many view addiction: the afflicted is addicted not to a specific substance or activity, but to the associated brain response.[105] Therefore, neurobiological similarities with commonly accepted addictions add further credibility to IVGA. Although substances of abuse and stimulating digital technology differ in how the input is received by the brain, both appear to stimulate a common pathway by which pleasure is experienced, reinforced, and regulated: the mesocorticolimbic dopamine system.[105–109] Dysfunction within this area is expected in all substance use disorders and behavioral addictions. A search of the international literature reveals a growing amount of research on the neurobiology of IVGA, using structural and functional imaging, electroencephalogram (EEG), and genetics. Here we review these studies to establish whether patterns of neurobiological functioning in IVGA resemble those found in substance use disorders, particularly in brain pathways involved in addiction.

The Dual Processing Model

One of the most comprehensive of established neurobiological models explaining how addictive behavior relates to dysfunction within the brain is the dual processing model. This paradigm describes addiction as an imbalance between the "go" network and the "stop" network.[110–113] The go network, also called the reactive system (RaS), mediates immediate outcomes from behavior. The stop network, also called the reflective system (RfS), provides inhibitory control based on long-term projections[114,115] (**Fig. 3**). Key structures involved in the go network are the bottom-up mesolimbic and mesocortical dopamine pathways (including the nucleus accumbens), other parts of the striatum, and the amygdala. Along the top of these pathways are key structures of the stop network, areas associated with control of impulses and attention, such as the ventromedial, dorsolateral, and anterior cingulate prefrontal cortices. Other vital stop network structures are associated with memory and affective states, such as

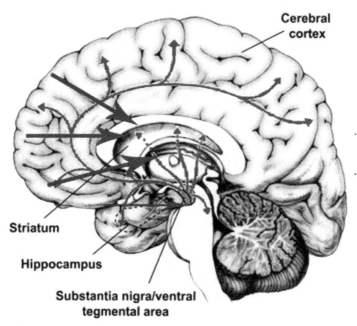

Fig. 3. Dual processing reward system model. The green arrows show the direction of the bottom-up "go" network (reactive) and the red arrows show the direction of the top-down "stop" network (reflective). An imbalance between these 2 systems is implicated in addiction. (*Adapted from* Dalley JW, Roiser JP. Dopamine, serotonin and impulsivity. Neuroscience 2012;215:46; with permission.)

the somatosensory cortex, the insula, and the hippocampus.[115] The dual processing model allows clinicians to understand addiction as an imbalance of 2 competing forces, which parallels the ambivalence that patients with addictions typically display. A stronger go network and weaker stop network have been found in patients with substance use disorders (SUDs) as well as ADHD. The adolescent brain has imbalance between the go and stop networks when compared with that of the adult brain, which may help explain why the onset of SUDs and IVGA often occurs in adolescence.[110]

The Go Network: Stimulation Seeking in Internet and Video Game Addiction

The "go" network, or RaS, is a bottom-up process involving the release of dopamine along the mesocorticolimbic dopaminergic pathway. Dopamine-agonist medication, often used to treat Parkinson disease, can stimulate the go network, causing addictive behaviors, such as gambling, binge eating, and hyper-sexuality.[116] Video gaming has been shown to cause dopamine release in the nucleus accumbens, the brain region that mediates pleasure, which is similar in magnitude to those created by recreational drug abuse.[116,117] Animal models have shown that the extent of dopamine release in this area is inversely related to the time between the initiating behavior and receipt of the reward. Therefore, the "rush" of dopamine release from using digital technology or drugs of abuse is related not only to the magnitude of reward received, but how quickly that reward is experienced.[118] This relationship becomes more relevant as digital technology evolves to be more immediately gratifying, more sophisticated applications and games are designed, solid state hard drives process ever faster, and Internet connections become more rapid. Through prolonged, excessive exposure to immediate rewards granted by engaging with video games and other digital entertainment, eventual downregulation of dopamine and glutamate receptors in the nucleus accumbens can occur, leading to tolerance, withdrawal, and compulsive stimulation seeking.[119–121]

Recent imaging studies demonstrate that go system changes occur in IVGA.[120] Researchers have found that patients with IGD have increased volumes of the caudate nucleus and nucleus accumbens, especially in the most severe cases.[121] PET scan studies indicate that excessive video game play is associated with downregulation of striatal dopamine receptors.[122,123] Patients with IVGA, including excessive "World of Warcraft" players, have been found to have a reward deficiency characterized by lower dopamine receptor density in these areas and lower physiologic responsiveness to rewards that are not game-related.[124] A recent study showed greater addictive behaviors in rats with genetic polymorphisms leading to decreased dopamine receptor density along the mesocorticolimbic pathway.[112] A similar study in human subjects found that excessive gamers with similar polymorphisms scored higher on a scale of reward dependence, a trait associated with addiction, than excessive gamers lacking these polymorphisms.[125]

Each of these studies suggests that the downregulation of dopamine receptors plays a key role in the pathology of IVGA, similar to that of SUDs.[126] Although SUD studies suggest that dopaminergic downregulation is reversible, estimates of recovery time vary widely.[127,128] It would be useful for providers to know whether dopaminergic downregulation is also reversible in IVGA, and if so, how long it takes. However, no applicable studies in IVGA could be found by these authors. Therefore, this area of clinical concern would benefit from research.

Prolonged stimulation of the go network and the resulting interaction between the amygdala and hippocampus leads to craving, which is often triggered by conditioned cues.[119] Functional MRI (fMRI) studies of addicts experiencing cue-induced cravings for video game play or pornography showed activation in these regions and throughout the mesocorticolimbic pathway (Gola and colleagues, 2017).[116,129–131] EEG research has shown that game-related cues occupy more attentional capacity in individuals with IGD than control groups.[54] These studies also parallel findings of similar processes in SUD.

The Stop Network: Impulsivity in Internet and Video Game Addiction

The "stop" network, or RfS, is a top-down process that inhibits the go network via glutamatergic pathways along the mesocorticolimbic regions, starting in the prefrontal cortex.[114,132] The stop network plays a major role in our ability to consciously resist impulses. Subjects with impairment within the stop network are more likely to be motivated by short-term versus long-term goals, compared with the general population.[107,133]

A 2014 meta-analysis of fMRI studies demonstrated that IGD is related to increased activation of known inhibitory, executive functioning, and working memory pathways in the prefrontal cortex, some of which increased along with time spent gaming. The investigators noted that this result, combined this with those of previous research, indicate a failure of self-regulatory processes in those with IGD.[134] A combined MRI and fMRI study found that patients with more severe Internet addiction have reduced gray matter in the right frontal pole, an area with increased functional connectivity to the left ventral striatum, resulting in "higher activation of the ventral striatum at rest." These investigators suggest that Internet addicts have reduced "ability to maintain long-term goals in face of distraction" due to diminished activity of the stop network. Another morphometry study demonstrated that patients with online gaming addiction have reduced gray and white matter integrity in the orbitofrontal and prefrontal cortex, areas integral to the stop network.[135] A genetic study found a target gene that modulates myelination in specific areas associated with the stop network (ie, the right frontal tracts and left cingulate gyrus, as well as the thalamus) to be protective against IGD.[136] In summary, imaging studies show that stop network regions, regulating impulse control and executive function, appear to be involved in regulating online habits, giving further weight to the dual processing model.

Numerous studies have explored the relationship between IVGA and impulsivity, using neurocognitive testing such as the Stroop test, go/no-go tasks, and delay discounting, often in combination with fMRI.[54,107,108,111,134,137,138] One showed that impaired ability to postpone rewards was associated with "problematic patterns" of play in multiplayer online games.[54] Another study found that individuals with IGD have poorer impulse control than nonaddicted recreational gamers, mirroring findings distinguishing dependent from recreational cocaine users.[54,139] Brains of individuals with IGD show less frontal cortical-striatal activation during testing, another indication of poor impulse control.[111] The brains of those with severe IGD showed weaker activity in the dorsolateral prefrontal cortex when experiencing risk, and greater activation in the ventral striatum (part of the go network), ventromedial prefrontal cortex, and orbitofrontal cortex when experiencing reward, also indicative of a failure in self-regulation.[140] Overall, research demonstrates that brain abnormalities associated with impulsivity are associated with a higher risk for IGD.

Long-Term Brain Effects

Imaging studies have also demonstrated how severity and duration of IGD cause changes in brain morphology similar to those caused by SUDs. Addiction duration, gaming duration, cognitive deficits, and severity of IGD correlate with disrupted gray and white matter integrity in the dorsolateral prefrontal cortex, orbitofrontal cortex, and striatum.[116,121,135] This may indicate that neuropathology along the mesocorticolimbic pathways is not only a cause of IGD pathology but also a downstream effect as well. These findings strongly support the theory that IVGA causes long-term changes in the brain, similar to those of substance abuse, but it is difficult to draw firm conclusions without a suitable animal model for IVGA. Newborn mice exposed to constant, variable multimedia exposure for 42 days entered a state of "overstimulation" after which they performed more poorly than controls on tasks measuring anxiety, hyperactivity, memory, and learning.[141] It is tempting to compare this overstimulated state to overuse of screen entertainment, but confounding variables contribute to problems in applying these results to humans. Nonetheless, studies like this one promise that the presence, quality, quantity, and reversibility of long-term brain changes from IVGA will be better illuminated by future research.[141,142]

SUMMARY

In spite of the lack of a consensus on diagnosis, and the resulting variations in epidemiologic, comorbidity, and neurobiological research, these studies provide overwhelming evidence of similarities between IVGA and SUD. Taken as a whole, the research presented here strongly suggests that IVGA is a clinically relevant and valid syndrome. Like other addictions, it is better understood when incorporating a neurobiological perspective. Our field must successfully address IVGAs to meet the needs of a society that is increasingly enmeshed in digital technology. Research in this area should continue to accelerate, allowing clinicians to better screen for, diagnose, psychoeducate, and provide multimodal treatment for our patients with IVGA. Treatment of IVGAs is explored in David N. Greenfield's article, "Treatment Considerations in Internet and Video Game Addiction: A Qualitative Discussion," in this issue.

Significant limitations in the current body of research include the difficulty in determining causality among many epidemiologic correlations, the limited knowledge of brain changes occurring in IVGA, including whether they are reversible, and the absence of animal model studies. These weaknesses will likely continue to encourage challenges to the validity of IVGA from critics. Some argue that digital technology use is so pervasive that the diagnosis may overpathologize behavior that is normative and acceptable in our culture.[105] On the other hand, modern society's excessive engagement with technology risks falsely normalizing addictions to technology, in what may be a culture of "functional tech-oholics." It seems difficult to walk down a public street without seeing multiple passersby engaged with smartphones, or to partake in a group conversation with no mention of digital media in some form. It seems evident that the human brain cannot evolve fast enough to adapt to the progress of digital technology, and that even the most powerful prefrontal cortex may be unable to resist the allure of instant stimulation in the ocean of digital screens that our world is becoming. Regardless of where we place the diagnostic cutoff for IVGA, our patients suffering the most profound dysfunction from their use of digital technology need better resources to recognize, understand, and treat their condition. If IVGA proves to be more abundant than a collection of a few extreme cases, it will be even more vital for our psychoeducational interventions to reach not only affected individuals, but their families and the communities as well. Ironically, social media and other forms of screen-based education may prove the best platforms for reaching out to those suffering IVGA without the insight, knowledge, and resources to address it.[a] This fact reminds us that learning more about the benefits of digital technology as well as its risks represents a challenge for modern providers and an opportunity for contemporary researchers.

---

[a] As an example of social media–based psychoeducation, the author has created an animated YouTube video designed to educate parents on how the brain responds to prolonged digital technology exposure. It can be accessed at www.cliffordsussmanmd.com by selecting the link "How Does Internet Use and Gaming Affect the Brain?"

REFERENCES

1. Common Sense Media I. The common sense census: media use by tweens and teens. 2015. Available at: https://www.commonsensemedia.org/research/the-common-sense-census-media-use-by-tweens-and-teens. Accessed January 5, 2017.
2. Young KS. Internet addiction: the emergence of a new clinical disorder. Cyberpsychol Behav 1996;1(3):237–44.
3. Weinstein A, Lejoyeux M. Internet addiction or excessive Internet use. Am J Drug Alcohol Abuse 2010;36(5):277–83.
4. Cash H, Rae CD, Steel AH, et al. Internet addiction: a brief summary of research and practice. Curr Psychiatry Rev 2012;8(4):292–8.
5. Weigle P. Internet and video game addiction: evidence & controversy. Adolesc Psychiatry (Hilversum) 2014;4(2):81–91. Available at: http://www.ingentaconnect.com. ezproxy.lb.polyu.edu.hk/content/ben/aps/2014/00000004/00000002/art00004.
6. Kuss DJ, Lopez-Fernandez O. Internet addiction and problematic Internet use: a systematic review of clinical research. World J Psychiatry 2016;6(1):143.
7. American Psychiatric Association. Diagnostic and statistical manual of mental disorders, fifth edition. Arlington (VA): American Psychiatric Publishing; 2013.
8. Kardefelt-Winther D, Heeren A, Schimmenti A, et al. How can we conceptualize behavioural addiction without pathologizing common behaviours? Addiction 2017;1–7. https://doi.org/10.1111/add.13763.
9. Rehbein F, Psych G, Kleimann M, et al. Prevalence and risk factors of video game dependency in adolescence: results of a German Nationwide survey. Cyberpsychol Behav Soc Netw 2010;13(3):269–77.
10. Achab S, Nicolier M, Mauny F, et al. Massively multiplayer online role-playing games: comparing characteristics of addict vs non-addict online recruited gamers in a French adult population. BMC Psychiatry 2011;11(1):144.
11. Ko CH, Yen JY, Chen CC, et al. Proposed diagnostic criteria of Internet addiction for adolescents. J Nerv Ment Dis 2005;193(11):728–33.
12. Ko CH, Yen JY, Chen SH, et al. Proposed diagnostic criteria and the screening and diagnosing tool of Internet addiction in college students. Compr Psychiatry 2009;50(4):378–84.
13. Kim D, Lee Y, Lee J, et al. Development of Korean smartphone addiction proneness scale for youth. PLoS One 2014;9(5):1–8.
14. Kwon M, Lee JY, Won WY, et al. Development and validation of a smartphone addiction scale (SAS). PLoS One 2013;8(2). https://doi.org/10.1371/journal.pone.0056936.
15. Kor A, Zilcha-Mano S, Fogel YA, et al. Psychometric development of the problematic pornography use scale. Addict Behav 2014;39(5):861–8.
16. Pearcy BTD, Roberts LD, McEvoy PM. Psychometric testing of the personal Internet gaming disorder evaluation-9: a new measure designed to assess Internet gaming disorder. Cyberpsychol Behav Soc Netw 2016;19(5):335–41.
17. Griffiths M. A "components" model of addiction within a biopsychosocial framework. J Subst Use 2005;10(4):191–7.
18. Orosz G, Bőthe B, Tóth-Király I. The development of the problematic series watching scale (PSWS). J Behav Addict 2016;5(1):144–50.
19. Orosz G, Tóth-Király I, Bőthe B, et al. Too many swipes for today: the development of the problematic tinder use scale (PTUS). J Behav Addict 2016;5(3):518–23.

20. Andreassen CS, Torsheim T, Brunborg GS, et al. Development of a Facebook addiction scale. Psychol Rep 2012;110(2):501–17.

21. Choi JS, Park SM, Roh MS, et al. Dysfunctional inhibitory control and impulsivity in Internet addiction. Psychiatry Res 2014;215(2):424–8.

22. Park J-S. Development of Internet addiction measurement scales and Korean Internet addiction index. J Prev Med Public Health 2005;38(3):298–306 [in Korean].

23. Romano M, Osborne LA, Truzoli R, et al. Differential psychological impact of Internet exposure on Internet addicts. PLoS One 2013;8(2):8–11.

24. King DL, Delfabbro PH, Zwaans T, et al. Clinical features and axis I comorbidity of Australian adolescent pathological Internet and video game users. Aust N Z J Psychiatry 2013;47(11):1058–67.

25. Rho MJ, Jeong J-E, Chun J-W, et al. Predictors and patterns of problematic Internet game use using a decision tree model. J Behav Addict 2016;5(3):500–9.

26. Moreno MA, Arseniev-Koehler A, Selkie E. Development and testing of a 3-item screening tool for problematic Internet use. J Pediatr 2016;176:167–72.e1.

27. Rafla M, Carson NJ, DeJong SM. Adolescents and the Internet: what mental health clinicians need to know. Curr Psychiatry Rep 2014;16(9). https://doi.org/10.1007/s11920-014-0472-x.

28. Chen YL, Chen SH, Gau SSF. ADHD and autistic traits, family function, parenting style, and social adjustment for Internet addiction among children and adolescents in Taiwan: a longitudinal study. Res Dev Disabil 2015;39:20–31.

29. Lam LT. Internet gaming addiction, problematic use of the Internet, and sleep problems: a systematic review. Curr Psychiatry Rep 2014;16(4):444.

30. Mihara S, Higuchi S. Cross-sectional and longitudinal epidemiological studies of Internet gaming disorder: a systematic review of the literature. Psychiatry Clin Neurosci 2017. https://doi.org/10.1111/pcn.12532.

31. Griffiths M, Pontes H, Kuss D. Clinical psychology of Internet addiction: a review of its conceptualization, prevalence, neuronal processes, and implications for treatment. Neurosci Neuroecon 2015;11. https://doi.org/10.2147/NAN.S60982.

32. Kilic M, Avci D, Uzuncakmak T. Internet addiction in high school students in Turkey and multivariate analyses of the underlying factors. J Addict Nurs 2016;27(1):39–46.

33. Király O, Griffiths MD, Urbán R, et al. Problematic Internet use and problematic online gaming are not the same: findings from a large nationally representative adolescent sample. Cyberpsychol Behav Soc Netw 2014. https://doi.org/10.1089/cyber.2014.0475.

34. Kawabe K, Horiuchi F, Ochi M, et al. Internet addiction: prevalence and relation with mental states in adolescents. Psychiatry Clin Neurosci 2016;70(9):405–12.

35. Shek DTL, Yu L. Adolescent Internet addiction in Hong Kong: prevalence, change, and correlates. J Pediatr Adolesc Gynecol 2016;29(1):S22–30.

36. Wartberg L, Kriston L, Kammerl R, et al. Prevalence of pathological Internet use in a representative German sample of adolescents: results of a latent profile analysis. Psychopathology 2015;48(1):25–30.

37. Bonnaire C, Phan O. Relationships between parental attitudes, family functioning and Internet gaming disorder in adolescents attending school. Psychiatry Res 2017;255:104–10.

38. Ač-Nikolić E, Zarić D, Nićiforović-Šurković O. Prevalence of Internet addiction among schoolchildren in Novi Sad. Srp Arh Celok Lek 2015;143(11–12):719–25.

39. García-Oliva C, Piqueras JA. Experiential avoidance and technological addictions in adolescents. J Behav Addict 2016;5(2):293–303.
40. Ha JH, Kim SY, Bae SC, et al. Depression and Internet addiction in adolescents. Psychopathology 2007;40(6):424–30.
41. Festl R, Scharkow M, Quandt T. Problematic computer game use among adolescents, younger and older adults. Addiction 2013;108(3):592–9.
42. Eichenberg C, Schott M, Decker O, et al. Attachment style and Internet addiction: an online survey. J Med Internet Res 2017;19(5):e170.
43. Ferguson CJ, Coulson M, Barnett J. A meta-analysis of pathological gaming prevalence and comorbidity with mental health, academic and social problems. J Psychiatr Res 2011;45(12):1573–8.
44. Przybylski AK, Weinstein N, Murayama K. Internet gaming disorder: investigating the clinical relevance of a new phenomenon. Am J Psychiatry 2017; 174(3):230–5.
45. Strittmatter E, Parzer P, Brunner R, et al. A 2-year longitudinal study of prospective predictors of pathological Internet use in adolescents. Eur Child Adolesc Psychiatry 2016;25(7):725–34.
46. Lau JTF, Wu AMS, Gross DL, et al. Is Internet addiction transitory or persistent? Incidence and prospective predictors of remission of Internet addiction among Chinese secondary school students. Addict Behav 2017;74:55–62.
47. Gentile DA, Choo H, Liau A, et al. Pathological video game use among youths: a two-year longitudinal study. Pediatrics 2011;127(2):e319–29.
48. Bessière K, Seay AF, Kiesler S. The ideal elf: identity exploration in World of Warcraft. Cyberpsychol Behav 2007;10(4):530–5.
49. Rodgers RF, Melioli T, Laconi S, et al. Internet addiction symptoms, disordered eating, and body image avoidance. Cyberpsychol Behav Soc Netw 2013;16(1): 56–60.
50. Dieter J, Hill H, Sell M, et al. Avatar's neurobiological traces in the self-concept of massively multiplayer online role-playing game (MMORPG) addicts. Behav Neurosci 2015;129(1):8–17.
51. Lemènager T, Gwodz A, Richter A, et al. Self-concept deficits in massively multiplayer online role-playing games addiction. Eur Addict Res 2013;19(5):227–34.
52. Subramaniam M, Chua BY, Abdin E, et al. Prevalence and correlates of Internet gaming problem among Internet users: results from an Internet survey. Ann Acad Med Singapore 2016;45(5):174–83.
53. Lemmens JS, Hendriks SJF. Addictive online games: examining the relationship between game genres and Internet gaming disorder. Cyberpsychol Behav Soc Netw 2016;19(4):270–6.
54. Nuyens F, Deleuze J, Maurage P, et al. Impulsivity in multiplayer online battle arena gamers: preliminary results on experimental and self-report measures. J Behav Addict 2016;5(2):351–6.
55. Eichenbaum A, Kattner F, Bradford D, et al. Role-playing and real-time strategy games associated with greater probability of Internet gaming disorder. Cyberpsychol Behav Soc Netw 2015;18(8):480–5.
56. Hilgard J, Engelhardt CR, Bartholow BD. Individual differences in motives, preferences, and pathology in video games: the gaming attitudes, motives, and experiences scales (GAMES). Front Psychol 2013;4:1–13. https://doi.org/10.3389/fpsyg.2013.00608.
57. Lukavska K. Time perspective as a predictor of massive multiplayer online role-playing game playing. Cyberpsychol Behav Soc Netw 2012;15(1):50–4.

58. Lukavská K, Hrabec O, Chrz V. The role of habits in massive multiplayer online role-playing game usage: predicting excessive and problematic gaming through players' sensitivity to situational cues. Cyberpsychol Behav Soc Netw 2016;19(4):277–82.

59. Weinstein A, Dorani D, Elhadif R, et al. Internet addiction is associated with social anxiety in young adults. Ann Clin Psychiatry 2015;27(1):4–9.

60. Caplan SE. Relations among loneliness, social anxiety, and problematic Internet use. Cyberpsychol Behav 2007;10(2):234–42.

61. Zadra S, Bischof G, Besser B, et al. The association between Internet addiction and personality disorders in a general population-based sample. J Behav Addict 2016;5(4):691–9.

62. Oberst U, Wegmann E, Stodt B, et al. Negative consequences from heavy social networking in adolescents: the mediating role of fear of missing out. J Adolesc 2017;55:51–60.

63. Kuss DJ, Griffiths MD. Social networking sites and addiction: ten lessons learned. Int J Environ Res Public Health 2017;14(3). https://doi.org/10.3390/ijerph14030311.

64. Meshi D, Morawetz C, Heekeren HR. Nucleus accumbens response to gains in reputation for the self relative to gains for others predicts social media use. Front Hum Neurosci 2013;7:1–11.

65. Jiang D, Zhu S, Ye M, et al. Cross-sectional survey of prevalence and personality characteristics of college students with Internet addiction in Wenzhou, China. Shanghai Arch Psychiatry 2012;24(2):99–107.

66. Jia R, Jia HH. Maybe you should blame your parents: parental attachment, gender, and problematic Internet use. J Behav Addict 2016;5(3):524–8.

67. Schimmenti A, Passanisi A, Gervasi AM, et al. Insecure attachment attitudes in the onset of problematic Internet use among late adolescents. Child Psychiatry Hum Dev 2014;45(5):588–95.

68. Beutel ME, Hoch C, Wölfling K, et al. Clinical characteristics of computer game and Internet addiction in persons seeking treatment. Z Psychosom Med Psychother 2011;57(1):77–90.

69. Kalaitzaki AE, Birtchnell J. The impact of early parenting bonding on young adults' Internet addiction, through the mediation effects of negative relating to others and sadness. Addict Behav 2014;39(3):733–6.

70. Wu X-S, Zhang Z-H, Zhao F, et al. Prevalence of Internet addiction and its association with social support and other related factors among adolescents in China. J Adolesc 2016;52:103–11.

71. Lam LT. Parental mental health and Internet addiction in adolescents. Addict Behav 2015;42:20–3.

72. Ding Q, Li D, Zhou Y, et al. Perceived parental monitoring and adolescent Internet addiction: a moderated mediation model. Addict Behav 2017;74:48–54.

73. Jelenchick LA, Hawk ST, Moreno MA. Problematic Internet use and social networking site use among Dutch adolescents. Int J Adolesc Med Health 2016;28(1):119–21.

74. Ge Y, Se J, Zhang J. Research on relationship among Internet-addiction, personality traits and mental health of urban left-behind children. Glob J Health Sci 2014;7(4). https://doi.org/10.5539/gjhs.v7n4p60.

75. Choi S-W, Kim D-J, Choi J-S, et al. Comparison of risk and protective factors associated with smartphone addiction and Internet addiction. J Behav Addict 2015;4(4):308–14.

76. Yu H, Cho J. Prevalence of Internet gaming disorder among Korean adolescents and associations with non-psychotic psychological symptoms, and physical aggression. Am J Health Behav 2016;40(6):705–16.

77. Wartberg L, Brunner R, Kriston L, et al. Psychopathological factors associated with problematic alcohol and problematic Internet use in a sample of adolescents in Germany. Psychiatry Res 2016;240:272–7.

78. Andreassen CS, Billieux J, Griffiths MD, et al. The relationship between addictive use of social media and video games and symptoms of psychiatric disorders: a large-scale cross-sectional study. Psychol Addict Behav 2016;30(2): 252–62.

79. Tang CSK, Koh YYW. Online social networking addiction among college students in Singapore: comorbidity with behavioral addiction and affective disorder. Asian J Psychiatr 2017;25:175–8.

80. Liu C-H, Lin S-H, Pan Y-C, et al. Smartphone gaming and frequent use pattern associated with smartphone addiction. Medicine (Baltimore) 2016;95(28): e4068.

81. Weinstein A, Yaacov Y, Manning M, et al. Internet addiction and attention deficit hyperactivity disorder among schoolchildren. Isr Med Assoc J 2015;17(12): 731–4.

82. Durkee T, Carli V, Floderus B, et al. Pathological Internet use and risk-behaviors among European adolescents. Int J Environ Res Public Health 2016;13(3). https://doi.org/10.3390/ijerph13030294.

83. Tan Y, Chen Y, Lu Y, et al. Exploring associations between problematic Internet use, depressive symptoms and sleep disturbance among southern Chinese adolescents. Int J Environ Res Public Health 2016;13(3):1–12.

84. Lim J-A, Gwak AR, Park SM, et al. Are adolescents with Internet addiction prone to aggressive behavior? The mediating effect of clinical comorbidities on the predictability of aggression in adolescents with Internet addiction. Cyberpsychol Behav Soc Netw 2015;18(5):260–7.

85. Melchers M, Li M, Chen Y, et al. Low empathy is associated with problematic use of the Internet: empirical evidence from China and Germany. Asian J Psychiatr 2015;17:56–60.

86. Tsimtsiou Z, Haidich A-B, Drontsos A, et al. Pathological Internet use, cyberbullying and mobile phone use in adolescence: a school-based study in Greece. Int J Adolesc Med Health 2017;2013–5. https://doi.org/10.1515/ijamh-2016-0115.

87. Gámez-Guadix M, Borrajo E, Almendros C. Risky online behaviors among adolescents: longitudinal relations among problematic Internet use, cyberbullying perpetration, and meeting strangers online. J Behav Addict 2016;5(1):100–7.

88. Braun B, Kornhuber J, Lenz B. Gaming and religion: the impact of spirituality and denomination. J Relig Health 2016;55(4):1464–71.

89. Lee S-Y, Lee HK, Jeong H, et al. The hierarchical implications of Internet gaming disorder criteria: which indicate more severe pathology? Psychiatry Investig 2017;14(3):249.

90. Kim DJ, Kim K, Lee H-W, et al. Internet game addiction, depression, and escape from negative emotions in adulthood: a nationwide community sample of Korea. J Nerv Ment Dis 2017. https://doi.org/10.1097/NMD.0000000000000698.

91. Reed P, Romano M, Re F, et al. Differential physiological changes following Internet exposure in higher and lower problematic Internet users. PLoS One 2017;12(5):1–11.

92. Shensa A, Escobar-Viera CG, Sidani JE, et al. Problematic social media use and depressive symptoms among U.S. young adults: a nationally-representative study. Soc Sci Med 2017;182:150–7.

93. Park S, Jeon HJ, Son JW, et al. Correlates, comorbidities, and suicidal tendencies of problematic game use in a national wide sample of Korean adults. Int J Ment Health Syst 2017;11(1):35.

94. Morrison CM, Gore H. The relationship between excessive Internet use and depression: a questionnaire-based study of 1,319 young people and adults. Psychopathology 2010;43(2):121–6.

95. Lehenbauer-Baum M, Klaps A, Kovacovsky Z, et al. Addiction and engagement: an explorative study toward classification criteria for Internet gaming disorder. Cyberpsychol Behav Soc Netw 2015;18(6):343–9.

96. Floros G, Siomos K, Stogiannidou A, et al. Comorbidity of psychiatric disorders with Internet addiction in a clinical sample: the effect of personality, defense style and psychopathology. Addict Behav 2014;39(12):1839–45.

97. Alpaslan AH, Soylu N, Kocak U, et al. Problematic Internet use was more common in Turkish adolescents with major depressive disorders than controls. Acta Paediatr 2016;105(6):695–700.

98. Ho RC, Zhang MW, Tsang TY, et al. The association between Internet addiction and psychiatric co-morbidity: a meta-analysis. BMC Psychiatry 2014;14(1):183.

99. Tateno M, Teo AR, Shirasaka T, et al. Internet addiction and self-evaluated attention-deficit hyperactivity disorder traits among Japanese college students. Psychiatry Clin Neurosci 2016;70(12):567–72.

100. Hu J, Zhen S, Yu C, et al. Sensation seeking and online gaming addiction in adolescents: a moderated mediation model of positive affective associations and impulsivity. Front Psychol 2017;8:1–8.

101. So R, Makino K, Fujiwara M, et al. The prevalence of Internet addiction among a Japanese adolescent psychiatric clinic sample with autism spectrum disorder and/or attention-deficit hyperactivity disorder: a cross-sectional study. J Autism Dev Disord 2017;47(7):2217–24.

102. Wölfling K, Beutel ME, Dreier M, et al. Bipolar spectrum disorders in a clinical sample of patients with Internet addiction: hidden comorbidity or differential diagnosis? J Behav Addict 2015;4(2):101–5.

103. Chuang C-WI, Sussman S, Stone MD, et al. Impulsivity and history of behavioral addictions are associated with drug use in adolescents. Addict Behav 2017;74: 41–7.

104. Baysan-Arslan S, Cebci S, Kaya M, et al. Relationship between Internet addiction and alexithymia among university students. Clin Invest Med 2016;39(6): S111–5.

105. Zastrow M. News feature: is video game addiction really an addiction? Proc Natl Acad Sci U S A 2017;114(17):4268–72.

106. Adinoff B. Neurobiologic processes in drug reward and addiction. Harv Rev Psychiatry 2004;12(6):305–20.

107. Jorgenson AG, Hsiao RCJ, Yen CF. Internet addiction and other behavioral addictions. Child Adolesc Psychiatr Clin N Am 2016;25(3):509–20.

108. Wang Y, Wu L, Wang L, et al. Impaired decision-making and impulse control in Internet gaming addicts: evidence from the comparison with recreational Internet game users. Addict Biol 2016. https://doi.org/10.1111/adb.12458.

109. Moschak TM, Carelli RM. Impulsive rats exhibit blunted dopamine release dynamics during a delay discounting task independent of cocaine history. ENeuro 2017;4:1–12.

110. Adisetiyo V, Gray KM. Neuroimaging the neural correlates of increased risk for substance use disorders in attention-deficit/hyperactivity disorder—a systematic review. Am J Addict 2017;26(2):99–111.

111. Dong G, Li H, Wang L, et al. Cognitive control and reward/loss processing in Internet gaming disorder: results from a comparison with recreational Internet game-users. Eur Psychiatry 2017;44:30–8.

112. Dobbs LK, Lemos JC, Alvarez VA. Restructuring of basal ganglia circuitry and associated behaviors triggered by low striatal D2 receptor expression: implications for substance use disorders. Genes Brain Behav 2017;16(1):56–70.

113. Blum K, Chen A, Chen TJ, et al. Activation instead of blocking mesolimbic dopaminergic reward circuitry is a preferred modality in the long term treatment of reward deficiency syndrome (RDS): a commentary. Theor Biol Med Model 2008;5(1):24.

114. Dalley JW, Everitt BJ, Robbins TW. Impulsivity, compulsivity, and top-down cognitive control. Neuron 2011;69(4):680–94.

115. Noël X, Van der Linden M, Bechara A. The neurocognitive mechanisms and loss of willpower. Psychiatry (Edgmont) 2006;3(5):30–41.

116. Weinstein A, Lejoyeux M. New developments on the neurobiological and pharmaco-genetic mechanisms underlying Internet and videogame addiction. Am J Addict 2015;24(2):117–25.

117. Koepp MJ, Gunn RN, Lawrence AD, et al. Evidence for striatal dopamine release during a video game. Nature 1998;393(6682):266–8.

118. Wanat MJ, Kuhnen CM, Phillips PEM. Delays conferred by escalating costs modulate dopamine release to rewards but not their predictors. J Neurosci 2010;30(36):12020–7.

119. Peraile I, Torres E, Mayado A, et al. Dopamine transporter down-regulation following repeated cocaine: implications for 3,4-methylenedioxymethamphetamine-induced acute effects and long-term neurotoxicity in mice. Br J Pharmacol 2010;159(1):201–11.

120. Kuss DJ. Internet gaming addiction: current perspectives. Psychol Res Behav Manag 2013;6:125–37.

121. Choi J, Cho H, Kim J-Y, et al. Structural alterations in the prefrontal cortex mediate the relationship between Internet gaming disorder and depressed mood. Sci Rep 2017;7(1):1245.

122. Kim SH, Baik S-H, Park CS, et al. Reduced striatal dopamine D2 receptors in people with Internet addiction. Neuroreport 2011;22(8):407–11.

123. Hou H, Jia S, Hu S, et al. Reduced striatal dopamine transporters in people with Internet addiction disorder. J Biomed Biotechnol 2012;2012. https://doi.org/10.1155/2012/854524.

124. Hahn T, Notebaert KH, Dresler T, et al. Linking online gaming and addictive behavior: converging evidence for a general reward deficiency in frequent online gamers. Front Behav Neurosci 2014;8:1–6.

125. Han DH, Lee YS, Yang KC, et al. Dopamine genes and reward dependence in adolescents with excessive Internet video game play. J Addict Med 2007;1(3):133–8.

126. Volkow ND, Chang L, Wang GJ, et al. Low level of brain dopamine D2 receptors in methamphetamine abusers: association with metabolism in the orbitofrontal cortex. Am J Psychiatry 2001;158(12):2015–21.

127. Volkow ND, Wang GJ, Smith L, et al. Recovery of dopamine transporters with methamphetamine detoxification is not linked to changes in dopamine release. Neuroimage 2015;121:20–8.

128. Pennay AE, Lee NK. Putting the call out for more research: the poor evidence base for treating methamphetamine withdrawal. Drug Alcohol Rev 2011;30(2): 216–22.

129. Gola M, Wordecha M, Sescousse G, et al. Can pornography be addictive? An fMRI study of men seeking treatment for problematic pornography use. Neuropsychopharmacology 2017;5:1–11.

130. Ko CH, Liu GC, Hsiao S, et al. Brain activities associated with gaming urge of online gaming addiction. J Psychiatr Res 2009;43(7):739–47.

131. Ko CH, Liu GC, Yen JY, et al. Brain correlates of craving for online gaming under cue exposure in subjects with Internet gaming addiction and in remitted subjects. Addict Biol 2013;18(3):559–69.

132. Bae S, Han DH, Kim SM, et al. Neurochemical correlates of Internet game play in adolescents with attention deficit hyperactivity disorder: a proton magnetic resonance spectroscopy (MRS) study. Psychiatry Res 2016;254:10–7.

133. Kühn S, Gallinat J. Brains online: structural and functional correlates of habitual Internet use. Addict Biol 2015;20(2):415–22.

134. Meng Y, Deng W, Wang H, et al. The prefrontal dysfunction in individuals with Internet gaming disorder: a meta-analysis of functional magnetic resonance imaging studies. Addict Biol 2015;20(4):799–808.

135. Weng C-B, Qian R-B, Fu X-M, et al. Gray matter and white matter abnormalities in online game addiction. Eur J Radiol 2013;82(8):1308–12.

136. Kim J-Y, Jeong J-E, Rhee J-K, et al. Targeted exome sequencing for the identification of a protective variant against Internet gaming disorder at rs2229910 of neurotrophic tyrosine kinase receptor, type 3 (NTRK3): a pilot study. J Behav Addict 2016;5(4):631–8.

137. Buono FD, Sprong ME, Lloyd DP, et al. Delay discounting of video game players: comparison of time duration among gamers. Cyberpsychol Behav Soc Netw 2017;20(2):104–8.

138. Van Holst RJ, Lemmens JS, Valkenburg PM, et al. Attentional bias and disinhibition toward gaming cues are related to problem gaming in male adolescents. J Adolesc Health 2017;50(6):541–6.

139. Fernandez-Serrano MJ, Cesar Peraleslopez J, Moreno-Lopez L, et al. Impulsivity and compulsivity in cocaine dependent individuals. Adicciones 2012; 24(2):105–13 [in Spanish].

140. Liu L, Xue G, Potenza MN, et al. Dissociable neural processes during risky decision-making in individuals with Internet-gaming disorder. Neuroimage Clin 2017;14:741–9.

141. Christakis DA, Ramirez JSB, Ramirez JM. Overstimulation of newborn mice leads to behavioral differences and deficits in cognitive performance. Scientific Reports 2012;2(546). https://doi.org/10.1038/srep00546.

142. Ravinder S, Donckels EA, Ramirez JSB, et al. Excessive sensory stimulation during development alters neural plasticity and vulnerability to cocaine in mice. eNeuro 2016;3:1–11.

Treatment Considerations in Internet and Video Game Addiction: A Qualitative Discussion

David N. Greenfield, PhD, MS[a,b],*

KEYWORDS

- Social media • Smartphone addiction • Online gaming • Internet addiction treatment
- Internet addiction • Process addiction • Video game addiction
- Child and adolescent addiction medicine

KEY POINTS

- This article reviews the etiologic and neurobiological antecedents to Internet and video game addiction.
- An understanding of patient readiness and motivational factors in Internet and video game addiction treatment is addressed.
- The unique aspects of Internet and video game use that contribute to its addictive nature are presented.
- Psychotherapeutic and pharmacologic treatment interventions are presented, along with a comprehensive treatment model.

INTRODUCTION

To address the myriad of potential treatment issues and strategies applicable to Internet and video game addiction (IVGA) and related use disorders, a working definition of addiction is first presented. All addictions have similar behavioral and neurobiological etiology and symptomatology, although the severity varies widely.[1]

ADDICTION MEDICINE DEFINED

Perhaps, the most comprehensive definition of addiction is one published by The American Society of Addiction Medicine,[1] which captures both the neurobiological and behavioral etiology of disruption in the mesolimbic reward circuitry of the brain and the impact of addictive behaviors:

Disclosure Statement: Dr D.N. Greenfield has nothing to disclose.
[a] Department of Psychiatry, University of Connecticut, School of Medicine, Farmington, CT 06030, USA; [b] The Center for Internet and Technology Addiction, 8 Lowell Road, West Hartford, CT 06119, USA
* The Center for Internet and Technology Addiction, 8 Lowell Road, West Hartford, CT 06119.
E-mail address: drdave@virtual-addiction.com

Child Adolesc Psychiatric Clin N Am 27 (2018) 327–344
https://doi.org/10.1016/j.chc.2017.11.007
1056-4993/18/© 2017 Elsevier Inc. All rights reserved.

Abbreviations	
ADHD	Attention deficit hyperactivity disorder
CBT	Cognitive–behavioral therapy
IVGA	Internet and video game addiction
OCD	Obsessive–compulsive disorder
SSRI	Selective serotonin reuptake inhibitor

Addiction is a primary, chronic disease of brain reward, motivation, memory and related circuitry. Dysfunction in these circuits leads to characteristic biological, psychological, social and spiritual manifestations. This is reflected in an individual pathologically pursuing reward and/or relief by substance use and other behaviors.

Addiction is characterized by inability to consistently abstain, impairment in behavioral control, craving, diminished recognition of significant problems with one's behaviors and interpersonal relationships, and a dysfunctional emotional response. Like other chronic diseases, addiction often involves cycles of relapse and remission. Without treatment or engagement in recovery activities, addiction is progressive and can result in disability or premature death.[1]

Although premature death is an infrequent consequence of IVGA, there are numerous psychological, behavioral, and physiologic consequences to protracted Internet and video game use.

Numerous anecdotal and clinical reports describe physiologic sequelae secondary to sedentary behavior, including elevated cortisol, hypertension, deep vein thrombosis, electrolyte imbalances leading to cardiac dysrhythmias, obesity, and metabolic disorders.[2,3] All addictions ultimately impact lifestyle, functioning, and behavior—and hence have similar functional deficits of variable severity.

Brain circuits implicated in the complex biobehavioral phenomenon of addiction include the ventral tegmental area/substantia nigra, amygdala, anterior cingulate, prefrontal cortex, and nucleus accumbens. These circuits are also implicated in IVGA.[4,5] There is some controversy in the addiction medicine as to the similarities and differences between substance-based and behavioral (or process) addictions.

The American Society of Addiction Medicine definition substantively captures the complex biopsychosocial interplay that defines addiction as a complex brain–behavior disorder. Research, clinical experience, and historical analysis of addiction by Hari[6] and Alexander[7] strongly suggest that social isolation is a strongly correlated factor for the development of an addictive pattern to a reinforcing behavior such as drug use or other behavioral addictions. We are hard-wired for social connection, and when deprived of it we are inclined to engage with a drug or behavior that medicates this need. The maxim that "the opposite of addiction is not abstinence but rather connection"[6] speaks volumes about the addictive nature of the Internet, video games and social media—all of which provide a pseudoconnection while often actually isolating the user socially.

A DIGITAL DRUG

Some disagreement exists regarding the appropriate nosology for IVGA, but considerable clinical and research data document the use of, abuse of, and potential addiction to the Internet and Internet-mediated gaming.[8–17] Internet content and video games are typically accessed easily via portable handheld and console computers, as well as on smartphones, making ease of access a factor[18] in their addictive potential. Ease of access (or threshold reduction) has a significant impact of the addictiveness of the Internet and video gaming, because shorter latency between substance ingestion or a mood-altering behavior and subsequent reinforcement, the more addictive that process is.[18,19] This is likely due to the operant and classically conditioned features of tolerance and extinction resistance characteristic of addictions, including Internet-related addictions.[18]

The marked phenomenological overlap between Internet addiction, substance addiction, and gambling suggests that a common neurobiological substrate involving an impairment of the "reward systems" underlies these disorders. The mesolimbic dopaminergic pathway represents the final common pathway for reinforcement and gratification induced by physiologic stimuli or psychotropic drugs. It follows that dopamine is considered to be the neurotransmitter mediating pleasure.[20]

Use of Internet entertainment, particularly via the smartphone, seems to hamper our ability to manage and balance time, energy, and attention, leading to lifestyle changes and behavioral deficits. IVGA impacts motivation, reward, memory, and various aspects of psychological functioning. There are numerous distinct psychological and cognitive processes that seem to contribute to the additive potential of the Internet. Numerous studies have found several key factors that are associated with the compulsive use of the Internet and video games, namely, disinhibition, ease of access, content stimulation, dissociation (time distortion), perceived anonymity, and the activation of neurobiological reward pathways.[8,9,16,18]

Disinhibition

Disinhibition allows users to express and experience themselves in manner that is less impacted by ego constraints, and take on a persona or alter-ego state. This may, in part, be due to less access to executive functions in the orbitofrontal area of the brain within which inhibitory circuits are organized. It seems the brain can become highjacked in it's inhibitory capacity during online access.

Content Stimulation

The Internet and its various portals are essentially delivery mechanisms for powerful and stimulating content. Video games, pornography, infotainment, social media, shopping, and gambling all have reinforcing properties unto themselves. The power of the Internet is in part due to its unique, interactive ability to rapidly deliver such content with greater ease of access, thereby creating a threshold reduction in experiencing said stimulating content.

The combination of stimulating content delivered with ever-decreasing latency produce synergistic amplification. Here, the whole is greater than the sum of its parts. The Internet experience can be thought of as a virtual hypodermic mechanism to deliver the digital-drug content in a highly efficacious manner.

Ease-of-Access

Ease-of-access is a well known contributory factor in all addictions; the ability to readily access intoxicating substances or behaviors clearly increases the likelihood of compulsive or addictive use. Internet and video game availability acts as a neurobiological trigger, facilitating activation of the mesolimbic brain pathways in a manner similar to kindling a fire. Once ignited, the neuropathways and behavior patterns become sensitized and essentially are on automatic pilot.

Dissociation (Time Distortion)

The experience of altered perception of time and space is a ubiquitous experience of the Internet medium.[9,18] The medium itself, along with the consumed content, alters the perception of time, and is therefore psychoactive and thus, mood and consciousness altering.

Perceived Anonymity

This curious phenomenon seems to be a significant marker for the Internet experience. As a communication and e-commerce modality: texting, instant messaging, chat, email, social media, shopping, stock trading, gambling, and pornography, and so on, are frequently experienced as anonymous or nearly anonymous, creating a unique commercial and communication interface. Users communicate and conduct business as if they are alone or as if they have a personal or private relationship with the person or business they are connecting to. Ironically, the Internet is perhaps the least anonymous of all communication mediums.

Activation of Neurobiological Reward Pathways

The Internet seems to activate the same mesolimbic reward pathways that are activated by psychoactive substances and other addictive behaviors.[21]

A VIRTUAL SLOT MACHINE

Use of the Internet functions as the "world's largest slot machine". The Internet operates on a variable ratio reinforcement schedule where there is unpredictability in what, when, and how desirable the content searched for, or received is. A slot machine operates similarly. Unpredictability keeps our brains tuned in and vigilant, and encountering pleasurable stimuli causes release of dopamine in the brain's reward circuits. This reward is variable and unpredictable, causing the related behavior of checking online accounts or accessing smartphones to be highly habit forming and resistant to extinction. Checking phones can reach compulsive levels, whether accessing stocks, sports, social media, web searching, text, email, gaming, or pornography. Numerous studies[5,22] suggest that addictive Internet and video game use is associated with excessive dopamine release in the mesolimbic system, which leads to a desensitizing reduction in dopamine receptor expression, reward deficiency syndrome, and hypofrontality.[18,22]

The smartphone adds another dimension to our Internet experience with its frequent use of notifications. Users may be constantly alerted via beeps, buzzes, and blips that inform users that information is waiting to be accessed. This leads to the anticipation of possibly desirable content, providing a significant increase in dopamine, analogous to that which keeps one pushing the handle on a slot machine. Preliminary evidence suggests that smartphone notifications and ringing stimulate release of the stress hormone cortisol, in turn triggering a self-medicating response to engage with the device.[2,3,23-25]

When the information accessed is perceived as pleasurable, the user receives another reinforcing dopamine surge. The smartphone can also be called the world's smallest slot machine fitting easily in one's purse or pocket.

Considerable research suggests that the stronger levels of dopamine occur in conjunction with anticipation of reward than with reward itself. Anticipation may occur when one is "triggered" by the sight of a computer device or to a greater degree when alerted by a notification.

Smartphones can keep users on "automatic pilot," responding to life on an automated, unconscious level, inhibiting one from making healthy choices. Users may socially isolate, become intolerant of boredom, and maintain constant distraction from their current situation. In short, users can become overstimulated and attention impaired.

The new digital culture places little value on real-time experiences that are not broadcast, as if our experiences do not actually occur unless witnessed and rated by others. This phenomenon further contributes to the experience of fear of missing out (FOMO), the concern that one must update via social media while monitoring the updates of peers, or one will fail to be noticed or included. Ironically, what we seem to be missing is the present-centered experience of our own lives. Excessive Internet use may cause health problems, including increased sedentary behavior, limited attention capacity, and stress from constant vigilance.

Compulsive smartphone use leading to elevated distractibility can also become a health threat; recent data[25,26] clearly demonstrate that excessive use often continues while users are driving their cars. Those who compulsively use smartphones while driving cause an alarming number of accidents, injuries, and deaths. Recent findings indicate that texting is not the only way smartphones distracts drivers, because users engage with a variety of smartphone functions while driving.

TREATMENT CONSIDERATIONS

The treatment of Internet addiction has not yet been standardized.[27–30] This factor is typical of addiction medicine, which is characterized by a lack of treatment standardization for most addictions.[31] A considerable lack of clarity remains regarding the exact definition of Internet addiction, what to label it, and whether to classify it via a unified diagnoses or distinct subdiagnoses.[32] Regardless, there is considerable public need for treatment services.[29]

A significant demand for treatment of Internet addiction exists in the United States; prevalence statistics suggest a range of 0.5% to 12%.[29,30] Even greater demand exists in China, Taiwan, and South Korea, where the estimated prevalence among adolescents ranges from 1.6%[33] to 11.3%.[34] Despite considerable overlap in current measures of diagnosis, a lack of agreed-upon criteria contributes to the difficulty in precisely determining prevalence. Treatment for addictions is often ultimately successful, which applies to both process and substance-based addictions.

SPECIFIC TREATMENT INTERVENTIONS

The first goal is to determine level of motivation of patient. Who is the "customer" and who is invested in the treatment process? In many cases, the patient may be a child, adolescent, or young adult, and treatment must involve parents as well. Try to structure interventions based on the motivation and resources of the patient and family. It is important to understand the developmental and psychosocial context of symptoms. Why is the patient presenting for treatment now? What developmental processes are ongoing for the patient? What stresses currently exist in patient's life? Are there social problems? Family re-education is critical, for re-empowering the parents to help set appropriate boundaries and expectations. Strategies include boundaries and limit setting, as well as management of family technology (parenting skills), modifying and controlling the use or abuse pattern, marital issues, medications, comorbidity, secondary gain, and incentive induction toward real-time living. Parental involvement in treatment is essential for successful outcome.

IMPLICATIONS OF CURRENT CLINICAL AND NEUROBIOLOGICAL RESEARCH ON THE TREATMENT OF INTERNET AND VIDEO GAME ADDICTION AND RELATED INTERNET USE DISORDERS

IVGA is part of a "reward deficiency syndrome" caused by a negative downregulation of dopamine after excessive dopamine release secondary to abnormal neurotransmitter interactions in the mesolimbic system.[35–38] Considerations include natural history, phenomenology, tolerance, withdrawal, comorbidity, attention deficit hyperactivity disorder (ADHD), overlapping genetic contribution, neurobiological mechanisms, and response to treatment strongly suggest that behavioral (process) addiction such as Internet addiction resemble substance addictions and that excessive Internet use is indeed an addiction. Winkler and colleagues[37] found that both pharmacologic and psychological treatments were effective in treating Internet addiction (time spent online, depression, and anxiety).

COGNITIVE–BEHAVIORAL THERAPY

Numerous studies have suggested cognitive–behavioral therapy (CBT) is an effective treatment for Internet addictions.[28,39–45] Patients are trained to recognize triggers that encourage self-medication using the Internet and video games, and how to alter thoughts and behaviors to promote abstinence.

A meta-review of Chinese Internet addiction studies[44] supported the relative efficacy of CBT. Most contemporary addiction treatments have a strong CBT component. As Greenfield[46] notes, many if not most psychotherapeutic and behavioral interventions have cognitive–behavioral components, but addiction medicine heavily relies on psychoeducational strategies and identifying the cognitive, emotional, and behavioral triggers and relapse antecedents.

Metaanaylses by King and Delfabbro[42] and others[43] found that cognitive–behavioral strategies are efficacious in managing IVGA. Similar results have been found in the treatment of substance abuse, especially for adolescents and young adults, for whom cognitive and psychoeducational approaches may be particularly effective.[47–49]

MOTIVATIONAL INTERVIEWING, MOTIVATIONAL ENHANCEMENT, AND HARM REDUCTION

Motivational interviewing and motivational enhancement are effective techniques to evaluate, establish, and increase motivation for abstinence as well as therapeutic alliance for treatment of addictions.[50] Patients seeking assistance for Internet-related disorders, like other addictions, have variable readiness for change,[51] and are frequently pressured into treatment by a family member. This factor is particularly relevant in treating Internet and gaming addictions, because these patients often lack an appreciation of the negative sequelae of their behavior. This barrier to successful treatment is exacerbated by a lack of clinicians experienced in treating IVGA and the variability of professional acceptance of the disorder as legitimate. These factors, along with the popular view of the Internet and video games as harmless entertainment, create roadblocks in the treatment process on many levels.

MOTIVATIONAL INTERVIEWING AND MOTIVATIONAL ENHANCEMENT

People are generally better persuaded by the reasons which they have themselves discovered than by those which have come in to the mind of others.
—*Blaise Pascal*

It is critical in the treatment of any substance or behavioral/process addiction that adequate treatment motivation exist. Typically, however, many patients do not arrive for treatment at the highest level of motivation; therefore, attempts must be made to enhance treatment readiness and motivation, and potentially enhance them in the early course of evaluation or treatment.[50]

It is important for the clinician to be aware of personal judgments, feelings, fears, and frustrations toward the Internet or video game addict and be conscious of our natural tendency to judge our patient's actions or behaviors. Be conscious of ascribing negative prognosis in the face of a chronic, relapsing disorder:

- Become familiar with the neurobiology of addiction both as a clinician and to help educate the patient to understand the process of IVGA. Many suffering with this issue do not know about the neurologic factors associated with their illness.
- Learn to assess your patient's readiness to change, so you can apply appropriate motivational interviewing and motivational enhancement[52] interventions; it is important to remember that readiness to change and motivation are not necessarily linear, and may wax and wane throughout the evaluation, treatment, and subsequent recovery process.
- Beware of cognitive dissonance, where we presume patient motivation and prognosis based on addiction-based behaviors.
- IVGA treatment and management can be challenging, but so are many chronic medical illnesses!
- View addiction as any other chronic medical condition that may have exacerbations, remissions, and relapses—as well as recovery periods. Educate your patient about this recovery process.
- Only 50% of the epidemiology for addiction seems to be genetic; the rest seems to be environmental/behavioral, and epigenetic, which is a large part of where we as clinicians need to work.
- The longer the patient is abstinent, the more likely sustainable and moderated Internet and video game will last.

READINESS FOR CHANGE AND TREATMENT

How many mental health or addiction clinicians does it take to change a light bulb? One, but the light bulb has to want to change.

The evaluation and management of patient motivation and readiness is as critical a feature of Internet addiction treatment as it is in other addictions. Patients' present at variable stages of readiness for change and recovery. The clinician must meet the patient with interventions appropriate to his or her particular level of motivation.[51] Stages of readiness for change are not linear; patients frequently move back and forth among varying stages, requiring clinicians to maintain a flexible treatment approach to remain effective. The stages of readiness and corresponding clinical goals are precontemplation, contemplation, preparation, action, maintenance, and relapse.

Precontemplation

In this stage, the patient is not currently considering change. The clinician should validate a lack of readiness. Clarify with the patient that the decision is theirs (although this is complicated when a parent is bringing a child or adolescent in for treatment). Encourage reevaluation of current behaviors and their consequences. Foster exploration for the patient, not actions. Explain and personalize the risks of excessive Internet use through psychoeducation, including the neurobiological underpinnings of addiction. Encourage questioning of whether the patient has a problem by highlighting that others (eg, parents, spouse, employer, friends) believe that they do.

Contemplation

In this stage, the patient is ambivalent about change, or "sitting on the fence." This patient is probably not considering changing within the next month. The clinician's goal is to validate their current lack of readiness and clarify that the decision regarding whether to change is theirs (as are the consequences). Encourage evaluation of the pros and cons of behavior change and help to identify and promote positive outcome expectations.

Preparation

Patients at this stage have some experience with change and are in the early stages of beginning to change addictive behavior: they are "testing the waters" and may planning to act within a month. Adolescents and young adults who are brought in for treatment by a family member are less likely to present at this stage. The clinician is to identify and assist in problem solving and helping them to remove obstacles to change. Help the patient to identify social supports for change. Encourage small, attainable initial steps in the recovery process. Affirm that patient has the ability to access or develop the necessary skills and behaviors to change their Internet and video game use patterns.

Action

Patients at this stage are practicing the new behavior. Clinicians should focus on restructuring cues and triggers, as well as strengthening social supports, including family relationships. Bolster self-efficacy for dealing with obstacles such as emotional challenges. Help to combat feelings of longing for the Internet and video gaming, and emphasize the long-term benefits of recovery and change. Highlight the positives of a balanced relationship with technology.

Maintenance

The patient has successfully changed behavior, and demonstrates a continued commitment to sustaining new behaviors. This outcome can occur at any point after treatment at 6 months to 5 years or more. Plan for supportive follow-up. Reinforce self-regulation including internal rewards for positive behavior. Discuss coping with potential relapse. It should be noted that all of these stages are not absolute or cumulative, and patients may move back and forth in their individual recovery readiness.

Relapse

This patient has resumed old addictive Internet and video game behaviors in a "fall from grace": clinicians should evaluate the triggers causing relapse including urges, cravings, and cognitions around relapse. Develop or reaffirm a clear relapse prevention plan. Reassess motivation and possible barriers to mindful and moderated use. Help the patient plan stronger coping strategies. Addiction is a chronic, relapsing disorder that can be progressive in severity as well as cumulative in its recovery. Relapse is a normal part of the IVGA recovery process.

Our greatest gift in medicine is the installation of hope. Sometimes it is difficult for us to feel hopeful, or to adequately convey it to our patients, especially when we see our patients relapsing and experiencing negative sequelae. Medical compliance and treatment adherence is about 50%, yet in the treatment of addictions we somehow expect better or higher compliance, and when we do not see it, we might interpret this as a lack of motivation, which can interfere with effective treatment.

ABSTINENCE VERSUS MODERATED OR MINDFUL TECHNOLOGY USE

It is indeed difficult to achieve abstinence with IVGA. Perhaps the best option is for moderated and mindful use and to remove the most problematic (triggering) content areas through external controls. Modified use via behavioral and neurobiological repatterning (identifying and changing the trigger or urge response pattern) can begin to repattern the neuropathways that have been established regarding the addictive pattern. The use of eye movement desensitization reprocessing has been helpful in reducing urges and triggers.[31,53] Treating concomitant social anxiety and social skills deficits (along with comorbid ADHD) may also be helpful.

Internet use disorder presents with a variety of unique characteristics in which addictive behaviors seem to be socially normative within the digital youth culture, further exacerbating denial.[46] Internet entertainment is an addictive behavior that seems to be acceptable within contemporary youth culture. As part of the youth digital culture, the smartphone has arguably become the dominant Internet access portal, and may be seen as a vital social and personal accessory, and may be personified as a digital member of the family.

A PRACTICAL ADDICTION MEDICINE TREATMENT OUTLINE FOR INTERNET AND VIDEO GAME ADDICTION AND RELATED USE DISORDERS

Greenfield[46] developed a 7-step treatment process for IVGA. The model was developed over a 20-year period of providing outpatient and intensive outpatient treatment for IVGAs. This model views the treatment in a manner analogous to standard treatment protocols for other addictions, with some unique variations. This outline is not a fixed treatment protocol as in most addictions. IVGA treatment must be modified with moderated and mindful use. Exacerbations, relapses, and treatment adjusts must be made throughout the process, and no 2 patients are alike. These are guidelines to help inform the clinician on how to begin to manage and treatment IVGA.

The Center for Internet and Technology Addiction[33] uses a combination of psychoeducation and neurobiological education, motivational interviewing and motivational enhancement, psychotherapy, pharmacotherapy, management of comorbid or concurrent psychiatric issues, eye movement desensitization reprocessing[53] using a modified addiction management protocol, and varied readiness for change[51] and harm reduction strategies as described herein.[52]

Patient Engagement

In this critical stage, a collaborative treatment relationship is developed for the management and treatment of IVGA. This first stage is the most critical component of successful treatment, because without a collaborative relationship, treatment motivation, adherence, and compliance will be greatly reduced. It is critical here to build the treatment relationship and, in accessing readiness for change, establishing motivational enhancement and patient support throughout the initial as well as subsequent phases of treatment.

Pattern Disruption

This phase is intended disrupt the behavioral aspects of the addiction and compulsive use patterns. The goal is to interrupt problematic coping, self-medication, and trigger–response loops and begin to allow new, more adaptive, healthier Internet and video game use to emerge. Sometimes it is necessary to prescribe a period of relative abstinence, with a particular focus on the problematic content, for example, video gaming, pornography, social media, or shopping; very problematic content may need to be blocked and/or monitors at this stage, in addition to other measures that can be taken. The patient begins to develop a more mindful use of the Internet, and in so doing, begins the process of breaking neural pathways associated with their maladaptive use pattern. Because all addictions involve both disruptions of the mesolimbic reward circuitry as well as antecedent and ritualistic behavioral patterns, we are attempting to access this brain circuitry through such pattern changes. We are counting on the neuroplastic and neurotrophic aspects of the brain–behavior relationship help to rewire the addiction behavior response pattern.

The goal is to begin to establish and strengthen new brain pathways, and to begin to decrease the pattern of dopamine post-synaptic receptor (downregulation) associated with addictive disorders. In doing so, we to begin to decrease the consequences of any reward deficiency syndrome by minimizing the excessive reward salience associated with addictive use, thus slowly encouraging other forms of rewarding behavior, possibly a novel experience after years of addiction. Hopefully, there will be more positive life consequences and rewards that are real time and naturalistic, as opposed to Internet or video game reward salience.

Trigger Identification

All addictions involve behavioral triggers, which themselves have antecedents. It is critical to identify emotional and situational triggers that exacerbate the additive cycle of behavior. Availability (ease of access), boredom, anxiety (particularly social anxiety), and academic/work avoidance are common triggers, but other triggers may be unique to the specific patient. The major treatment goal of this phase is to help the patient identify the triggers for their addictive use, and establish more mindful, moderate technology habits. Patients must increase self-awareness and then develop new trigger management skills in anticipation of posttreatment triggers.

Management of Urges, Cravings, and Compulsions (Pharmacologic and Other Therapeutic Interventions)

In this stage, psychoeducational and cognitive–behavioral strategies are most useful. The management of cravings to engage in Internet use involves an increased awareness of one's inner mood state and external environmental triggers.

Internet addicts are typically hyperfocused on screen content and unaware of their internal process, and are, therefore, disconnected from themselves and others. This lack of mindfulness impairs social connection, which further exacerbates a desire to self-medicate. In-person social connection can be a partial antidote to IVGA. The absence of in-person contact contributes to social isolation, dissociation, and time distortion that coincides with Internet addiction. Addicts have little awareness of how much time they are spending online, and this further inhibiting self-reflection, examining contributing triggers, and the monitoring of physiologic symptoms and experiences.

PHARMACOTHERAPY AND MEDICALLY AUGMENTED THERAPIES

A number of recent studies have addressed the use of pharmacotherapy in the treatment of IVGA.[54–61] Antidepressants[54,56,58] and antipsychotics[54] have both been used with varying degrees of success, along with other pharmacologic agents. Evidence-based addiction medicine has repeatedly demonstrated the need to use a combination of psychotherapeutic and psychoeducational approaches as the primary treatment of addiction, even when using medications adjunctively. Pharmacotherapies seem to have promising usefulness as adjunctive treatment of IVGA, as well as for management of comorbid symptomatology.

Several psychopharmacologic agents may be useful in medically augmented treatment for Internet addiction and related disorders, although research evidence regarding medication strategies is limited in both depth and breadth. Efficacy has been demonstrated to some degree for various antidepressants, opioid receptor antagonists and partial agonists, mood stabilizers, antipsychotics, glutametergic drugs, N-methyl-D-aspartate receptor antagonists, and psychostimulants.[54–63]

The medication that has been studied most extensively for the treatment of IVGA is bupropion. A 6-week open- label trial of buproprion sustained release in 11 patients with IVGA was related to decreased craving for video games and cue-induced brain activity, Internet addiction scores, and time spend online.[60] It seems that the drug was effective, but the study noted limitations by its small sample size. A randomized, double-blind trial compared bupropion plus psychoeducation with placebo plus psychoeducation in 50 participants with excessive online gaming and major depressive disorder.[61] During the 8-week trial, those treated with bupropion showed improvement in depression and video game addiction, and spent less time online than those treated with placebo. Bupropion seemed to be an effective adjunctive treatment for both depression and video game addiction in this study. A third open-label clinical trial of 65 adolescents with comorbid major depressive disorder and video game addiction compared bupropion with combined bupropion plus group CBT.[41] After 8 weeks, both groups showed improvement, but the combination group showed greater benefit for video game addiction severity and life satisfaction compared with the medication-only group. This finding suggests that bupropion treatment for depression and video game addiction may be most effective when combined with CBT.

One case report indicated that a patient with an Internet gaming addiction who was treated with escitalopram 30 mg for 3 months resulted in improved mood and a significant reduction in the drive to play online gaming, with a complete functional recovery.[56] An open-label trial of escitalopram (20 mg/d for 10 weeks) on 19 Internet addicts found significant decreases in weekly hours spent online and improvements in global functioning in 11 patients (64.7%).[56] At the end of the trial, subjects were blindly randomized either to continued escitalopram treatment or to placebo; both groups maintained gains made in the initial open-label treatment, but at the end of the double-blind phase there were no significant differences between the 2 groups. Larger controlled trials are clearly needed to investigate the efficacy of escitalopram and other selective serotonin reuptake inhibitors (SSRIs) for the treatment of IVGA.[58]

SSRIs may suppress inhibitory responses and the control of compulsive repetition, which likely explains their effectiveness in treating obsessive–compulsive disorders (OCDs). There also seem to be data indicating a high lifetime prevalence of major depression in Internet addicts. Clinical studies have also suggested a close relationship between dysregulation, impulsivity, and symptoms of the obsessive–compulsive spectrum, for which serotonergic drugs are known to be effective.[59,64,65] However, although definitely effective in treating OCD, SSRIs have shown mixed results in some impulse control disorders, namely, pathologic gambling, kleptomania, and compulsive shopping (as well as Internet addiction).[57,62,63,65]

The augmentation of SSRIs with atypical antipsychotics for the management of refractory OCD is gaining increasing acceptance. IVGA has some features in common with OCD, but appears to be a unique and distinct disorder. It has been hypothesized that quetiapine might be particularly useful for OCD,[59] and may also be a safe and effective augmenting medication in cases with problematic Internet use. Atypical antipsychotics have been successfully used to remediate address behavioral issues associated with drug abuse, including impulsivity. In a review article Camardese and colleagues[57] proposed that SSRIs may potentially efficacious in the treatment IVGA and related disorders.[57]

The role of psychostimulants may be confounded by the frequently observed co-morbidity of ADHD seen in IVGAs. Indeed, it is uncommon for a patient to present with Internet addiction without preexisting or concomitant ADHD symptomatology Pharmacologic interventions are often used in addiction medicine as an adjunct for managing comorbid psychiatric symptoms, and less frequently than for the pharmacologic management of urges, cravings, and triggers, which also likely seems to be the case for psychostimulant management of IVGA.

In an 8-week trial of methylphenidate treatment for children with ADHD who played online video games, Internet addiction score and Internet use times were significantly decreased. The changes in Internet addiction scores between the baseline and 8-week assessments were correlated positively with the changes in inattention scores and performance on the Visual Continuous Performance Test. This finding suggests that Internet video game play is directly related to ADHD severity, and might be a means of self-medication for children with ADHD. This reflects the high rates of ADHD in patients with IVGA[18,65]

Opioid receptor antagonists inhibit dopamine release in the nucleus accumbens and ventral pallidum, and other brain areas that mediate gratification, reinforcement, compulsion, and perseveration. Agents such as naltrexone have shown some clinical usefulness in the treatment of substance use disorders, gambling disorder, and kleptomania, and have also been considered for use in some behavioral addictions. However, research evidence regarding their effectiveness in are currently limited case reports.[62]

This case described a successful treatment of online pornography addiction with naltrexone.[20,62] By blocking the capacity of endogenous opioids to trigger dopamine release in response to reward, naltrexone may block the reinforcing nature of compulsive Internet and video game use.[64] Internet sexual activity and theoretically other IVGA behaviors. Future research is needed to better assess the effectiveness of these and other pharmacologic agents in treating IVGA. However, for the time being medication treatment remains adjunctive to more effective psychotherapeutic remedies, as described elsewhere in this article.

Blocking, Monitoring, and Filtering

When dealing with substance-based addictions, addiction medicine typically espouses abstinence from all substances of abuse. This goal is appropriate for substance use disorders. However, in cases of IVGA it is generally unrealistic to avoid all Internet use. It seems that many aspects of everyday work and personal life are conducted online, and this perhaps is further complicated by modern society's dependence on smartphones. It is possible to achieve absence from specific problematic areas of Internet use (such as video games, pornography, social media) while continuing to use the Internet in more mindful and conscious ways.

An important goal for the treatment of Internet addiction should be to limit, monitor, and possibly block specific triggers, such as problematic content websites and Internet or video game content that serve as gateways to pathologic use. The initial goal is to detox from the most problematic sites and content, and then to relearn mindful technology use. It is sometimes possible to later reintroduce some of the problematic content in a limited way with less risk of relapse. However, in the case of an addiction to specific video games or pornography, it may be necessary to maintain ongoing abstinence. Many Internet and video game users have specific games, apps, or content that quickly lead to addictive use and may need to be avoided.

It should be noted that patients with an addictive video game habit often substitute gaming with watching videos of gaming on YouTube or other sites. This activity stimulates the addict's brain and may trigger a craving to play, creating opportunities for potential relapse. A qualified IT expert can block such triggering sites on the addict's computers, providing a buffer against triggering access to the most problematic sites and content, while allowing use of safer Internet content that may be useful for daily living. This measure creates a delay that allows for lithe inhibitive orbitofrontal circuits to be more easily accessed, preventing instant gratification via addictive content. We have seen how the addictive Internet content, once accessed, operates on a variable ratio reinforcement schedule, but such blocks can minimize potential relapse by creating disruptive extinction resistance.

An IT specialist can also set up monitoring software, providing the clinician with weekly reports detailing the patient's Internet use; in essence, this is an Internet abuse "toxicology screen," similar to a urine toxicology screen for substance-based addictions.

Care needs be taken not to assume that blocking, monitoring, or filtering a patient's online behavior will, on its own, be sufficient to treat Internet addiction. Often, a patient's family members attempt to manage their loved one's addiction via blocks and filters, but such IT strategies alone will likely fail unless part of a comprehensive treatment plan. The Internet addict is frequently more technologically sophisticated than their family, and may easily sabotage such efforts.

Many video game addicts, if blocked from playing their favorite games, switch to other media modalities (eg, YouTube) to watch others' gaming and experience game-play vicariously. Studies imply that video game addicts undergo a similar mesolimbic reward activation from simply observing other people's play as when playing the games themselves.[20]

Real-Time Living Strategies

A hallmark of successful treatment of any addiction is the instillation or reinstallation of normalized life skills and behaviors. The Real-Time 100 involves a treatment strategy where the patient develops list of 100 real-time behaviors (non–screen-based) that are introduced and used when urges or cravings are noted; the idea is to slowly reintroduce "normal living" and reward saliency back into the patient's life. Addiction creates an imbalance in functional and developmental tasks where the addictive behavior becomes the primary source of dopaminergic stimulation in the nucleus accumbens and other reward brain structures. In the case of Internet and video game addicts, the inherit need for social competence, self-efficacy, accomplishment, and skills mastery becomes subsumed by Internet activities.

In such cases, we see desensitization (upregulation of postsynaptic dopamine receptors). This process results in the weakening of circuits related to naturalistic rewards (eg, food, sex, socializing, accomplishment in work or academics, etc). The Internet or video game addict has a diminished capacity to enjoy such everyday pleasures, and the redevelopment of naturalistic reward stimulation is essential in recovery. Nature abhors a vacuum, and as we decrease desensitized reward circuitry, it is necessary reestablish more naturalistic reward behaviors.

REWARD DEFICIENCY SYNDROME

Addictions are, in part, maintained by a reward deficiency syndrome, in which normal life seems tedious compared with highly stimulatory addictive behaviors. This desensitization (dopamine receptor upregulation) involves a weakening of circuits related to naturalistic rewards (eg, food, sex, social activities, work/academic reward, and delayed gratification for long-term goals). Once an addict enters this state, previously reinforcing behaviors decrease and excessive amounts of time become devoted to Internet use. Addictions are typically accompanied by a degree of developmental arrest with manifested impairment of typical social, occupational, and academic milestones. Patients typically need to resume healthy real-time living strategies to substitute dopaminergic reinforcement that addiction creates with the typical joys and satisfactions balanced living provides.

RELAPSE PREVENTION

The goal of IVGA treatment is to maximize realistic sustainable recovery and maintain mindful moderation of technology use. For moderated use to continue even after treatment has completed, the clinician must help to inoculate the patient from relapse. The irony of relapse prevention is to acknowledge and assume potential relapse triggers and situations and to rehearse how these will be address not "if" they occur, but rather, "when" they will occur.

INTERNET AND VIDEO GAME ADDICTION: A NEW DRUG OF CHOICE

Although a variety of therapeutic techniques have been presented for the treatment of IVGA, they are only at the beginning stage of validation and standardization. Although many of the general psychiatric and psychological treatments for Internet addiction are derived from an addiction medicine perspective, others are wholly novel. Internet addiction treatment should be seen as a distinct subspecialty of addiction medicine requiring specialized skills. Misdiagnosis is common, because many patients present for Internet addiction treatment only after numerous unsuccessful treatments failing to address the primary problem and instead focusing on general psychiatric symptomatology.

A common tenet in addiction medicine states that unless addictive behavior is addressed, treating comorbid psychiatric symptoms and disorders tends to be ineffective. Psychiatric conditions such as ADHD, depression, anxiety disorders, and autism spectrum disorder are typically premorbid and ensuing sequelae of the addiction, as with all addictions. The treatment of Internet addiction has not yet attained the benchmark of evidence-based criteria, but research evidence continues to mount, and better designed and implemented research is on the horizon.

An important perspective in treating Internet and video gaming addiction is that there is no need reinvent the wheel. Many well-established addiction treatment protocols and techniques have proven effective in correcting similar disruptions of the reward pathways of the brain, with or without psychiatric comorbidities. Internet use disorder may be new as a "drug of choice," but numbing and self-medicating addictively are by no means new. We can draw from established substance use, alcohol use, and gambling disorder treatment protocols and therapies in helping our patients who suffer from an addiction to the Internet and video games; we know what can work in addiction medicine, and we know that addiction treatment is an ongoing recovery process. With adequate patient motivation and ongoing, targeted clinical care, healthier and sustainable technology use can be achieved and maintained over time.

ACKNOWLEDGMENTS

The author acknowledges the patients over the last 25 years who have guided this journey toward treating this addiction; the author admires their courage to heal. The author also acknowledges Dr Kimberly Young, who saw this disorder early on, and dedicates this article to a dear friend and colleague, Dr Alvin Cooper, with whom the author conducted early research and writings; God bless his soul.

REFERENCES

1. Ries RK, editor. The ASAM principles of addiction medicine. 5th edition. Philadelphia: Wolters Kluwer; 2014.
2. Bibbey A, Phillips C, Ginty AT, et al. Problematic internet use, excessive alcohol consumption, their comorbidity and cardiovascular and cortisol reactions to acute psychological stress in a student population. J Behav Addict 2015;4(2): 44–52.
3. Reed P, Vile R, Osborne LA, et al. Problematic internet usage and immune function. PLoS One 2015;10(8):e0134538.
4. Kuss DJ, Griffiths MD. Internet and gaming addiction: a systematic literature review of neuroimaging studies. Brain Sci 2012;2(3):347–74.
5. Kim SH, Baik S-H, Park CS, et al. Reduced striatal dopamine D2 receptors in people with Internet addiction. Neuroreport 2011;22(8):407–11.
6. Hari J. Chasing the scream. New York: Bloomsbury; 2015.
7. Alexander BK. Addiction: the urgent need for a paradigm shift. Substance Use Abuse 2012;47:1475–82.
8. Greenfield DN. The nature of internet addiction: psychological factors in compulsive Internet use. Paper presented at the 1999 American Psychological Association Convention, Boston, August 20, 1999.
9. Greenfield DN. Psychological characteristics of compulsive internet use: a preliminary analysis. Cyberpsychol Behav 1999;2(5):403–12.
10. Greenfield DN. The nature of internet addiction: psychological factors in compulsive internet behavior. Journal of e.Commerce and Psychology 2001;Vol 1.
11. Beard KW. Internet addiction: a review of current assessment techniques and potential assessment questions. Cyberpsychol Behav 2005;8:7–14.
12. Davis RA. A cognitive–behavioral model of pathological internet use. Comput Human Behav 2001;17:187–95.
13. Griffiths MD. Does internet and computer "addiction" exist? Some case study evidence. Cyber Psychology & Behavior 2004;3(2):211–8.
14. King DL, Delfabbro PH. Understanding and assisting excessive players of video games: a community psychology perspective. Aust Community Psychol 2009;18: 62–74.
15. Young K. Caught in the net. New York: John Wiley; 1996.
16. Griffiths MD, Kuss DJ, Billieux J, et al. The evolution of internet addiction: a global perspective. Addict Behav 2016;53:193–5.
17. Griffiths M. Does internet and computer "addiction" exist? Some case study evidence. Cyberpsychol Behav 2000;3(2):181–8.
18. Greenfield DN. What makes internet use addictive?. In: Young K, Abreu CN, editors. Internet addiction: a handbook for evaluation and treatment. New York: Wiley; 2010. p. 135–53.
19. Allain F, Minogianis EA, Roberts DCS, et al. How fast and how often: the pharmacokinetics of drug use are device in addiction. Neurosci Biobehav Rev 2015;56: 166–79.
20. Jovic J, Dindic N. Influence of dopaminergic system on Internet addiction. Acta Med Medianae 2011;50(1):66.

21. Duven E, Müller KW, Wölfling K. Internet and computer game addiction—a review of current neuroscientific research. Eur Psychiatry 2011;26:416.
22. Matthias E, Young KS, Elaier C. Prefrontal control and internet addiction: a theoretical model and review of neuropsychological and neuroimaging findings. Front Hum Neurosci 2014;8:375.
23. Kaess M, Parzer P, Mehl L, et al. Stress vulnerability in male youth with internet gaming disorder. Psychoneuroendocrinology 2017;77:244–51.
24. Lemieux A, Mustafa A. Stress psychobiology in the context of addiction medicine: from drugs of abuse to behavioral addictions. Prog Brain Res 2016;223:43–62.
25. Greenfield D. AT&T—it can wait survey of distracted driving. 2014. Available at: http://www.prnewswire.com/news-releases/are-you-compulsive-about-texting–driving-survey-saysyou-could-be-281586711.html; http://about.att.com/newsroom/compulsion_research_drivemode_ios_availability.html. Accessed October 17, 2017.
26. Greenfield DN. Driven to distraction: why we can't stop using our Smartphone's when driving. Keynote address at the 2017 Michigan Traffic Safety Summit, Michigan State University, East Lansing (MI), March 23, 2017.
27. Przepiorka AM, Blachnio A, Miziak B, et al. Clinical approaches to treatment of Internet addiction. Pharmacol Rep 2014;66(2):187–91.
28. King DL, Delfabbro PH, Griffiths MD, et al. Assessing clinical trials of Internet addiction treatment: a systematic review and CONSORT evaluation. Clin Psychol Rev 2011;31(7):1110–6.
29. Byun S, Ruffini C, Mills JE, et al. Internet addiction: metasynthesis of 1996–2006 quantitative research. Cyberpsychol Behav 2009;12:203–7.
30. Griffiths MD. Internet and video-game addiction. In: Essau C, editor. Adolescent addiction: epidemiology, assessment and treatment. San Diego (CA): Elsevier; 2008. p. 231–67.
31. Greenfield DN. Internet use disorder: clinical and treatment implications of compulsive internet and video game use in adolescents. Child & Adolescent Psychiatric Society of Greater Washington Spring Symposium, Addictions and the Adolescent Brain, Suburban Hospital, Bethesda (MD), March 7, 2015.
32. Cash H, Rae CD, Steel AH, et al. Internet addiction: a brief summary of research and practice. Curr Psychiatry Rev 2012;8(4):292–8.
33. Kim K, Ryu E, Chon M, et al. Internet addiction in Korean adolescents and its relation to depression and suicidal ideation: a questionnaire survey. Int J Nurs Stud 2006;43:185–92.
34. Geng Y, Su L, Cao F. A research on emotion and personality characteristics in junior 1 high school students with Internet addiction disorders. Chin Ment Health J 2009;23:457–70.
35. Blum K, Chen AL, Braverman ER, et al. Attention-deficit-hyperactivity disorder and reward deficiency syndrome. Neuropsychiatr Dis Treat 2008;4(5):893–918.
36. Grant JE, Potenza MN, Weinstein A, et al. Introduction to behavioral addictions. Am J Drug Alcohol Abuse 2010;36:233–41.
37. Winkler A, Dörsing B, Rief W, et al. Treatment of Internet addiction: a meta-analysis. Clin Psychol Rev 2013;33:317–29.
38. Du Y, Jiang W, Vance A. Longer term effect of randomized, controlled group cognitive behavioral therapy for Internet addiction in adolescent students in Shanghai. Aust N Z J Psychiatry 2010;44:129–34.
39. Jorgenson AG, Hsiao RCJ, Yen CF. Internet addiction and other behavioral addictions. Child Adolesc Psychiatr Clin N Am 2016;25(3):509–20.

40. Jäger S, Müller KW, Ruckes C, et al. Effects of a manualized short-term treatment of internet and computer game addiction (STICA): study protocol for a randomized controlled trial. Trials 2012;13(1):1.
41. Kim SM, Han DH, Lee YS, et al. Combined cognitive behavioral therapy and bupropion for the treatment of problematic on-line game play in adolescents with major depressive disorder. Comput Hum Behav 2012;28(5):1954–9.
42. King DL, Delfabbro PH. The cognitive psychology of internet gaming disorder. Clin Psychol Rev 2014;34:298–308.
43. Young KS. CBT-IA: the first treatment model for internet addiction. J Cogn Psychother 2011;25:304.
44. Liu C, Liao M, Smith DC. An empirical review of internet addiction outcome studies in China. Res Soc Work Pract 2012;22(3):282–92.
45. King DL, Delfabbro PH, Griffiths MD, et al. Cognitive-behavioral approaches to outpatient treatment of internet addiction in children and adolescents. J Clin Psychol 2012;68(11):1185–95.
46. Greenfield DN. Internet and Technology Addiction: Are we controlling our devices or are they controlling us? Keynote address at the National Association of Social Workers, South Dakota Conference, Sioux Fall (SD), March 17, 2016.
47. Young K. Cognitive behavior therapy with Internet addicts: treatment outcomes and implications. Cyberpsychol Behav 2007;10:671–9.
48. La Salvia TA. Enhancing addiction treatment through psychoeducational groups. J Subst Abuse Treat 1993;10:439–44.
49. Botvin GJ, Baker E, Filazzola AD, et al. Cognitive-behavioral approach to substance abuse prevention; a one-year follow up. Addict Behav 1990;15:4743.
50. Miller WR, Rollnick S. Motivational interviewing: helping people change. New York: The Guilford Press; 2013.
51. Prochaska JO, DiClemente CC, Norcross JC. In search of how people change: applications to the addictive behaviors. Am Psychol 1992;47:1102–14.
52. Marlatt GA. Taxonomy of high-risk situations for alcohol relapse: evolution and development of a cognitive-behavioral model. Addiction 1996;91(Suppl):37–49.
53. Shapiro F. Eye movement desensitization and reprocessing: basic principles, protocols, and procedures. 2nd edition. New York: The Guilford Press; 2001.
54. Atmaca M. A case of problematic internet use successfully treated with an SSRI-antipsychotic combination. Prog Neuropsychopharmacol Biol Psychiatry 2007; 31(4):961–2.
55. Moreira FA, Dalley JW. Dopamine receptor partial agonists and addiction. Eur J Pharmacol 2015;752:112–5.
56. Camardese G, De Risio L, Nicola Di, et al. A role for pharmacotherapy in the treatment of internet addiction. Clin Neuropharmacol 2012;35(6):283–9.
57. Camardese G, Leone B, Walstra C, et al. Pharmacological treatment of Internet addiction. In: Montag C, Reuter M, editors. Internet addiction. Studies in neuroscience, psychology and behavioral economics. Switzerland: Springer International Publishing; 2015. p. 151–65.
58. Dell'Osso B, Hadley S, Allen A, et al. Escitalopram in the treatment of impulsive-compulsive Internet usage disorder: an open-label trial followed by a double-blind discontinuation phase. J Clin Psychiatry 2008;69(3):452–6.
59. Goddard AW, Shekhar A, Whiteman AF, et al. Serotoninergic mechanisms in the treatment of obsessive-compulsive disorder. Drug Discov Today 2008;13(7–8): 325–32.
60. Han DH, Hwang JW, Renshaw PF. Bupropion sustained release treatment decreases craving for video games and cue-induced brain activity in patients

with Internet video game addiction. Exp Clin Psychopharmacol 2010;18(4): 297–304.

61. Han DH, Renshaw PF. Bupropion in the treatment of problematic online game play in patients with major depressive disorder. J Psychopharmacol 2012; 26(5):689–96.

62. Bostwick JM, Bucci JA. Internet sex addiction treated with naltrexone. Mayo Clin Proc 2008;83(2):226–30.

63. Grant JE, Kim SW, Hollander E, et al. Predicting response to opiate antagonists and placebo in the treatment of pathological gambling. Psychopharmacology (Berl) 2008;200(4):521–7.

64. Besson M, Belin D, McNamara R, et al. Dissociable control of impulsivity in rats by dopamine D2/3 receptors in the core and shell subregions of the nucleus accumbens. Neuropsychopharmacology 2010;35:565–9.

65. Bernardi S, Pallanti S. Internet addiction: a descriptive clinical study focusing on comorbidities and dissociative symptoms. Compr Psychiatry 2009;50(6):510–6.

The Interplay Between Digital Media Use and Development

Roslyn L. Gerwin, DO[a],*, Kristopher Kaliebe, MD[b],
Monica Daigle, DO[c]

KEYWORDS

- Media • Development • Social media • Television • Mobile • Video game • Family
- Advertising

KEY POINTS

- Today's children and adolescents spend their lives immersed in a digital media world.
- Surveys have consistently shown increased, earlier, and more diverse use of digital media.
- Media preferences and their effects depend greatly on cognitive, physical, and social-emotional development.
- Youth should be considered a vulnerable population to lurid content, consumer culture, advertising, media overuse, and addictive behaviors.

INTRODUCTION

The meaning of the word media has evolved over time. In short, media characterizes the way people communicate information, and is often a direct reflection of a society and its present culture. However, looked at more closely, media is a deceptively simple term that describes a vast and heterogeneous set of technologies and the content transmitted by these mediums.

Digital media has become an increasingly powerful influence on the lives of both adults and children. Modern technologies afford an almost limitless and instantaneous ability to be connected around the globe. The normal way of life increasingly both relies on, and draws people to, being able to access media quickly. It often involves simultaneous use of various devices, including televisions, computers, consoles,

Disclosure Statement: The authors having nothing to disclose.
[a] Pediatric Psychiatry Consultation Service, Department of Child and Adolescent Psychiatry, Barbara Bush Children's Hospital, Maine Medical Center, 66 Bramhall Street, Portland, ME 04103, USA; [b] Department of Psychiatry, University of South Florida Medical School, 3515 East Fletcher Avenue, MDC 14, Tampa, FL 33613, USA; [c] Department of Mental Health and Detox, St. Mary's Health System, 93 Campus Avenue, Lewiston, ME 04240, USA
* Corresponding author.
E-mail address: rlevine.gerwin@gmail.com

Child Adolesc Psychiatric Clin N Am 27 (2018) 345–355
https://doi.org/10.1016/j.chc.2017.11.002
1056-4993/18/© 2017 Published by Elsevier Inc.

childpsych.theclinics.com

mobile telephones, and tablets. These devices enable streaming video, apps, video chat, games, texting, e-mail, and browsing the Internet.

Today's youth will spend their entire lives immersed in a complex web of online and digital technologies. Children and adolescents are tasked with fast adaptation. In 1970, children began to regularly watch television at 4 years of age, whereas in 2012 the average child was 4 months old when they first watched a television.[1] There have been escalations in overall daily use in the past decade, likely based on both preference and necessity. Specific use for tweens and teens is shown in **Fig. 1**.[2]

The overall data are clear: children and adolescents spend more time with media, have earlier use, and use digital media in more social and interactive ways. Leaders, scholars, and professionals entrusted with child welfare frequently provide a negative perspective. A quote from a recent publication regarding media and youth stated " enthusiasm and technological progress goes hand and hand with fear or even aversion of the same progress."[3] Risks regarding the introduction of new digital media into children's lives will always be opaque: controlled experiments will not occur for practical and ethical reasons. Similarly, the downfield benefits of such use are unknown. Thus it is unlikely that professionals tasked with promoting child welfare will ever be to predict precisely how new technologies and changing use patterns will affect development.

A balanced approach regarding the positive and negative effects of electronics and the media content is to first examine the individual child's cognitive, physical, and social-emotional development. Both risks and benefits need to be examined, with attention paid to what needs the use of digital media fill. The effects of electronic media on individual youth are highly variable.[3]

CHANGES IN YOUTHS' MEDIA DIET

A media diet encompasses many activities and ways of interacting with media.[4] The use of more established older media, such as reading, radio, watching television, is categorized as mainly passive. Today's children and adolescents continue to consume large amounts of passive digital media content.[5] However, electronics and media usage now includes highly social and interactive options and more

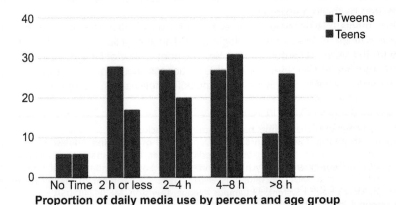

Fig. 1. Comparison of daily media use by age group. (*Data from* Common Sense Media. The common sense census: media use by tweens and teens. Available at: https://www. commonsensemedia.org/research/the-common-sense-census-media-use-by-tweens-and-teens. Accessed May 6, 2017.)

consumer-created content, such as digital artwork and music mixing, maintaining and updating Web sites, blogging, sharing photos and videos, online commentary, online book publishing, and social media.[6] Many youth report at least weekly postings of original videos, essays, or poems, fulfilling needs for creative expression and social exploration.[7]

Currently unknown, but worth considering, is the possibility that are there critical developmental periods in which skill acquisition or activities need to be accomplished for ideal development. Both environmental input and the child's behavior guide the course of development of vision, hearing, ambulating, and so forth. Lack of expected biomechanical pressure or repeated movement patterns can deform the body, causing so-called tech neck or hip dysplasias. Similarly, sensory overload, such as fast-moving visual cues, bright artificial lights, and excessive noise could also cause problems. Just as repeated use of near vision via reading over time distorts the lens, causing myopia, it is unknown what problems may occur in generations with early high intensity and duration digital media habits. This is especially concerning if digital media displace the developmentally expected variety of activities.

CHILDREN (0–8 YEARS)
Infants and Toddlers

Infants are quite capable of attending to screen media content, being most naturally drawn to media that uses different pitched voices and bright, bold contrasting colors.[8] Should infants be exposed to screens, or how much and what type of content, and what types of use will result in harm? There continues to be debate and evolving guidelines.[3] In 2016, American Academy of Pediatrics updated their screen use guidelines. The guideline previously set in 1999 recommended no screens before the age of 2 years. This is now 18 to 24 months because children younger than 18 months do not comprehend what they are viewing but instinctually engage with their senses in keeping with the sensorimotor stage of development.[3,9]

By the age of 2 years, a child typically begins to recognize familiar content patterns and establish programming preferences.[10] Toddlers are attracted to television media that is slow paced and depicts familiar contexts, which is consistent with the moderate-discrepancy hypothesis that theorizes a preference to view objects that are only modestly dissimilar to what a child knows or is capable of understanding.[3,11] Children younger than 2 years may also mimic observed behaviors and reactions, both those on the digital devices and of those using the device. These children can also establish beliefs in response to how advertising affects their parents and at 1 year old may emulate the emotions seen on television.[10] As such, families should be aware that digital media exposures affect young children, even if comprehension of content is incomplete and evolving. In general, younger children use games for education and creativity, consistent with their developmental capabilities and their dependence on caretakers to enable use of digital media.

Preschool Children (2–8 Years)

By preschool age the preferred content is faster and more adventurous. The draw toward fantasy is consistent with the correlating developmental stage of an unclear demarcation between fantasy and reality. Research on television in this age group shows small amounts of developmentally appropriate educational programming can have benefits for young children. At 2 to 4 years, children have some physical abilities for changing channels or navigating simple apps, but media exposure is generally curated by caretakers. Perhaps for this reason, children ages 2 to 4 years are most likely to play educational games, at 52%, across all platforms, and popular television programming tends to have a prosocial and educational focus. Yet this group is also exposed to programming for older children and even for adults. Mixed evidence suggests faster paced programming could be disorienting and contribute to attention or learning problems.[12] In addition other studies have shown preschool children guided to watch educational programming became less aggressive and had healthier social behaviors than children who watched violent programming.

Larger amounts of programming correlated with several harms. For example, children with large amounts of television exposure at 29 months are less likely to play outside, are less fit, and have decreased classroom engagement at 53 months.[13] Research on television can be extrapolated to more engaging and interactive media available to the current generation, thus supporting concerns that media can displace exercise, academic engagement, and outdoor activities. This research also supports the idea that children exposed to electronics tend to develop the desire for continued electronics use, creating a potentially harmful cycle.

Yet more concerning are the effects from digital media on young children via interruption of the parent and child interaction.[3,9] Disrupted parent–child dyads can arise through both parent's involvement in their own media and the child's media exposure. Distracted parents are a significant concern because many parents are unaware that parent–child dyads are fundamental to promote healthy emotional and cognitive development.

Preschool age children's orienting reflex draws them to new things, including novel digital media content, and at this stage of development they enjoy exploring outlets for creative expression. During this preoperational developmental stage, they remain largely unable to evaluate content and the consequences of time spent using media. At this age they are developing the physical ability to access and use digital devices without their caretakers.

The recent proliferation of inexpensive and powerful tablets, video games, and digital devices has enabled caregivers in all social economic groups to choose to allow their children their own devices. Most children by age 4 years are capable of independently managing electronics or touch screens, and many are allowed these devices in their rooms.[10,14] This independent engagement with digital media leads to more challenging parental monitoring.

TRANSITION FROM CHILD TO TEEN (8–12 YEARS)

Traditionally, this period of development has been referred to as preadolescence. Contemporary use of the term tween emerged, at least in part, less as a comment on development, and more as a marketing term.[15] It signified the growing commercial presence and influence of this age group on technology, retail, and media use.

Life becomes much more complex for tweens as they transition out of the latency stage. Their cognitive and social-emotional development allows for more sophisticated perspectives and social interactions. As they near adolescence, and Piaget's formal operational stage, abstract thought and metacognition emerge. Identity, both as an individual and within a group, further develops. Tweens mix the desire for family connections while retaining many of their childhood preferences and family connections.

Tweens exhibit increased autonomy and self-sufficiency. The following typical trends can be observed:

- Hero worship of public figures
- Emulating the behavior of idealized older adolescents.

- Strong group affiliation
- Attraction to more realistic and personally meaningful media content.

Differences within the progression of this developmental stage remain heavily influenced by the media habits of their families. Technology is deeply ingrained in the cultures of certain families, whereas others remain less digital. As they reach adolescence, they will become primarily influenced by their peer groups, and family use becomes a less prevalent predictor of individual media habits.

ADOLESCENCE (13–18 YEARS)

Adolescence is developmental period marked by a desire for autonomy, identity exploration, and the prioritization of social relationships. The adolescent brain has a less developed ability to delay gratification, and seeks novelty and sensation, making modern media very attractive. As their brain matures, cognitive abilities advance, and they become invested in questioning their environment, particularly authority figures. This is typical of the formal operational period and results in the rebellion seen against adult values and customs, which parallels the increased need for peer relationships and acceptance. Teens' draw to both mobile and digital media for teens is, therefore, developmentally appropriate. Digital media provides an almost limitless capacity to connect with others across numerous platforms. This can, of course, have both positive and detrimental effects.

Reasoned analysis media content and usage is impeded by the social and emotional instability of the teen years along with less frontal lobe regulatory ability. The need to both cooperate and compete with others becomes intensified. Some have argued that modern teen lives have become more disconnected, often highly scheduled, and without safe and easily assessable skill building and leisure options. If offline opportunities are limited, this may contribute to a vulnerability for overdependence on media.

Thus a variety of different risks present themselves. Media content can take on an importance and an emotional weight in a teen that it would not necessarily impart to a fully developed adult psyche. Role models within media have long been a source of life lessons for teens, but they now have access to options such as reality television shows, which provide often unrealistic and risky examples to follow. By late adolescence, ideally, there is more overall stability and consolidated identity, and media choices reflect this transition into young adulthood.

GENDER DEVELOPMENT AND MEDIA

Gender differences begin to emerge at an early age, on average between ages 2 and 3 years but can be noted even younger. Media preferences between children identifying as male or female gender can be quite distinct and stereotyped. Younger boys will trend toward content with more action, sports, and science fiction. Girls seek out stories with relationships, and seek out princesses, dancers, and fairies. Favorite character preferences become more masculinized or feminized.[3]

In response, the external world serves to both reinforce and capitalize on gender preferences. Products are developed for children across rigid gender lines, and are similarly advertised. Video games characters have been found to enable stereotyped gender roles with male characters more likely portrayed as more aggressive than female characters, who are more commonly objectified.[16] So, although gender identity is a naturally occurring process, society also exerts influence, media being one modality. This creates an area of concern for caregivers and clinicians hoping to create environments accepting of all gender preferences and discouraging of binary and traditional standards.

As children get older, gender still drives media preferences, though the definition becomes less concrete. For example, girls are still more typically drawn to content with relatable characters and storylines, but boys also begin show similar interest. By adolescence, all youth are working toward general identity formation, including but not limited to their gender. Media preferences return to being a more specific reflection of that individual's ideal.[3]

MEDIA TYPES AND USAGE TRENDS ACROSS DEVELOPMENT
Text and Messaging

Tweens are now frequently using group texts and messaging apps, via telephones and Internet-connected devices. By adolescence, messaging is typically a preferred means of peer communication through texts, apps, or social media:

- Of teens with cellphones, 33% use messaging apps.
- The number of text messages sent or received by cell phone-owning teens (directly through phone or on apps on the phone) on a typical day is 30.
- If calling does take place, almost half of teens report they enjoy talking over video connections, such as Skype or Facetime, which can be easily accessed through their mobile device.[17]

Mobile Media

Access to mobile media and applications has dramatically increased over the past decade across all ages.[2,3,14] From 2011 to 2013, a Common Sense Media study showed:

1. Of children aged 0 to 8 years, 40% had access to a tablet device, up from 8%.[2,18,19]
2. Smartphone access increased from 41% to 63%.
3. Smartphone use increased from 38% to 72%.

Additional research has shown:
- The age of mobile media has also shifted downward.[2,3,14]
- Mobile devices has allows many tweens and teens to be constantly connected.
- Tweens and teens prefer mobile media consumption.[17,20,21]

Television

For all ages, television viewing in rooms is shifting in favor of streaming on mobile devices.[22] What is viewed can often go unsupervised, especially with older ages. New technology compounds the challenge of parents monitoring of duration and timing of viewing, as well as content:

- More devices in a family and for individuals increase the likelihood of solitary viewing. This undermines the benefits of viewing programming together.[9,18]
- Expert guidelines have long recommended televisions should be publicly located in the household, regardless of age. These guidelines are not widely followed.
- A survey done on children born between 1995 and 2012, reflecting older children, showed that 70% preferred streaming video over cable or commercially supported shows.[23]
- The draw of streaming is multifactorial, including fewer commercials, instant access to varied programming, the ability to binge watch, and the ability watch on multiple platforms.

Video Games

Children play video games for creativity, learning through play, testing limits in a safe environment, and recreation. As they age, gaming tends to become more social:

- As of 2015, 72% of teens reported playing video games either online or on their phone.
- As of 2015, 81% have, or have had, access to a game console.[17]
- Video games tap into child or teen's inherent desire for a feeling of mastery.
- Video games present players with tasks within the scope of their abilities. Players feel empowered by their success in a manner that may not be mirrored by their real-life activities.
- Video games frequently include a social component and are a major social activity in many tween and teen subcultures.
- The gaming social milieu can lead to bonding experiences but can also foster toxic exchanges.

Video Sharing

Video sharing sites are one of the first sites youth visit when they gain Internet access:

- YouTube reports a 200% growth in their family entertainment sector,[24] with thousands of channels for children alone.
- Myriad of other developers also offering child-safe applications.
- YouTube and Vine, in which content is created by their peers and well-known online personalities, are popular with teens and tweens, and have also risen in popularity.
- You Tube stars or Viners are often regaled more than Hollywood stars.[25]
- The emotional attachment tweens and teens feel for YouTube stars is often greater than toward a traditional celebrity. Their ordinary just-like-us image and casual but intimate postings likely makes them so attractive.
- Teens and tweens seek answers through video sharing sites. There are thousands of instructional videos, ranging from makeup and fashion, to an entirely separate YouTube gaming channel.
- Of teens and tweens, 77% reported subscribing to a YouTube channel, 63.5% watch YouTube daily.[26]

Social Media

School-age children may begin to show interest in being part of social groups. There are online networking sites geared toward children, most beginning around age 7 years. All sites require parent permission and supervision, and may also include external monitors. By preadolescence, they start to prioritize peer acceptance, and their developmental pace drives their engagement in social media. By the time they reach adolescence, investment in their peer group becomes clearly defined:

- Many teens are spending more than 2 hours per day on social media.
- In 2016, it was estimated that 17.5 million teens between 12 and 17 years would use a social network at least monthly.
- By 2020, it was expected 18.2 million teens between 12 and 17 years would use a social network at least monthly.[17]
- Of 13- to 17-year-old teens, 60% have at least one profile.

Online profiles can satisfy the need to explore different identities and personalities, and many teens will have specific profiles for a particular platform. Most teens split their attention across multiple platforms, identifying friends or followers on sites such as Facebook, Twitter, or Instagram (**Fig. 2**).[21] Teens typically either compartmentalize various networking sites for specific purposes or have specific reasons for trending away from certain sites. For example, certain teens shared that Facebook had become drama central, leading them to favor sites they thought were more supportive or encouraging, such as Instagram.[27]

For teens who want to feel less pressure for longer term consequences of their posts or want to easily hide their communication from parents, Snapchat fills that need. It is an application that quickly deletes content once it is sent, providing both fast transmission and an avenue for silly, embarrassing, or sometimes risky content to a limited audience. There is less worry on appearing perfect, because there is no intention for the image to endure. Adding to that is the option for discussion boards and anonymous sharing apps or sites.[17]

As teens take to social media and online communication in greater numbers, there are potential benefits and pitfalls. Some of these have already been recognized. Social networks and communication via various electronic means allow teens to identify and connect with communities that share their interests and/or struggles, even if they are physically or socially isolated offline. However, with this newfound ability to connect online come myriad risks, some of which are unique to the medium, whereas others are longstanding but perhaps enhanced or altered by the method of communication. Online bullying and shaming are well-known problems, perhaps contributed to by the inherent reduction of empathy that online anonymity can bring. This coincides with the development of more sophisticated social and emotional skills and awareness, and subsequent concern about public opinion. In addition, social skill formation could be altered for better or worse when large portions of a teen's interactions occur without the ability to judge body cues and vocal intonation. Research is currently mixed on how a predominance of communication through media effects adolescent's social abilities and empathy. It should be noted that the current generation are the first generation to grow up with these capabilities, likely changing how they process the world, and adapting them for a future replete with communication options.

Advertising and Consumerism Across Platforms

Selling to children is big business. Young people represent both present consumers, great influences on their families purchasing, and future adult consumers. However,

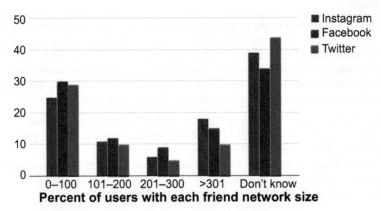

Fig. 2. Comparison of friend networks. (*Data from* Lenhart A. Teens, Social media & technology overview 2015. Pew Research Center. Available at: http://www.pewinternet.org/2015/04/09/teens-social-media-technology-2015/. Accessed April 29, 2017.)

unlike adults, young children are "cognitively and psychologically defenseless against advertising."[28] Due to the ubiquity of media use among youth, advertising targets them everywhere they go and within all forms of media, which now includes tweet, text message, corporate-created games, or Web sites with product placement. As a rule, the purpose of marketing is to target people who are vulnerable to persuasion and suggestion, and youth represent a susceptible market. The United States has very limited regulation of advertising to children, thus primarily economic forces determine what is for children. Let the buyer beware will likely continue to be the default societal response to new technologies and their use by children and adolescents:

- Industry prioritizes sales, and has limited concerns for children's health, privacy, or emotional-social development.
- Youth are routinely exposed to, and affected by, ads for adult or developmentally inappropriate products, including tobacco, alcohol, medications, food, and adult video game and R-rated movies.[28]
- Most advertised foods do not meet the federal government's nutrition guidelines, such as sugary drinks, fast food, candies, and highly sugared cereals.[29]
- Many children now experience social pressure to adopt technologies at even earlier ages.
- Purveyors of tablets, smartphones, and video games have made little effort to warn about the dangers of their products or to keep their product out of the hands of youth who are not capable of understanding the risks of these devices.
- Social media companies, search purveyors, and digital content providers are aware large numbers of children younger than 13 years access their products in violation of the Children's Online Privacy Protection Act, yet have not taken any substantial steps to stop this practice.[30]

SUMMARY

How can clinicians best guide, influence, and empower children in their use of technology and media? Parents, and the medical professionals they look to for guidance, would benefit from becoming more conversant with all aspects of available devices and content. However, individual parents or practitioners cannot stay ahead of ever-changing trends in use patterns and digital devices. Collective knowledge and rules of thumb are needed to guide action.

Understanding children's needs at various developmental stages can inform what a healthy digital media diet. For infants and toddlers, evidence for benefits of media is limited, and caretakers should be mindful of their paramount needs: a supportive and active parent–child dyad, sensory motor exploration, and rest to avoid overstimulation. By late teen years, today's adolescent should be able to fully regulate their relationship with digital media. Understanding the developmental stage and unique characteristics of the individual can assist parents and professionals helping to guide youths navigate the peril and promise of today's digital media landscape.

REFERENCES

1. Bucholz L. Child care doubles TV time for some kids. Reuts Health. 2009. Available at: http://www.reuters.com/article/us-tv-time-idUSTRE5AN3GA20091124. Accessed May 28, 2017.
2. Rideout V. Zero to eight: children's media use in America 2013. Common Sense Media. 2013. Available at: https://www.commonsensemedia.org/research/zero-to-eight-childrens-media-use-in-america-2013. Accessed May 6, 2017.

3. Valkenburg P, Piotrowski J. Plugged in: how media attract and affect youth. New Haven (CT): Yale University Press; 2017.

4. Defy Media. Youth video diet. Acumen Report. 2015. Available at: http://www.defymedia.com/acumen/acumen-report-youth-video-diet/. Accessed May 3, 2017.

5. O'Keefe G. Overview: new media. Pediatr Clin North Am 2012;59:589–600.

6. Odden L. "What is Content? Learn from 40+ definitions." TopRank Online Marketing Blog. 2013. Available at: http://www.toprankblog.com/2013/03/what-is-content/. Accessed May 28, 2017.

7. Kleinschmidt M. Generation Z characteristics: 5 infographics on the Gen Z lifestyle. Vision Critical Web site. 2015. Available at: https://www.visioncritical.com/generation-z-infographics/. Accessed May 28, 2017.

8. American Academy of Pediatrics. Media use by children younger than 2 years. Pediatrics 2011;128(5):1–8.

9. American Academy of Pediatrics. Media and young minds. Pediatrics 2016; 138(5):1–8.

10. PBS Parents. TV and kids under age 3. Children and Media Web site. 2006. Accessed June 17, 2017. Available at: http://www.pbs.org/parents/childrenandmedia/article-faq.html. Accessed December 12, 2017.

11. Valkenburg P, Vroone M. Developmental changes in infants' and toddlers' attention to television entertainment. Communication Research 2004;31(3):288–311.

12. Lillard AS, Peterson J. The immediate impact of different types of television on young children's executive function. Pediatrics 2011;128(4):644–9.

13. Pagani LS, Fitzpatrick C, Barnett TA, et al. Prospective associations between early childhood television exposure and academic, psychosocial, and physical well-being by middle childhood. Arch Pediatr Adolesc Med 2010;164(5):425–31.

14. Kabali HK, Irigoyen M, Nunez-Davis R, et al. Exposure and use of mobile media devices by young children. Pediatrics 2015. [Epub ahead of print].

15. Levasseur M. Familiar with Tweens? You Should Be. The Tourism Intelligence Network Web site. 2007. Available at: http://tourismintelligence.ca/2007/02/09/familiar-with-tweens-you-should-be/. Accessed May 6, 2017.

16. Dill KE, Thill KP. Video game characters and the socialization of gender roles: young people's perceptions mirror sexist media depictions. Sex Roles 2007; 57(11–12):851.

17. Lenhart A. Teens, Social media & technology overview. Pew Research Center. 2015. Available at: http://www.pewinternet.org/2015/04/09/teens-social-media-technology-2015/. Accessed April 29, 2017.

18. Rideout V. Zero to eight: children's media use in America. Common Sense Media 2011. p. 1–48. Available at: https://www.commonsensemedia.org/research/zero-to-eight-childrens-media-use-in-america. Accessed May 6, 2017.

19. Reid Chassiakos YL, Radesky J, Christakis D, et al. Children and adolescents and digital media. Pediatrics 2016;138(5) [pii:e20162593].

20. Rainie L. 13 Things to know about teens and technology. Pew Research Center. 2014. Available at: http://www.pewinternet.org/2014/07/23/13-things-to-know-about-teens-and-technology/. Accessed May 6, 2017.

21. Rideout V. The common sense consensus: media use by teens and tweens. Common Sense Media 2015. p. 1–104. Available at: https://www.commonsensemedia.org/research/the-common-sense-census-media-use-by-tweens-and-teens. Accessed May 5, 2017.

22. Parker-Pope T. A one-eyed invader in the bedroom. New York Times 2008. Available at: http://www.nytimes.com/2008/03/04/health/04well.html. Accessed May 28, 2017.

23. Dixon C. 70% generation Z kids prefer streaming to cable. nScreenMedia Web site. 2016. Available at: http://www.nscreenmedia.com/70-generation-z-kids-prefer-streaming-to-cable/. Accessed June 8, 2017.

24. Perez S. Hands on with "YouTube Kids," Google's newly launched, child-friendly YouTube app. TC Sessions Robotics Web site. 2015. Available at: https://techcrunch.com/2015/02/23/hands-on-with-youtube-kids-googles-newly-launched-child-friendly-youtube-app/. Accessed June 3, 2017.

25. Ault S. Survey: YouTube stars more popular than mainstream celebs among U.S. teens. Variety Web site. 2014. Available at: http://variety.com/2014/digital/news/survey-youtube-stars-more-popular-than-mainstream-celebs-among-u-s-teens-1201275245/. Accessed May 6, 2017.

26. Teen Trend Report. Statistics about teenagers and You Tube. 2014. Available at: Stagesoflife.com. https://www.stageoflife.com/StageHighSchool/TeenYouTubeStatistics.aspx#Survey Results. Accessed May 28, 2017.

27. Madden M, Lenhart A, Cortesi S, et al. Teens, social media & privacy. Pew Research Center. 2013. Available at: http://www.pewinternet.org/2013/05/21/teens-social-media-and-privacy/. Accessed May 29, 2017.

28. Shifrin D, Brown A, Dreyer B, et al. Children, adolescents, and advertising. Pediatrics 2006;118(6):2563–9.

29. Schermbeck RM, Powell LM. Peer reviewed: nutrition recommendations and the children's food and beverage advertising initiative's 2014 approved food and beverage product list. Prev Chronic Dis 2015;12:140472.

30. Minkus T, Liu K, Ross KW. Children seen but not heard: When parents compromise children's online privacy. 24th International Conference Web site. 2015. Available at: http://cse.poly.edu/~tehila/pubs/WWW2015children.pdf. Accessed July 31, 2017.

Printed and bound by CPI Group (UK) Ltd, Croydon, CR0 4YY

07/10/2024

01040501-0005